LPN to RN Transitions

Achieving Success in Your New Role

4th Edition

LPN to RN Transitions

Achieving Success in Your New Role

4th Edition

Nicki Harrington, RN, MAEd, MSN, EdD

CHANCELLOR
Yuba Community College District
Marysville, California

Cynthia Lee Terry, RN, MSN, CCRN, CNE

ASSOCIATE PROFESSOR
Health Sciences Division
Lehigh Carbon Community College
Schnecksville, Pennsylvania

OUTDOOR EMERGENCY CARE INSTRUCTOR
National Ski Patrol
Blue Mountain Ski Area
Palmerton, Pennsylvania

Wolters Kluwer | Lippincott Williams & Wilkins
Health
Philadelphia · Baltimore · New York · London
Buenos Aires · Hong Kong · Sydney · Tokyo

Senior Acquisitions Editor: Elizabeth Nieginski
Product Manager: Eric Van Osten
Editorial Assistant: Jacalyn Clay

Design Coordinator: Joan Wendt
Manufacturing Coordinator: Karin Duffield
Production Services: SPi Global

4th edition

Library of Congress Cataloging-in-Publication Data
Harrington, Nicki.
 LPN to RN transitions : achieving success in your new role / Nicki Harrington, Cynthia Lee Terry. — 4th ed.
  p. ; cm.
 Includes bibliographical references and index.
 ISBN 978-1-60913-691-8
 1. Nursing—Vocational guidance. 2. Practical nurses. I. Terry, Cynthia Lee. II. Title.
 [DNLM: 1. Nursing—Examination Questions. 2. Career Mobility—Examination Questions.
3. Nurse's Role—Examination Questions. 4. Nurses psychology—Examination Questions.
WY 18.2]
 RT82.H37 2012
 610.7306'9076—dc23

2011022764

Care has been taken to confirm the accuracy of the information presented and to describe generally accepted practices. However, the authors, editors, and publisher are not responsible for errors or omissions or for any consequences from application of the information in this book and make no warranty, expressed or implied, with respect to the currency, completeness, or accuracy of the contents of the publication. Application of this information in a particular situation remains the professional responsibility of the practitioner; the clinical treatments described and recommended may not be considered absolute and universal recommendations.

 drug selection and dosage set forth in this text are in accordance with the current recommendations and practice at the time of publication. However, in view of ongoing research, changes in government regulations, and the constant flow of information relating to drug therapy and drug reactions, the reader is urged to check the package insert for each drug for any change in indications and dosage and for added warnings and precautions. This is particularly important when the recommended agent is a new or infrequently employed drug.

 Some drugs and medical devices presented in this publication have Food and Drug Administration (FDA) clearance for limited use in restricted research settings. It is the responsibility of the health care provider to ascertain the FDA status of each drug or device planned for use in his or her clinical practice.

LWW.com

To my father, whose spirit is still with me, and to my mother, who continues to believe in me and support me. I thank you for the values you have modeled and instilled in me throughout my life. My greatest appreciation goes to Jim, my husband, partner, and best friend in life, for his enduring love and support; and Cayden Chance, our beautiful son, who always keeps me focused on the most important things in life—God's gifts of love and life.

—NICKI HARRINGTON

To my husband, Dale Robert Terry. You are a calming, quiet factor in a crazy, chaotic world. I love you, and this book is dedicated to you, my soulmate.

—CINDY TERRY

REVIEWERS

Mary Cornell, RN MSN
Clark State Community College
Springfield, Ohio

Sandra Baker, DNP, RN, CNE
Riverside Community College
Riverside, California

Janis Simpson, RN, BSN, MA, EdS
Tennessee Technology Center
Athens, Tennessee

Donna M. Bys, RN, BSN, MPA, LHNA
Stone Academy
Springfield, Massachusetts

Deborah Burton, RN, MSN
San Bernardino Valley College
San Bernardino, California

Nancy Hutchison, RN, MSN
North Metro Technical College
Acworth, Georgia

Susan Mullaney, Ed.D. RN CNE
Framingham State University
Framingham, Massachusetts

Carolyn Buancore, MN, RN, CNE
Our Lady of the Lake College
Baton Rouge, Louisiana

Dawn Adkins, ADN, PN
Southwest Wisconsin Technical College
Fennimore, Wisconsin

Michele Dickson, RN, BSN, MSN
Prince George's Community College
Largo, Maryland

Beth Hensley, EdD, MEd, BSN
Southside Regional Medical Center
 Professional Schools
Petersburg, Virginia

Lisa Gutierrez, RN, MSN
Blinn College
Bryan, Texas

Denise Marshall, EdD, MEd, BSN
Wor-Wic Community College
Salisbury, Maryland

Mary Alice Schuster, BSN, MSN
North Metro Technical College
Acworth, Georgia

Daisy Hines, RN, MSN, EdD
Long Beach City College
Long Beach, California

PREFACE

Reentering the rigors of academic life is a monumental decision for any LPN/LVN returning to school. It is both a personal and financial investment, fraught with extreme highs and lows. This new path will challenge the aspiring Associate Degree Nurse to operate in a sometimes chaotic new world that requires nonlinear thinking, balancing many simultaneous challenges, and a global perspective. It also requires the nurse to be an independent practitioner, while functioning collaboratively within an expanded and more specialized health care team. The revised fourth edition of *LPN to RN Transitions: Achieving Success in Your New Role* serves as a guide to prepare students for a successful journey on this new path.

We have retained those features of the third edition that former students and educators found most helpful, such as the vignettes, the "Thinking Critically" feature, student exercises, sample NCLEX-RN questions, the personal education plan (PEP), and additional print, electronic, and web resources. We have left the vignettes of real student experiences at the beginning of each chapter as they continue to assist the reader in realizing that the journey to associate degree nursing is not an isolated one, but one that is shared by other students. Students may see their own situations portrayed in one or more of these vignettes and recognize that others have experienced the same challenges.

Interactive student exercises and development of a PEP are strategies used throughout the text to help the student with role transition to the ADN program, taking into consideration the student's own experience and the program's philosophy, curricular framework, and student learning outcomes. The "Thinking Critically" feature provides students with the opportunity to reflect on material presented, to examine application of theoretical content to the clinical practice setting and to share perspectives in a group setting. This text is designed to be used by students in a variety of adult learning modes, including independent study, classroom collaborative work groups, and online discussions.

Chapters have been revised to include evidence-based practice strategies where indicated. Tables and displays have been condensed and supplemented to help clarify important concepts. Updated resources, professional documents, and websites (including new audiovisual sites) will be of interest to returning students and will afford them the opportunity to further explore individual topics.

The first several chapters have incorporated numerous college success strategies, and have been revised in this fourth edition to address a more diverse, multicultural student population. The addition of student learning outcomes to nursing curricula, as required by accrediting bodies, has been described in this edition. Students are given the opportunity to assess their preferred learning styles, and more information is provided on emotional intelligence, study skills, writing professional papers for college courses, and time management/organizational skills. Success strategies for English language learners and for those with alternative lifestyles have also been included. More support and resource information is provided for male nursing students, students of color, and those with cross-gender sexual orientation.

The concepts of "role overload" and "role transition" have been expanded in this fourth edition. Students today are experiencing more financial problems, working longer hours due to the economic downturn, and facing personal challenges within their own social structures in today's economy. The increased use of faculty web pages, threaded discussions, and social networking may pose additional challenges for those re-entry students who are not at ease with these media. Returning veterans entering nursing programs, coping with not only the transition to the student role, but also the transition to civilian life, may experience additional difficulties. Strategies for coping with such challenges of "role overload" and "role transition" are discussed.

Therapeutic communication techniques and the nurse's role in collaborative practice with other health care providers continue to be stressed in this edition. The SBAR (Situation-Background-Assessment-Recommendation) communication tool has been added as a suggestion to enhance successful communications between health care providers. Today, nurses do much more than care for individuals and families; they also have the responsibility of making ethical decisions and advocating social policy. Therefore, we have included content on the international code of ethics and ethical decision-making for the nurse as an integral part of a health care industry that is dealing with such issues as reportable information, bioterrorism, genetic re-engineering, cloning, stem cell research, cryogenics, and other technological advances. The role of today's nurse in evidence-based research and establishment of nursing diagnoses and best practices is also examined.

The challenges of the LPN/LVN returning to school to seek a career in professional nursing are many. However, as more nurses venture into such specialized areas as nursing informatics, disaster preparedness, homeland security, holistic nursing, spiritual nursing, and entrepreneurism, the opportunities for careers in professional nursing practice continue to increase. We have expanded Chapter 4's content on evidence-based practice and the impact of emerging societal trends on the practice of nursing. The world has become a different place in the past decade, and students are asked to think critically about their personal and professional viewpoints, values, and patient care interventions in the context of these societal trends, which contribute to the constantly evolving role of the professional nurse. Additionally, continued increased health care costs, patient acuity, and pressures on the health care system to maximize efficiency and productivity through greater nurse-patient ratios and the use of paraprofessionals place new demands on today's nurse. Critical thinking is encouraged throughout the text as each nurse confronts these challenges as a critical member of the health care team.

Chapters 4 and 8 provide updates on legal and regulatory changes in nursing and nursing education. The Nurse Compact and licensure issues are examined as nurses become more mobile working in multiple states, and telecommunications and portable medical records become more available. Other issues explored include informatics and HIPAA requirements, issues of homeland security and immigration, the impact of terrorism and disasters on nursing, and the increased tension between Eastern healing and preventative health methods and Western medical treatment and reimbursement policies. Changes in the health care delivery system, including managed health care, benefit and reimbursement programs, changes in Social Security, the national health care agenda, and quality outcomes are also discussed as the profession of nursing continues to "reshape" its agenda for the future.

The concept of "cultural proficiency" is introduced, including the six stages of developing cultural proficiency as a nurse. Cultural proficiency will be critical as today's nurse both models and leads others on the health care team to serve changing demographics. Today's healthcare team must grapple with issues of immigration, caring for a multicultural clientele that may include many undocumented community members, and caring for domestic partners and same-sex married couples.

We believe that all of the features, revisions, and additions to this fourth edition will meet the needs of a diverse student population with varied adult learning styles and experiential backgrounds. It is our desire to provide students with useful tools to successfully balance career, school, and personal lives while pursuing their educational and professional goals.

Nicki Harrington, RN, MAEd, MSN, EdD
Cynthia Lee Terry, RN, MSN, CCRN, CNE

ACKNOWLEDGMENTS

I would like to continue to thank my students, both LPN and RN. Many minds paint perspectives on ideas and concepts that one individual could never consider alone. I would like to thank Aurora Weaver, MEd, MSN, RN. Your counsel and encouragement have meant a lot to me over these past years. I would like to thank the faculty of the Adult Education Program at Harrisburg's Pennsylvania State University. Thank you also to my editor, Rebecca von Gillern, for your guidance and support.

—CINDY TERRY

I would like to thank the many individuals who supported me in the writing of this book. To the many LVN-to-RN students in the past with whom I shared learning experiences in the classroom as their teacher, I thank you for your inspiration, which continues with me today. It was the memory of your struggles that kept me focused on your needs throughout my writing. To my co-author, Cindy Terry, thank you for your hard work, patience, perseverance, and continuing contributions to the profession of nursing. Thanks also to Rebecca von Gillern, our editor, who patiently supported us through the project. To my family, thank you for allowing me the time to complete this text when I wanted instead to be with you those many long nights and weekends. Thank you for your ongoing support.

—NICKI HARRINGTON

CONTENTS

UNIT

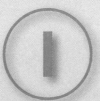

The Transition Process

1

Lifelong Learning: Returning to School

● **LEARNING OUTCOMES**

By the end of this chapter, the student will be able to:

1 Describe the importance of lifelong learning in nursing.

2 Describe the process of re-entry into the role of student.

3 Outline the stages of the return to the student role.

4 Describe diverse learning styles.

5 Compare personal learning style with those described by theorists.

6 Develop beginning strategies for being successful in college.

7 Summarize learning resources that enhance the student's ability to be successful.

8 Discuss methods to manage time effectively.

9 Give examples of effective study skills and strategies.

10 Apply positive approaches to the educational process.

abstract	disintegration	re-entry process
conceptualization	diverse learning styles	reflective observation
active	diversity	reintegration
experimentation	educationally mobile	resolution
active learning	evidence-based	returning to school
assertiveness	nursing	syndrome (RTSS)
best practice	honeymoon	teaching–learning
concrete	learning outcomes	environment
experimentation	learning style	time management
creative thinking	lifelong learning	VAK system
critical thinking	portfolio	win/win agreement
curriculum threads	program philosophy	

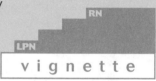

v i g n e t t e

Sandy Martin has been an LPN for 10 years. Although she has always wanted to go back to school for her RN, marriage and a full-time job at a skilled nursing facility have kept her more than busy since graduation. In addition to raising two children, she has a mortgage and all the trappings that come with life. She has never seemed to have time for herself. Finally, with her two children now in middle and high school, and the nursing shortage at its highest in years, Sandy has decided to reduce her full-time work schedule and go back to school part time to seek an ADN. However, as Sandy waits to talk to the nursing advisor about class requirements and prerequisites, she begins to worry. Can she really meet her current obligations and earn her degree? It is going to take her at least 3 to 5 years to finish her degree, which is a bit discouraging. Also, will she have retained enough after all these years? She remembers the struggles she had with anatomy, physiology, and pharmacology, as well as her fear of clinical rotations and assignments. These struggles and fears will be revisited. She also worries about whether she will "fit in" with the younger students. She hopes the nursing advisor will be able to help alleviate her concerns and help her through all this.

Remember when you first made the decision to be a nurse? For many people, the desire to be a nurse revolved around wanting to help people who could not help themselves and putting caring into action. However, with your experience in the world of nursing as a licensed practical nurse/licensed vocational nurse (LPN/LVN), your vision and opinions of nursing may have changed somewhat. Perhaps your view of nursing differs from the views of other nurses. Your reasons for returning to school reflect changes in your life. Your reasons may include the desire to have more job opportunities, increase your job satisfaction, or expand the scope of your responsibilities, or you may be seeking self-improvement.

The fact that you are returning to school reflects the positive impact of the many changes that have occurred in your life and in society. At one time, a diploma from a school of practical/vocational nursing was seen as a terminal process; an

LPN/LVN would not seek higher education. If an LPN/LVN wanted to continue her or his nursing education, it often meant starting over. Conversely, changes in the educational system have enhanced your ability to further your education, building on your prior knowledge, skills, and experience. Chandler (2010) notes that the attrition rate of registered nurses (RNs) is high, with many leaving in the first year of practice as they "enter a resource-poor environment with staffing shortages and an increase in patient acuity" (p. 22). However, your foundation as an LPN/LVN has given you a preview to what Registered Nursing practice will be, and your choice to pursue professional registered nursing licensure and an associate or baccalaureate degree in nursing has been made with this basis of knowledge of the workplace. Such experiential knowledge is already a foundation for your success in the ADN or BSN program you are entering in pursuit of a higher, professional degree. It must be noted that this too will not be a "terminal process." As MacIntosh (2003) identified in a research study of practicing professionals, "becoming professional involves more than graduating and earning the legal title 'nurse.' They [practicing professionals] indicate the need to work consciously over a career to develop and maintain their professional identity" (p. 740).

● LIFELONG LEARNING IN NURSING

Participation in lifelong learning has been identified by the National League for Nursing as 1 of 51 assumptions about the practice of the associate degree nurse of the future (National League for Nursing, 2000). The National Council of State Boards of Nursing (2009), in its development of the new National Council Licensure Examination for Registered Nurses (NCLEX-RN) implemented in April 2010, stated, "Nursing is a dynamic, continually evolving discipline that employs critical thinking to integrate increasingly complex knowledge, skills, and technologies and client care activities into evidence-based nursing practice" (p. 2).

Today's nurse must be committed to lifelong learning and the use of new evidence and best practices to continuously provide high-quality care to patients. Lippincott Williams & Wilkins (2007), in its text *Best Practices: Evidence-Based Nursing Procedures*, states "Best practice refers to the clinical practices, treatments, and interventions that result in the best possible outcome for the patient and the health care facility providing those services" (p. 1). Evidence-based nursing is further defined as "the term used to describe nursing practice based on information obtained from research" (p. 2). As you embark on your registered nursing educational path, lifelong learning and evidence-based research will be essential not only to your ability to exercise best practices but also to the ongoing revitalization of your professional identity.

Advances in the health care industry, technological advances, societal trends, and nursing research for best practices all require nurses to continually update their knowledge and practices. In establishing the *Scope and Standards of Practice for Nursing Professional Development*, the American Nurses Association (2000) stated the belief that "Lifelong learning is the responsibility of the nurse and is essential to maintain and increase competence in nursing practice" (p. 1). As you

display **1.1**	**Basic Skills and Competencies for a Lifelong Learning World**

Information handling	Problem solving
Presenting–communicating formally	Self-esteem, self-management,
Discussing–communicating informally	self-awareness
Learning to learn	Empathy, tolerance for others
Listening, memorizing	Creativity, a sense of humor
Entrepreneurial skills	Meditation skills
Making-practical skills	Flexibility, adaptability, versatility
Critical judgment, reasoning	Thinking, vision, planning
Decision making	

Adapted from Longworth, N. (2003). *Lifelong learning in action: Transforming education in the 21st century* (p. 140). London, UK: Routledge/Falmer.

return to school, you will likely find a new learning environment where faculty use teaching strategies to develop your competencies as a lifelong learner. Such skills and competencies include those identified by Longworth (2003) and shown in Display 1.1.

• THE RE-ENTRY PROCESS: OVERCOMING BARRIERS AND FEARS

Although you may be as hesitant as Sandy Martin about the prospect, your return to school is important. It is also a challenge and an adventure. Arnoldussen (2006) sorts fact from fiction regarding the profession of nursing today, reviews dozens of nursing specializations both inside and outside the hospital setting to spark your enthusiasm about future goals, and shares tips for success from other students including how to thrive in the clinical setting. Whether you have been out of school for only a brief time or for many years, you will probably have fears; however, these should diminish after a few months. Returning to academic life is not easy. The thought of new risks or the return to old roles may be frightening. Dunham's (2008) *How to Survive and Maybe Even Love Nursing School* covers a wide array of topics from academic to personal, including how to cope with the fear of clinical rotations. Other factors may relate to your desire to be highly successful in the educational process, while also wanting to be successful in other roles, such as an employee, a parent, or a spouse. Each person has individual issues as he or she returns to school, but you may find you have many things in common with others. It is important to examine what it means to return to school and to determine what strategies will best help you cope, succeed, and achieve satisfaction in the process.

Returning to the role of student nurse involves more than taking a deep breath and mustering the courage to face both the familiar and the completely unknown. There may also be barriers and fears to overcome. For some returning students, this section will not apply. You may not have experienced any apprehension about the re-entry process and be well prepared to accept the challenges that lie ahead. However, for most students, some or all of this will be familiar. For this reason, common barriers and fears that are seen with the re-entry process are presented. The Thinking Critically activity in this section provides you with the opportunity to examine your own issues.

Age

One perceived barrier in returning to school may be your age. You may believe that it has been too many years since you were in school. You may also fear that the other students will be much younger and that you might have little in common with them; you will find that this is almost definitely not the case. You may think that your academic ability is less than what is needed and worry because you have not had to study intensively for a long time. Attaining a college degree may seem like an out-of-reach dream. The mystique that surrounds college course work can be intimidating. As an older student, you may fear that you do not have the intellectual skills to succeed, that the math and science knowledge you once had has diminished over time, or that younger students will think you are inferior or out of place. Steele, Lauder, Caperchione, and Anastasi (2005) found that the two most prominent concerns of mature students entering nursing programs were financial difficulties and the re-entry process itself. Three coping mechanisms they identified to overcome these concerns were (a) using support networks, (b) prioritizing and organizing, and (c) having positive expectations and attitudes for the future. Curry (2008) stresses the need for both short- and long-term goals, noting that "achieving … short-term goals provides a sense of satisfaction, which can energize and increase motivation" (p 16). She further notes, "Goals are powerful entities that can provide a focus, sustain commitment, reinforce priorities, and provide a framework for current and future decisions" (p. 16). In Chapter Six you will be developing a Personal Education Plan (PEP) and individualizing it for your success. Establishing short- and long-term goals will both motivate and inspire you in your return to school.

Ethnicity, Gender, Sexual Orientation, and Cross-Gender Issues

Another barrier may be related to ethnic, gender, or sexual orientation issues. You will be joining an academic community that may differ from that of your LPN/LVN program. It can be emotionally difficult to look, feel, or be different than other students, particularly in a setting in which you may already be uncomfortable. Again, you may fear that you will have little in common with your classmates. However, nursing in general has become much more diverse. Ethnic, cultural, and other diversity, as well as the addition of greater numbers of men, have caused the profession of nursing to more closely "mirror" the general population. Academic settings have also benefited from such diversity because students have more opportunities to learn from each other's experiences and worldviews, and to relate to a more diverse client population. You may also find that faculty and staff in academic settings have become more diverse and that this diversity is more greatly valued than it was at the time of your LPN/LVN training.

The percentage of nurses who are men increased from less than 1% in 1966 to 5% in 1996, with 12% to 13% of nursing students in 1996 being male

(Katz, Carter, Bishop, & Kravits, 2000). Over the past decade, these male nursing students have now entered the workforce and many have pursued higher degrees and have assumed nursing faculty positions as well. Likewise, today's college classroom has a wider diversity of students than ever before. Crews, North, and Thompson (2001) stated, "In its broadest sense, diversity includes the following: ethnicity, racial background, economic status, physical and mental ability, and the aspects of culture that include nuances of language, heritage, personal behavior, and self-identification" (p. 97). The Latino population has grown tremendously in the past two decades. Gandara and Contreras (2009) state, "In 2025 one in four students in the United States will be Latino, and in California 48% of all students and the majority of kindergarteners are Latino" (p. 305). Within this diverse environment, you will likely find other students with whom you will have cultural values and interests in common.

If you are a male nursing student, you may want to subscribe to *Men in Nursing*. This journal, launched in February 2006, provides information and support for male nurses and their colleagues in four areas: clinical, technological, career, and personal. Articles deal with such topics as overcoming gender bias in educational programs, overcoming gender-related obstacles to professional growth, and strategies for collaboration with other health care team members. A number of Web sites for male nurses are also included at the end of this chapter.

Various journal articles, associations, and Web sites (such as www.minoritynurse. com) can be found through any online search engine for a wide array of diverse issues that may be of interest to you. Your faculty advisor, counselor, and college librarians are also good resources to assist you in finding literature on your specific areas of concern. These individuals, with greater representation of diversity themselves, have also participated in professional development activities to expand their understanding of and support for students of diverse backgrounds. In their text *Academic Advising: New Insights for Teaching and Learning in the First Year*, Hunter, McCalla-Wriggins, and White (2007) devote a whole chapter to lesbian, gay, bisexual, and transgender (LGBT) students, and another on first-generation college students.

Fear of Nursing Faculty, Technology, and Today's Classroom

A common fear of returning students is a dread of nursing faculty. This may be related to previous experiences with nursing instructors or stories you may have heard from other students. However, nursing faculties are also increasingly diverse. As with other professionals, each instructor has various strengths and weaknesses. Some may intimidate you or expect you to know more than you do. Some may treat you as a novice, whereas others will treat you as the adult learner that you are. You will undoubtedly find that you relate well with some of the faculty and have difficulty relating to others. Nursing faculty members are similar to you—unique and imperfect but dedicated to their profession as nurses and nurse educators.

You may also be intimidated by today's technology and classroom environment. Perhaps your LPN/LVN program theory content was delivered in an all-lecture format. Today's registered nursing students are active participants in teaching–learning environments that use computer technology, Internet research, collaborative work groups, Web-based "chat rooms" and "threaded discussions," case studies, learning contracts, role playing, debates, and other interactive processes to foster critical and creative thinking and to develop the lifelong learning skills already presented in this chapter.

The teacher's role is to facilitate learning, ensure relevance and inclusiveness of the diversity of learners, and assist students with attitudes and techniques to strengthen their motivation to learn. Cerbin (2000) noted:

> I am suggesting that what is important is not just what students know, but how they think with what they know. A teacher who is attuned to students' thinking will make different decisions about what to tell students and how to support the development of their understanding, than a teacher who simply lectures according to pre-planned and inalterable syllabus (p. 17).

As a returning student, this "new" classroom environment and associated technology may make you uneasy, and it could take you several months to become comfortable in this more active student role. Becoming familiar with today's technology, conducting research online using Web-based search engines, developing computer literacy, learning how to write professional papers, and working in teams with classmates on group projects will all be important skills for today's new classroom environment as an active learner. In *Your Guide to College Success: Strategies for Achieving Your Goals*, Santrock and Halonen (2010) provide tips for success, including emphasizing gaining experience with different teaching and learning methods to diversify your learning styles.

Financial and/or Family Constraints

Another barrier to your return to school may be financial and/or family constraints. The student role may require financial sacrifices. Tuition, books, student uniforms, and commuting costs are large burdens. The necessity to remain employed and/or find and finance child care may add to these pressures. The current recession in the United States has exacerbated financial constraints for returning students, who are often single-family breadwinners and/or caretakers. The economic downturn has caused families to "double-up" in housing, with extended family members and/or multigenerational households becoming more prevalent. Financial obligations have expanded, credit standards have tightened, and accessing loans has become more difficult. This may cause you additional strain as you return to school, and may also cause you to have to work more hours, impeding your ability to devote study time needed to be successful as a returning student. Fortunately, there is a great deal of assistance available for students, and many scholarships for nursing students in particular.

In addition to financial constraints, returning students at times experience family constraints. Children or other family members may need your time and support. Although supportive of your desire to return to school, they may also want life to remain unchanged. Another related factor is that life does not stop while you are in school. Illnesses, life events, and crises may occur. Although you may have planned for many things, the unexpected and unplanned may occur over the next months and/or years as you pursue your degree. College campuses have many resources for students, including scholarships and programs targeted to assist first-generation college students, students of color, and students who are socioeconomically disadvantaged. Federal, state, and community-based support programs of which you may not yet be familiar, such as TRIO, Student Support Services, Puente, and MESA, are often available. Gandara and Contreras (2009) describe barriers many Latino students encounter and provide strategies for success. Talk to your nursing advisor or college counselor if you find you are in need of financial or other support services.

Fear of Failure

A last barrier to returning to school is fear of failure. You have invested a lot of time and effort to be where you are today. Taking exams and being observed in the clinical area can be frightening. You may have developed shortcuts to clinical skills or bad habits that will need to be corrected. The fear of not being successful as a student nurse can be overwhelming. Some of this may stem from previous school experiences or from lack of self-confidence. You may also find yourself hesitant or uneasy in new clinical settings. Adult learners are typically hard on themselves because they not only want to be successful but they often also want to be perfect. It takes frequent reminders that the learning and transition processes need not be perfect, only positive. In addition, many factors are involved as a student progresses through a nursing program, including learning at a professional practice level that will require nursing diagnosis, critical thinking, and judgment not required at the LPN/LVN level.

Later in this chapter, some strategies for success and minimizing fears are presented. Remember that the barriers and fears you may be experiencing are real and are shared by others who are also returning to school. For instance, as you get to know your classmates, you will find that your age, experience, and unique qualities are valuable to other class members. It may be advantageous to have had the experience of raising a family or to be of a particular culture or ethnicity. Your concerns about studying may be the same as those of your fellow students; you may find that you will be able to assist each other. You may also find that your study skills did not disappear. In fact, you may be more organized and better able to complete the assigned work than you anticipated. Other students may provide insight into particular courses or instructors. Financial concerns are experienced by many, and so you may find that you can share commuting costs, child care, or other resources. It is beneficial to identify your fears and concerns as you return to school. You may find that they are common to other students and that together you can find answers and solutions. It may also be reassuring to know that you are not alone. As you develop your individual educational plan and discuss these issues with your advisor, success strategies will emerge.

thinking critically

After reading the previous section, you may have found yourself nodding your head in recognition or wondering why your fears and concerns were not voiced. At this point, identify the barriers and fears that you face as you return to school. Include all of them, regardless whether they have been mentioned. If you have determined some solutions, include those as well. As a next step, talk with a fellow student or another nurse at work who returned to school to determine whether you share common concerns. You may also find it useful, as did the student in the vignette, to share these concerns with your nursing advisor. This is a beginning step in preparing for success on returning to school.

• RETURNING TO THE STUDENT ROLE: "RETURNING TO SCHOOL SYNDROME"

Donea L. Shane (1983) identified the process of re-entry as the "returning to school syndrome" (RTSS). In studying educationally mobile nursing students as they returned to school, she was able to identify stages that comprise an entire syndrome. Educationally mobile nurses are those who are returning to school or at least contemplating such a return. Shane's work was derived from stories and data collected during a 6-year period from those studying to become RNs. Those students were able to "share their insecurities, sorrows, failures, and anxieties as well as their triumphs, humor, and joy" (p. vii). The results of her work remain valuable today.

Shane (1983) defined RTSS as up-and-down emotional swings that are experienced by nursing students who are returning to school. These swings occur because returning students are familiar with their nursing roles within the work setting, yet are taking on a different role by becoming nursing students again. The RTSS model depicts a series of sequential stages. "However, an individual nurse may not proceed through these phases in a linear fashion. The usual progression is an irregular one, with relapses, detours, and expressways through certain stages" (p. 73). Shane identified three major stages within the RTSS syndrome (Table 1.1).

Stage 1: Honeymoon

Typically, the shortest and most benign stage is called the honeymoon stage. It is a somewhat blissful time in which the reality of a situation has not quite been

table 1-1   RETURNING TO SCHOOL SYNDROME

Stage	Description
Honeymoon	Individual is happy and delighted about being back in school; does not see any problems with the process.
Conflict	Characterized by high anxiety: individual feels conflict about educational process and role changes.
a. Disintegration	a. Individual represses feelings of anger and hostility; may become depressed and sullen.
b. Reintegration	b. Person becomes outwardly hostile and angry, particularly with nursing faculty; individual is frustrated with the educational program.
Resolution a. Chronic conflict	There are various forms in the process of resolving conflicts. a. The student nurse maintains angry feelings and fails to see anything worthwhile or valuable in the educational process.
b. False acceptance	b. Individual pretends to accept the changes in role but actually does not understand or see any difference.
c. Oscillation	c. The educationally mobile nurse vacillates between stages; generally involves regression if a stressful event occurs; once the stressor is resolved, the person moves to a more positive resolution.
d. Biculturalism	d. A positive resolution in which the individual accepts the differences and role values and is challenged to grow within the professional role.

absorbed. Individuals are generally happy about being in school and see the experience as congenial. The end of the honeymoon usually occurs when the educationally mobile nurse is enrolled in her or his first clinical nursing course. At this point, the student may become intimidated and begin to fear that her or his experience is no longer of value. In particular, the dreaded clinical evaluation looms ahead, causing the individual increasing anxiety.

Stage 2: Conflict

Shane (1983) suggested that the longest and most intense phase is conflict. It is a difficult time that can be emotionally exhausting and overwhelming. In general, the educationally mobile nurse experiences conflicts with beliefs, family roles, work roles, prior knowledge versus new knowledge, and nursing faculty. Such nurses may believe that there is no difference in the educational programs, that they already know what they need to know to be RNs, or that they are already better than the graduates of this program, and thus, nothing will change by continuing the educational process. Work role conflicts arise from realism versus idealism. Working nurses know and understand the real work world, and so they dispute the idealistic presentations or experience guilt at not being able to practice idealistically. Other conflicts also arise, such as stressful relationships with clinical faculty, dealing with various teaching styles, and adjusting to new ways of learning in the nursing program.

The conflict stage is subdivided into two parts: disintegration and reintegration. Disintegration is characterized by a state of anxiety in which the individual turns her or his anxious feelings inward. This can result in several negative feelings that are potentially harmful: depression; sadness; withdrawal from friends, family, and others; and attitudes of obstinacy and gloom. It is remarkable that significant people who have contact with this person are able to overlook these behaviors or do not notice them.

Reintegration is marked by outwardly intense feelings of frustration and hostility that are directed toward those around the individual, especially the faculty. This anger is the result of the individual's frustrations with the nursing program or with the whole educational process. Although these outbursts are difficult to handle, they are healthier than the repression of feelings that is seen in disintegration (Shane, 1983).

Stage 3: Resolution

The third and final stage, resolution, is a variable phase because each individual experiences different lengths of time and outcomes. Shane (1983) presented a few of the forms that resolution can take.

1. **Chronic conflict.** This resolution is the least effective because these nurses become stuck in a quagmire of anger. They may continue with their nursing education, but they fail to recognize the value of that education or the inherent worth of the role change. They spend valuable energy and time being angry and belligerent, with little energy put into creating a positive outcome.

2. **False acceptance.** This resolution is also not considered particularly positive. Educationally mobile nurses play games of deceit and pretense. They may claim to accept the differences in the former work role and the present educational role, and the value of the new role, but do not actually recognize any difference. They cannot also perceive the positive aspects of education and transition. In some regard, they become their own victims by not realizing any difference or usefulness in the process.
3. **Oscillation.** Individuals who fall into this category vacillate between the various resolutions. To some degree, their oscillation occurs because they have experienced each resolution in various forms. Fortunately, oscillation is reversible. An oscillation (most frequently a regression to a more negative state) usually occurs because of some unusual stressor, such as failure on an exam, an illness at home, or an unfortunate interchange with a faculty member.
4. **Biculturalism.** This resolution is the most positive. These educationally mobile nurses have positive feelings about their previous educational experiences. They also value their current education and their growth within the nursing profession. It is important to them to be challenged and to develop their professional roles.

The RTSS presents an interesting way to view the re-entry process. You may recognize the various emotional states. However, Shane (1983) also found that some educationally mobile nurses deny that any of the RTSS concepts apply to them. These nurses resent being analyzed and categorized. Behavior and role changes are not uniformly valued in the educational process. It is even more difficult to identify your own emotions and feelings. The value of understanding this syndrome is that it provides you with some insights into the conflicts and concerns that can arise when you are dealing with role change and changes in your own beliefs and it can affirm that these are normal responses.

• DIVERSE LEARNING STYLES

The process of learning often seems formidable, particularly if the learner has not been engaged in formal learning activities for several years or if previous experiences were not especially positive. Adults have long been occupied with the tasks of returning to educational settings in pursuit of further educational degrees. Many adults fear that they will not be capable of learning new information or that they

thinking critically

After reading about the RTSS, consider how these phases apply to you in your own LPN/LVN-to-RN role transition. For example, recall your practical/vocational nursing education experience. Was it positive or negative? In thinking about the role change from LPN/LVN to RN, what do you value about this process? Have you experienced any of the emotions described in the explanation of RTSS? As you consider these questions, write down what you are experiencing and why. You may find it helpful to keep a journal as you progress through this role transition, or make a note on your calendar to review this material again after taking your first clinical course.

NCLEX–RN *Might Ask*

The student nurse is studying about theories of adjustment to nursing school. The stage of Shane's theory that describes developing family conflicts, conflicts between the real and ideal nursing world, and feelings of being exhausted and overwhelmed is the _____ stage of the returning to school syndrome.

    A.   Honeymoon
    B.   Disintegration
    C.   Reintegration
    D.   Resolution

• *See Appendix A for correct answer and rationale.*

will not be able to focus on their educational program due to other commitments or interests that demand their attention. However, for most adults, it is a pleasant surprise to find that not only are they still able to learn but that they are also more focused and dedicated than in previous educational endeavors.

Much research has been conducted over the past few decades to determine how people learn and what learning styles exist. One categorization of learning styles is to examine one's preference for learning through visual, auditory, or kinesthetic delivery mechanisms. Ellis (2011) called this the "VAK" system. For example, some of us learn faster, or retain more, when information is accessed in an auditory manner. Some individuals learn better when information is provided visually. Use of graphs, charts, visual aids, DVDs, Internet, or video streaming modes of delivery is more effective for these individuals. Acquiring information through a lecture, DVD, or other method where listening is involved is another common learning style. A third learning style is the preference for "doing" things to learn new information and concepts. Assembling three-dimensional objects, building conceptual models, role playing, and "learning by doing" all align with this learning style. Identifying your own learning style and using study techniques that address that style will maximize your success as you return to school.

Adult Learning Styles

Learning styles of adults differ from those of children. Adults have a different and clearer sense of themselves, what their purpose is in a particular educational endeavor, and what is worthwhile and what is not. Adults are able to draw on their experiences to gain a deeper and more meaningful understanding, and therefore, have a greater capacity to apply theoretical concepts to practical situations. Adults pursue educational opportunities because there is a desire or need to attain new learning for job acquisition, career advancement, or personal gratification or self-actualization. Covey (2004) noted that finding meaning and your own voice (ie, why you are going back to school, your true aspirations) will yield greater success. Achievement will also be stronger if motivation is intrinsic, coming from within yourself rather than from external forces.

Learning from experience changes what we do and how we view things. You may find differences between what you have learned from experience as an LPN/LVN and what you read in preparation for class assignments. This is to be expected because patients bring with them a unique array of personal attributes, and you as an adult learner also bring with you various life experiences. Your learning in the RN program will involve an active process in which you will engage in activities that provide knowledge, practice, and abstract skills. Styles of learning are the methods that the learner prefers to use for perceiving and processing new information (Ellis, 2011).

Perceiving and Processing Tasks

It is advantageous to be aware of diverse learning styles to recognize that there are differences, to use strengths, and to adapt when the learning styles of others are predominant. Ellis (2011) identified styles of learning as involving two tasks: perceiving and processing. He summarized two methods of perceiving.

Some people perceive by

> Using concrete experimentation
> Dealing with situations with an intuitive ability to problem solve
> Sensing and feeling
> Taking the initiative in unstructured settings

Other people perceive by

> Using abstract conceptualization
> Thinking about things completely and analytically
> Using a scientific approach to problem solving
> Functioning well within structured settings

> Along with styles of perception, Ellis also delineated two styles of processing.

Some people process new information by

> Using active experimentation
> Applying new information in practical situations
> Seeing results despite potential risks

Others process by

> Using reflective observation
> Considering various points of view
> Presenting different ideas about a specific situation

As Ellis (2011) emphasized, these categories are not absolute, and successful learners benefit from participating in all four styles of learning. Refer to Display 1.2 for a review of terms used in this section.

Four Styles of Learning

When considering the different styles of perceiving and processing, four distinct styles of learning emerge (Ellis, 2011). The following material has been adapted from Ellis's *Becoming a Master Student*. Each learning style is intended to serve as a guide for you to begin thinking about your own learning preferences. There is no hierarchal design in the four learning styles; each has validity and usefulness.

---

display 1.2   **Review of Terminology**

Abstract conceptualization: a mode of perceiving new knowledge that entails an ability to analyze, think through, and organize theoretical material in a logical way
Active experimentation: a method to process information that involves a hands-on approach to be able to apply new information; implies that an individual wants to work with an idea or concept to determine if it makes sense
Concrete experimentation: a means to perceive new information in a more passive way; involves approaching situations in a more observational manner, preferring to look at a situation from several viewpoints and ponder various ideas
Experiential learning: a process of learning that evolves and is evolving as an individual matures and has a wider range of experiences: involves adaptation and growth, and increased self-awareness
Learning style: preferred methods to perceive and process new information
Reflective observation: a method of processing information that involves careful observation and a pondering about those observations, judgments occur after the individual has contemplated several alternatives

---

It is helpful to review each style and identify the characteristics that best describe your own learning preferences. This is intended to assist you in increasing your self-awareness. You will discover that you probably draw from all four categories and that it often depends on the particular situation, the context, or your experiences.

STYLE 1 LEARNERS

Perception of new information is best accomplished with concrete experiences. These learners prefer to find examples of how particular information applies to their world. They use reflective observation to process new learning. Characteristics may include the following:

- Viewing concrete situations from different points of view
- Approaching events as observers
- Reflecting on situations rather than taking action
- Enjoying experiences that necessitate creation of ideas
- Using imagination
- Working for harmony and developing support
- Placing importance on concerns, caring, and trust in others

   Goals: being involved in important issues, bringing harmony
   Favorite questions: Why? Why do I need to know this? Why should I attend this class? How do these concepts relate to my life?
   Skills: valuing—brainstorming, listening, speaking, interacting, feeling, data gathering, imaging
   Preferred skill: problem identification

STYLE 2 LEARNERS

These learners perceive best through abstract conceptualization. Explanations through lecture style are favored, particularly if a theoretical base is included. They process new information generally by reflective observation. Characteristics may include the following:

- Understanding a broad range of information
- Compiling information in a concise and logical form
- Being interested more in abstract ideas and less in people
- Favoring theory that is logical as opposed to practical
- Preferring traditional learning settings that include lectures and reading assignments and do not include open-ended tasks
- Being industrious and goal oriented with attention to detail

    Goal: understanding things on an intellectual level
    Favorite questions: What? What is important to learn from this particular class?
    Skills: thinking—observing and analyzing; classifying, theorizing, organizing, conceptualizing, and testing theories
    Preferred skill: solution identification

STYLE 3 LEARNERS

Perceiving knowledge is best done through abstract conceptualization. Traditional modes of lecture and listening to theory are most preferred. New learning is best processed through active experimentation. Characteristics may include the following:

- Being skilled at applying ideas and theories for practical use
- Answering questions and demonstrating problem-solving and decision-making skills
- Enjoying technical tasks, as opposed to contemplating social issues
- Discovering how things work, including experimentation and tinkering
- Preferring plans and schedules

    Goal: putting new information into use in their work and daily living tasks
    Favorite questions: How does this thing operate? How can I use this information to make a positive difference in my life?
    Skills: deciding—manipulating, tinkering, improving, applying, experimenting, goal setting
    Preferred skill: selecting a workable solution from all possibilities

STYLE 4 LEARNERS

These learners perceive information by using concrete experience. They also use active experimentation to process new information. They prefer to explore ideas to determine if they can make sense of them or apply them in a practical way. Characteristics may include the following:

- Learning best from hands-on methods
- Carrying out plans
- Being involved in new and different experiences
- Relying on gut feelings, as opposed to logical analysis
- Taking risks

- Feeling comfortable in new situations
- Encouraging others to be independent thinkers
- Drawing conclusions without necessarily having logical reasons

Goals: bringing action to ideas; encouraging creativity
Favorite questions: What if? If I am learning important and accurate information, how does it apply to my own life? What else does it mean?
Skills: activity—modifying, adapting, risking, collaborating, committing, influencing, leading
Preferred skill: implementing a selected solution

Being aware of your learning preferences will help you have a greater understanding of your learning needs and strengths. By appreciating your own individuality and recognizing that there are many learning styles, you should be open to situations that are not conducive to your style of learning. You will be exposed to different modes of education and instruction. You also will care for a range of clients who will have educational needs and styles of learning that are different from yours. Having the knowledge that there are various learning styles provides you not only with flexibility but also with an ability to meet your own needs and the needs of others. The following example illustrates this truth.

EXAMPLE

A student nurse is assigned to care for a client who has recently been diagnosed with hypertension. The client has begun a regimen of antihypertensives and a low-sodium diet. The student observes the dietitian reviewing diet pamphlets and a list of low-sodium foods with the client. She instructs the client to read the materials and jot down any questions. After the dietitian leaves, the client tells the student nurse that he is totally confused: None of this makes sense. Although the student nurse believes that the instructional methods were appropriate, he asks the client what would help him learn the information. The client tells him that it would be much easier to see the information than to read about it: "I don't learn well when I just have to read about it." The student recognizes that a more visual method of instruction might be beneficial to this client and arranges for him to view a video and to learn to recognize low-sodium foods by reading their labels.

For a more in-depth discussion of learning styles, including the VAK system, multiple intelligences, and a learning style inventory to assess your own learning style preference, refer to Ellis's (2011) *Becoming a Master Student.*

thinking critically

After reading the preceding material and determining which characteristics apply to you, list your preferred learning styles. Identify which of the four styles is the most predominant for you. Give several examples of why that style is the most preferred. You may use examples that demonstrate when you have enjoyed or deplored a particular learning situation. Share this information with a partner, and discuss observations about yourself and each other that back your selection of a learning style. It also may be helpful for you to share this with your faculty advisor.

• STUDENT ROLE: STRATEGIES FOR SUCCESS

The key to being a successful student rests with you. Although methods and techniques to assist you in your endeavors are available, only you can make them work. This will require that you assume responsibility for your academic efforts and use assertive behavior to meet your goals. Assertiveness is a positive skill because it provides you with the courage and stamina to meet your needs. Assertiveness does not mean confrontation or aggression; rather, it implies that you are able to communicate in a positive and constructive manner. Assertive behavior assists you in exploring possibilities, asking for more information and clarification, considering various viewpoints, and making informed decisions. It will be important that you are assertive in building a relationship with faculty and in seeking their feedback on what you are doing well and where you need to improve. This will assist you in setting clear goals for yourself for success.

College Success Courses

Colleges today provide you with many opportunities to sharpen your academic skills. For instance, you may find it helpful to take a course that provides you with study skills, test-taking skills, or an improved ability to write professional term papers. If you have been away from an academic setting for a while or were overwhelmed by previous academic experiences, it may be extremely beneficial to enroll in a course designed for college success. In addition, computer literacy and library research courses may be helpful. Many colleges require or strongly suggest that you take these courses. Again, you may be pleasantly surprised that some of the obstacles that you believed had prevented you from being successful were not as much of a problem as you anticipated, given the right tools and college success strategies. You may also discover that the relearning of various academic and study skills was not especially difficult and was more rewarding than it was in prior experiences.

On your return to school, take advantage of any courses that are available to assist you in being more successful in your nursing program. Research shows that students who take college success courses as they enter or re-enter college do better in their course work. In a study of mature students entering registered nursing programs, Fleming and McKee (2005) found that students who took courses focused on socializing the student into college life and developing study skills progressed better in the nursing program. They found that students recommended that these courses should also include an overview of the nursing courses, more in-depth study and computer technology skills, and time management techniques. If you are not able to take a course in these areas, there is also a wide array of college success texts on these subjects. This chapter and the bibliography identify several excellent texts, and more are available in your college library and through online search engines.

Working With a Faculty Advisor

Once enrolled in a program of nursing, you will be assigned to a faculty advisor, most likely a member of the nursing faculty. You should introduce yourself to your advisor as early as possible so that both of you get to know each other.

Exchanging telephone numbers and e-mail addresses will help you keep in closer contact and can be invaluable in the event of illness or a personal emergency. Your faculty advisor is available to you throughout the length of the program. Many students have primary contact with their advisor when it is time to register for the next term's classes. This contact may consist of getting a signature on the registration or add-drop form. However, there are many other reasons to have contact with a faculty advisor. Students often consult with their advisors when they are experiencing academic difficulties. Faculty advisors are knowledgeable about finding appropriate resources for students to improve their academic performance. For example, if a student finds that she or he is having trouble taking multiple-choice exams, the advisor may refer the student to college resources that can teach the student ways to be successful with that type of exam or to someone who can review past exams with the student and develop methods for taking future exams. Some faculty advisors are skilled in these methods and assist the student directly.

Some students also seek assistance from faculty advisors if they believe that they are not skilled at taking notes in class or grasping material from text and/or online assignments. Again, discussing these issues with an advisor may help the student focus on topics that are outlined in the study guides or that are main themes in a text or Web source. The advisor may also refer the student to other college resources for improving study and note-taking skills.

Other reasons that students go to see advisors are related to personal problems at home or in the college environment. Advisors are generally skilled at listening to problems and, although they are not trained counselors, will be able to refer the student to an appropriate resource. If the problem involves another faculty member, the advisor may choose not to hear that issue completely but may suggest that the student speak directly with the faculty person, counselor, or program administrator.

An advisor can be most helpful if you meet him or her as soon as possible, instead of waiting until you have an insurmountable or overwhelming situation. It is highly advantageous to schedule an individual appointment at the start of the term to develop a rapport with your advisor. Advisors can be many things, but they are not mind readers, miracle workers, or saviors. If you begin to experience academic problems, you are expected to proactively seek help early in the process so that the difficulty can be remedied before failure. Advisors can help only as much as you are willing to seek help. Advisors are not always immediately available because of other academic commitments. In most instances, you will have to make an appointment to meet with your advisor. If you have an urgent issue, other faculty members may need to be involved if the advisor is not available. If you find that you have difficulty relating to your advisor, you may be able to change advisors by speaking with the program administrator.

Resource Materials

As you begin your nursing program, many different resources are available to you that will enhance your success. The following is a brief summary of some of these resources.

STUDENT HANDBOOK

A student handbook or pamphlet is designed specifically for students at the college or university and is often available to those in the nursing program. Within these handbooks is information about student policies, grading procedures, and resources available on campus. When you receive a copy of the handbook, it is important that you familiarize yourself with its contents so that you will know how to obtain pertinent information and use campus resources. This will avoid conflict and issues during the program that can occur if you do not know college or program policies and procedures. When a question arises, refer to your handbook rather than asking a fellow student, who may give you inaccurate or incomplete information.

PROGRAM PHILOSOPHY

Faculties for each nursing program have developed a program philosophy that presents the concepts, themes, and curriculum threads for the nursing program. Generally, nursing education philosophies are composed of beliefs about nursing, the education of nurses, and the various recognized levels of nursing education. They may include philosophical approaches to the education of adults and the responsibilities of adult students. In many instances, the program philosophy carries out the principles stated in the college or university philosophy. It is also helpful to explore this in terms of your own evolving philosophy about nursing.

LEARNING OUTCOMES

The nursing program will also have identified Student Learning Outcomes for students as they progress through the course work. Additional learning outcomes for all students earning a degree from a particular college or university are required by accrediting bodies for the institution and can often be found in the college catalog. Learning outcomes portray the knowledge, skills, and abilities expected of all program participants as they graduate and proceed to higher educational degrees or enter the workforce. Individual courses and their learning activities are designed to facilitate the student achieving these learning outcomes upon completion of the program. College success courses often provide an overview of these learning outcomes and identify resources to assist students as they progress through their course work.

COURSE SYLLABUS

A course syllabus is an outline and summary of material that will be covered in a particular course. Students find this extremely useful because a brief description of the course is provided, along with expected outcomes, course objectives, teaching methods, learning activities, required texts, Web-based resources, and course requirements, such as tests, papers, projects, reading assignments, and other activities. The syllabus becomes a study guide by defining the focus, direction, and expected outcomes of the course. You must become well acquainted with the syllabus to understand the course requirements, to concentrate on the most important aspects of the course, to achieve its expected outcomes, and to be aware of how your progress and performance in the course will be assessed and evaluated.

FACULTY AND COURSE WEB PAGES

Many faculties now maintain a home page online with e-mail addresses, other contact information, announcements, reminders, and other important information for students. Many courses have associated online chat rooms, shared spaces for threaded discussions, and other helpful tools vital to student success in the course. If you are unfamiliar with these learning technologies, talk to your faculty advisor for assistance in locating an orientation session, class, or other forum for becoming familiar with these online resources.

PERSONAL PROFESSIONAL LIBRARY

Collecting nursing texts, resources, and Web-based materials can be confusing, overwhelming, and expensive. Students returning to school are often tempted to purchase all the books they can, with the hope that each book might be helpful. There are many excellent resource books, but you do not need all of them. The course syllabus generally lists required and recommended texts. The faculty members usually select recommended texts to assist you in acquiring more knowledge about a particular topic. In general, students should be required to attain a comprehensive medical dictionary, a drug resource manual, a laboratory manual, and possibly a text that assists with the nursing process and the development of care plans. Computer-based resources in these areas are also available. Other resources that students may want to purchase are those about a particular subject in which they have a strong interest. The nursing textbooks and other resources you acquire will be valuable after completing the program when you prepare for the NCLEX-RN. Although they eventually become outdated, the information has merit for a long time. Other resources that may be helpful are pharmacology and nutrition texts, state board review books, CDs, DVDs, and computerized programs. Before purchasing anything, you may find it helpful to discuss your choices with faculty and recent graduates of nursing programs. Your college's library will have additional resources, and many more are available via interlibrary loan and online.

PERIODICAL SUBSCRIPTIONS AND WEB RESOURCES

Many nursing journals are available both by subscription and online. It is often difficult to choose which journals are appropriate for you. Again, talking with faculty and other students may assist you. Many nursing journals are available on campus, in hospital libraries, and online, which is a cheaper and easier way to become familiar with nursing journals as resources of information. As a student nurse, you will have many opportunities to read journal articles as part of course requirements. This will help you decide whether you want to subscribe to a particular journal. If you use an online resource, make sure it is reputable. Not all information on the Web is accurate; therefore, if you are unsure of the accuracy of a Web site, consult your instructor or the college learning resource center.

Resources for Updating Your Research Skills

Web resources have greatly expanded over the past decade. In completing your general education and nursing course requirements and writing professional papers, you will find general resources, such as a dictionary, thesaurus, encyclopedia, and standards for writing professional papers, readily available online. Search engines and directories are abundant, including those available in other languages if English is not your first language. You will need to become skilled at using these resources, and many students enhance their abilities in this area via a college success or library use course, or by working with the college library staff. Although it may take some time for you to become comfortable in this environment, you will find your time saving is extensive once you are adept at online research. Examples of Web resources are available at the end of this and other chapters.

If you have not been in an academic setting recently, you will discover that performing research for assignments and term papers has also become a more technical process because most libraries now have computerized records. There also are several sources from which to obtain particular articles, journals, and books, depending on what you are researching. You must become familiar with using the college's library and its computer system to research a topic properly. As part of your initial orientation to academic life, make sure that a library orientation is provided or independently orient yourself to the college's library. While you may feel "technologically challenged" initially, you will find that technology actually expedites and expands your research capability, and often allows you to do your research at times and places more convenient to you. Hardesty (2007) notes how important effective library research skills are in increasing motivation and decreasing anxiety, and thereby enhancing student success. Once you begin to use the library, do not be afraid to ask the library staff for assistance. You will soon be able to access many resources, which will enable you to research a topic thoroughly. These skills will be critical to your lifelong learning as an RN, as well as to your pursuance of advanced degrees and/or clinical certification.

Valuing Prior Learning

As stated previously, adults often return to school with the fear that they will not do well, that they will appear foolish, or that the rest of the students will be more advanced. For the LPN/LVN, it is also difficult to be removed from an environment that values clinical skills and to be placed in an environment that values skills necessary for academic success. However, the value of your experiences as an LPN/LVN and your life experiences in general is immeasurable. You will probably find that your view of the world and of nursing has been greatly influenced by your many experiences.

Adult educators have long recognized the value of prior learning. You will find that your experiences enable you to perceive course work in a different way and to place a higher value on your efforts. Ellis (2011) states, "Being an older student puts you on strong footing. Having a rich store of life experiences equips, you to ask meaningful questions and make connections between course work and daily life" (p. 13).

Valuing who you are and your life, work, and educational experiences provides you with a foundation for continued growth and development in your career as a nurse and as a person. You remain capable of acquiring new knowledge and of adapting to the educational process. Everything that you have learned before returning to school will serve you well. Instead of despairing about what you may not know or understand, rejoice in the knowledge that you can achieve your goals with hard work and a reliance on the skills and knowledge that put you where you are today.

Campbell, Cignetti, Melenyzer, Nettles, and Wyman (2011) stress the importance of students in professional careers developing personal portfolios. They define a portfolio as "a collection of documents that provides tangible evidence of the wide range of knowledge, dispositions, and skills that you possess as a growing professional" (p. 3). Furthermore, they note that since documents in your portfolio are self-selected, they reflect your individuality, autonomy, and unique attributes. A portfolio can be used with your nursing advisor to introduce yourself, and to identify strengths and areas where you may need further mentoring or development. Items that may be useful to assemble for your portfolio when meeting with your nursing advisor include sample nursing care plans, clinical skills checklists, papers you have written, case study projects, and other documents or projects you have completed as an LPN/LVN and/or returning student that demonstrate your critical thinking ability and work as a health care professional.

Time Management

BALANCING PERSONAL, CAREER, AND STUDENT ROLES

One of the biggest obstacles that returning students face is the lack of time to perform all roles adequately. There never seems to be enough time to manage everything and to do it well, but developing a plan will assist you in managing your time more effectively. McCarey, Barr, and Rattray (2006) found that nursing students older than age 26 with high absenteeism experienced poor academic achievement. Good time management will ensure you have strong attendance and thereby support your success in nursing school.

It is particularly helpful to plan a weekly schedule to see the entire picture. Some blocks of time are inflexible, such as work and class schedules. You must also remember to make time for other activities, such as sleeping, eating, exercising, family time, and studying. Once you have the weekly plan in place, it is helpful to formulate a daily to-do list to keep yourself organized and to be realistic about your time commitments.

It is not necessary that you do everything as you did before you started school. Involve your significant others in your scheduling plan. Delegate some tasks or hire others to help. Give up some tasks until there is time to do them, and learn to be flexible so that you can take care of unexpected things. Let your family and friends know your schedule so that they have a better understanding of your needs. This may need to be the year you decline roles you may have held in the past as the organizer of events or activities in your personal life.

Do not give up all your exercise and recreation activities; you may need to modify what you do or when you do it, but continue to find time for yourself. Exercise is not only healthy but also reduces your stress level. Some students find it helpful to walk or jog between classes, plan a physical activity with a friend, or take a physical education class. You also will find it beneficial to designate some periods of quiet time for reflection and/or meditation. Students often feel guilty about taking time for a walk or quiet time, but it can actually rejuvenate you and cause your work and study time to be more productive. Reading for pleasure, watching television or a movie, listening to music, meditating, or even just taking a walk may help you regroup and recharge.

Returning students need to be prepared to spend 2 to 3 hours of studying for every hour spent in class. If you are carrying a full-time student load, you will need to plan 20 to 30 hours per week for reading, studying, and completing assignments. This does not need to be done in huge blocks of time; most people generally study best in 1- to 2-hour blocks of time spent at the library or another quiet place without distractions. The benefits will be realized at exam time or when a project is due because you will not have to have marathon study times to prepare or complete the work. Retention of information is also improved when you avoid "cramming" at the last minute. For some students, carrying a full academic load is not feasible, and so they choose to attend school on a part-time basis. This will reduce both the workload and stress of multiple role responsibilities.

It is also helpful to communicate early with your employer regarding your needs and potential scheduling difficulties. Although most employers will support your decision to return to school, they also have to manage an entire staff, multiple work schedules, and many other details. Most students find that it is advantageous to reduce the number of work hours to the least number that is absolutely necessary to maintain financial commitments. With a full course load, it is recommended that you work only 1 to 2 days/shifts per week. Salamonson and Andrew (2006) examined the influence of part-time employment on nursing students. They found that those who worked more than 16 hours per week experienced a detrimental impact on their academic performance. Students who complete their general education and science course work before entering the nursing program, however, may find that they can work half time while attending college. In Display 1.3, Simon (2009) summarized suggestions from adult students such as you, providing 10 hints for time management.

REASSESSING COMMITMENTS

When you are rationing your time, consider also creating a "not-to-do" list. This list should include tasks that are not a priority and those that can be done by others while you are in school. For instance, if you serve on a committee at your child's school, consider resigning and letting someone else have the opportunity to serve. If you volunteer for a local nursing home, you may decide to take a leave of absence. When you finish school, there will always be opportunities to be a member of a board or committee or a chance to do volunteer work. One student who returned to school referred to his time in school as "the years to say 'no.'"

thinking critically

Track your time commitments for 1 week. Think in terms of 15-minute blocks of time so that you can account for short activities. Account for all 24 hours of a day, and include adequate personal time and study time to avoid cramming assignments and exams. Carry the plan with you, and at the end of the week, examine what you did, and modify your plan for the following week so that you are organizing and using your time more efficiently.

---

display 1.3   **Ten Hints for Time Management**

1. Be realistic.
   Don't overestimate what you can take on, how long it will take, or schedule
   yourself so tightly that you cause stress for yourself.
2. Build in "safe time."
   Give yourself some "wiggle room" to allow for computer down time, car problems,
   or other realities of life that can cause you to get behind, miss deadlines, or be
   underprepared for a test.
3. Keep a planner.
   Develop a plan for the week, with time allotted for each of your roles (student,
   spouse, parent, worker, community service member, and, most important,
   yourself).
4. Find a space.
   Find a quiet, uncluttered space for reading, studying, writing papers, and working
   on projects, and let others know not to bother you when you are in that space.
5. Look at the big picture.
   Balance time among your courses and other development needs. Celebrate your
   accomplishments as well as focus on your "to-do" list.
6. Speak out about your concerns and commitments.
   Maintain open communication with your family, friends, employer, and faculty
   advisor. Make agreements ahead of time as you anticipate problems or high
   stress times.
7. Work a little every day.
   Break things into "small bites" in order to maintain a positive outlook, make progress, and gain a sense of accomplishment.
8. Make a checklist each week.
   Identify tasks to be accomplished for the week and spread them out so as not to
   forget any and not to end up with too many tasks on a particular day. Postpone
   tasks that are not essential for your success.
9. Just say "no!"
   Learn how to say "no" or propose an alternative that will be more expedient. Offer
   to volunteer for things in a year or two when you have finished the program.
10. Get a "study buddy."
   Find someone to be your "study buddy" who will be honest and challenge you so
   that you can keep each other on track and quiz each other on course content.

Adapted from Simon, L. (2009). *New beginnings: A guide for adult learners and returning students*
(pp. 42–46). Upper Saddle River, NJ: Prentice-Hall.

USING THE WIN/WIN AGREEMENT

Stephen Covey (1989, 2004) formulated a method to reach agreements in which
there is mutual benefit or satisfaction from the agreement for all involved. Win/win
agreements create an environment in which each party thinks in terms of cooperation, as opposed to competition. Win/win is conceived on the idea that "there is
plenty for everybody, that one person's success is not achieved at the expense or
exclusion of the success of others" (p. 207). Such agreements are useful in working
out arrangements with significant others while you are in nursing school.

Covey (2004) identified five dimensions that are interdependent and relational:

1. Character: This is the foundation of win/win and consists of three traits:
   a. Integrity: the value you place on yourself; a commitment to yourself and
      others

    b. Maturity: the maintenance between the ability to express your opinions and attitudes and the respect for the opinions and attitudes of others

    c. Abundance mentality: the notion that there is enough or plenty for everyone; requires the individual to have strong integrity and maturity

2. Relationships: Win/win involves a level of trust in the process and in the person(s) that are involved with the formulation of an agreement. It also involves an ability to listen and to communicate with respect for the person(s) and the various points of view.

3. Agreements: Win/win requires that each party have a clear understanding of the limits and scope of the process. The agreements include an understanding of the desired results, any guidelines that are needed, an awareness of all available resources, accountability by all those involved in the agreement, and an evaluation of the process with possible consequences.

4. Systems: For win/win agreements to work there must be support for the process. Each individual involved must feel equal responsibility for achieving goals and results, and therefore, solutions.

5. Processes: Win/win solutions are best achieved if each person looks at the problem from the other's perspective; this gives the other person a chance to be heard. It is then essential to name the concerns and issues that are involved. Each person next presents possible results that would be acceptable solutions to the problem. As a last step, various options could be determined for achieving the specific results.

Win/win agreements do not need to be elaborate or lengthy. The process can actually be simple, particularly if each person is committed to the process. An example of a win/win agreement within a family is illustrated in the following example.

EXAMPLE

When Sandy, an LPN, returned to school, she recognized that her time would be more restricted because she would be in class for 6 hours a week and clinical practice for 15 hours a week. Her study and preparation time would require 20 to 30 hours a week. She also needed to work two 8-hour shifts per week to pay certain bills and maintain benefits and seniority. Her husband works full time (Monday–Friday, 9 AM–5 PM). Their son and daughter are 10 and 16 years old, respectively. Historically, Sandy has taken care of many of the household chores, particularly housecleaning, preparing meals, and the majority of errands. The other family members helped, but not on a regular basis and often only with much persuasion. With classes and studying, Sandy realized that she could no longer be responsible for all of these tasks. Sandy's family developed the following win/win agreement:

    Sandy will do the housecleaning in the living room, dining room, and kitchen. The son and daughter will be responsible for the bedrooms, and the husband will be responsible for the bathrooms. They agree that these jobs will be done without reminders and in a timely manner. The daughter will have Sandy's car 2 days a week, and for that privilege will be responsible for doing most of the weekly errands and transporting her mother to and from school. The son and husband will do the weekly grocery shopping. Everyone will share in meal preparation and cleanup, with assigned days for those tasks. The children will receive compensation for their work, and the parents will put aside an equal amount so that they can have an occasional evening out. On Sunday evenings, they will have a brief family meeting to plan for the coming week and evaluate how things are going based on the agreement.

The wins for Sandy are more time to devote to classes and studying and fewer responsibilities at home. The wins for the family members are that Sandy will have some time to spend with them, and everyone benefits from sharing responsibilities without having to be reminded or badgered. There are financial and social benefits for all. The consequences of failure are also made clear: If a person does not uphold his or her responsibilities, he or she will not receive the agreed-on compensation. They have built in some flexibility by planning ahead each week to account for special activities and needs. At the end of this chapter, you have an opportunity to develop a win/win agreement to assist you in developing methods to manage your time more effectively.

Developing Study Skills

Forming study habits and developing good study skills can be big challenges for returning students. The difficulty is often related to previous experiences in which adequate study skills were not formed or because there are many other distractions for adult learners. Another difficulty may be that past study skills involved rote memory, whereas you now will be asked to analyze, synthesize, and think critically about the material presented.

TIME AND PLACE FOR STUDY

A first step in developing good study habits is to create study time. The specific time will depend on your other demands, but it will be most helpful if you can select a time of day in which you learn best or when you can be assured of minimal or no interruptions. Plan to study in short blocks of time (1 hour) with 5- to 10-minute breaks. Many students also plan study time between classes or other activities.

A place to study is also essential. It is not a good idea to try to read while reclining on the sofa. Instead, try to find a quiet area in your home or go to the library. Your family and friends need to be aware that your study time and place are off-limits so that you can study without interruption. Turn off your cell phone and plan to return calls on breaks or after the study time.

Another useful study skill is to plan your time so that you know what you want to accomplish each day. Short-term goals are often less intimidating than long-term goals. Once your overall weekly plan is established, break up large or lengthy assignments into "small bites" that can be accomplished in 1- to 3-hour time blocks. You will be surprised at how much progress you will make using this strategy.

Last, a common challenge for adults returning to school is procrastination. As an LPN/LVN, your time outside of work hours has been filled with family time and/or other interests. You may find you procrastinate when faced with heavy reading assignments, writing papers and nursing care plans, and other assignments. Hamachek (2002) described common causes of procrastination, including fear avoidance, self-doubt, self-delusion, blame, sympathy, and manipulation.

Identifying the cause of your procrastination is the first step in overcoming it. An effective strategy to prevent it, however, is breaking down tasks into smaller "doable bites" that can be built into your weekly and daily planning timeline as described previously.

READING AND NOTE-TAKING SKILLS

Other study habits are related to those that assist you to improve or strengthen your abilities. For example, in reading textbooks there are a few methods that will help make your reading time more productive. Many educators recommend that you take a few minutes to scan a reading assignment before reading it. This enables you to get a feel for the subject and to identify the main themes of the material. You can also decide how much time is needed to complete the assignment. Some material requires in-depth concentration, whereas other texts can be skimmed. In addition, focus on reading with the course objectives in mind. The objectives are a valuable tool to help pinpoint information mastery.

Other strategies involve taking notes while you read. This can be in the form of an outline, or it can be more elaborate if the material is complex. Some students find it helpful to highlight or underline so that when they review the material, they can focus on these sections. It may also be useful to make notes in the margins or to write questions. Instructors usually start their lectures by asking for student questions; this would be a perfect time to ask for clarification of your reading materials. Make use of the chapter objectives, terminology list, summaries, and review questions. These help clarify and reiterate certain concepts. Some students find it helpful to read aloud to maintain their focus. Finally, review your readings frequently so that the material will not look new just before an exam.

Note taking in class is another necessary skill to master. One of the most useful note-taking skills is to complete the reading assignments before attending class. Thus, the material will not sound foreign, and you might be able to reduce or simplify the notes you take. It also helps you focus on the class content, ask questions, and synthesize information attained from multiple resources rather than worrying that you are missing something. Another important aspect of note taking is to sit where you will not be distracted and where you can focus on what you need to do. Maintaining your concentration is also related to having sufficient supplies, having everything in good working order, and running on a "full battery." If an instructor is agreeable, you may want to record her or his classes as an adjunct to note taking; you can use the recording to clarify certain points or as a way to review if you have a long commute. Some faculty videostream their lectures, and/or post them to their Web sites so that students may review them again later for this same purpose. If you have solid keyboarding skills, taking a portable laptop to class may expedite your note-taking ability.

Other tips for note taking are related to format and responding to clues. Note taking can be done in many forms; you have probably seen various methods. Generally, whether you outline or write in narrative form, it is best to be as brief as possible. It does not matter whether you use complete sentences or words as long as you write in a way that you can decipher later. Be consistent with the abbreviations that you use. Underline or star important points; instructors often emphasize or state what is particularly important and may repeat a key issue. It is useful to copy information from overheads, slides, computer presentations, or white boards, although the information does not need to be verbatim. Develop your own system of shortcuts, abbreviations, and coding. Many computer software programs now provide notetaking, highlighting, and other editing features that will assist you in organizing your notes. Lastly, it is also important to review your notes within 1 to 2 days, rather than waiting until time for an exam.

PREPARATION FOR TESTS

Developing study skills also includes preparing for tests and exams. This can be stressful for many students, and so it is beneficial to use methods that will aid the process. Reading assignments and notes should be reviewed on a regular basis to keep familiar with the course content. This does not substitute for the big review before a test, but it does enhance the process. It can help to review your previous exams to learn from your mistakes and to get a feel for how the instructor asks questions.

Developing study skills is an important component of student success. Again, the process depends on you. Being a proactive student means that you accept responsibility for achieving your goals. If you are having difficulty studying or taking exams, or if you experience test anxiety, you must seek help from appropriate sources. Asking for help is not a weakness; rather, it is strength. Your advisor, counselor, and many text- and computer-based programs can all be resources to support your success. For those who specifically are having difficulty with math or who have Math anxiety, Ooten and Moore (2009) offer strategies for success in their text *Managing the Mean Math Blues: Math Study Skills for Student Success.*

CULTIVATING STUDY GROUPS AND MENTORS

It can be rewarding to form a study group. The group needs to have a spirit of cooperation, as opposed to competition, to be beneficial. The group's meeting cannot be a social gathering because the purpose must be to study. It is best to join a group with students who have similar goals and study habits and who seem to have the same focus in classes. If the group is larger than five or six people, it will probably be too unwieldy. A "study buddy" can also be helpful in motivating you during times of procrastination.

The format of study group meetings should include reviewing material, comparing class notes, testing each other with review questions, or asking questions based on the readings or notes. A study group can be used for developing projects or reviewing members' written work. Nursing students find it useful to develop nursing care plans to help each other understand the process and to strengthen the comprehensiveness of such plans.

It may also be helpful for you to develop a mentor as you enter the program. A mentor is generally defined as a wise and trusted counselor. It is a person for whom you have respect and admiration, and from whom you feel you will receive guidance and support. As you begin the nursing program, you may find that a faculty member, a nurse where you work, or even a more advanced student is someone with whom you are able to consult or use as a role model. This relationship may provide you with the courage to explore other options or discuss new ideas. More information on developing mentors is presented in Chapter 6.

• CONCLUSION

Returning to school as an adult is not easy. For as many reasons as there are for returning, there are undoubtedly as many to postpone or deny the experience. However, the strategies presented in this chapter provide you with a means to facilitate the educational process and to make the journey more successful and enjoyable; they also put you in the driver's seat.

At this point, you should not be intimidated by the process. Your prior learning and work experiences have provided you with a wonderful foundation. As an adult learner and a returning student, you have a wealth of knowledge and experience that will support your efforts. Now, you must continue to maximize your skills and abilities. Remember Sandy Martin? She involved her job and family to meet her needs. She met with her nursing advisor and took a proactive approach to her learning experience. Together, they have built a strong foundation on which she can build her continued success.

student exercises

Consider the relationship you have with family and significant others from whom you will need support in your return to school. Develop a win/win agreement that encompasses the following:

1. Who needs to be involved with determining the win/win agreement?

2. What are the desired results of the agreement?

3. What perspectives would you anticipate that each individual has of how he or she contributes to reaching the results desired?

4. What perspective do you have?

5. What guidelines can you identify to guide the agreement?

6. What resources might be necessary to carry out the agreement?

7. What is the win for each individual?

8. What are the consequences if the agreement is not followed?

Capture what you have identified in writing and review it together. Make adjustments as needed. An effective agreement will be extremely helpful in managing your time and commitments as you return to school.

References

American Nurses Association. (2000). *Scope and standards of practice for nursing professional development.* Washington, DC: Author.

Arnoldussen, B. (2006). *Changing your career: Nursing as your new profession.* New York: Kaplan.

Campbell, D. M., Cignetti, P. B., Melenyzer, B. J., Nettles, D. H., & Wyman, Jr., R. M. (2011) (5th ed.). *How to develop a professional portfolio: A manual for teachers*. Boston: Pearson.

Cerbin, W. (2000). Investigating student learning in a problem-based psychology course. In P. Hutchings (Ed.), *Opening lines: Approaches to the scholarship of teaching and learning* (Case study 1, pp. 11–22). Menlo Park, CA: Carnegie Foundation for the Advancement of Teaching.

Chandler, G.E. (2010). *New nurse's survival guide*. New York: McGraw-Hill.

Covey, S. (1989). *The seven habits of highly effective people*. New York: Simon & Schuster.

Covey, S. R. (2004). *The 8th habit: From effectiveness to greatness*. New York: Free Press.

Crews, T. B., North, A. B., & Thompson, S. L. (2001). Diversity today: Challenges and strategies. In B. J. Brown (Ed.), *Management of the business classroom*. Reston, VA: National Business Education Association.

Curry, B.D. (2008). Coping with returning to school. In *Advancing your career: Concepts of professional nursing* (Chapter 2). Philadelphia: F.A. Davis.

Dunham, K.S. (2008). *How to survive and maybe even love nursing school* (3rd ed). Philadelphia: F.A. Davis.

Ellis, D. (2011). *Becoming a master student* (13th ed.). Boston: Wadsworth, Cengage Learning.

Fleming, S., & McKee, G. (2005). The mature student question. *Nurse Education Today*, 25(3), 230–237.

Gandara, P., & Contreras, F. (2009). *The Latino education crisis: The consequences of failed social policies*. Cambridge, MA: Harvard University Press.

Hamachek, A. L. (2002). *Coping with college: A guide for academic success* (2nd ed.). Upper Saddle River, NJ: Prentice-Hall.

Hardesty, L. (2007). *The role of the library in the first college year* (Monograph No. 45). Columbia, SC: University of South Carolina, National Resource Center for the First-Year Experience and Students in Transition.

Hunter, M. S., McCalla-Wriggins, B., & White, E. R. (Eds.). (2007). *Academic advising: New insights for teaching and learning in the first year* (Monograph No. 46 [National Resource Center]; Monograph No. 14 [National Academic Advising Association]). Columbia, SC: University of South Carolina, National Resource Center for the First-Year Experience and Students in Transition.

Katz, J. R., Carter, C., Bishop, J., & Kravits, S. L. (2000). *Keys to nursing success*. Upper Saddle River, NJ: Prentice Hall.

Lippincott Williams & Wilkins. (2007). *Best practices: Evidence-based nursing procedures* (2nd ed.). Philadelphia: Author.

Longworth, N. (2003). *Lifelong learning in action: Transforming education in the 21st century*. New York: Routledge/Falmer.

MacIntosh, J. (2003). Reworking professional nursing identity. *Western Journal of Nursing Research*, 25(6), 725–741.

McCarey, M., Barr, T., & Rattray, J. (2006). Predictors of academic performance in a cohort of pre-registration nursing students. *Nurse Educator Today*, 27(4), 357–364.

National Council of State Boards of Nursing. (2009). *NCLEX-RN examination: Test plan for the National Council Licensure Examination for Registered Nurses*. Chicago: Author.

National League for Nursing. (2000). *Educational competencies for graduates of associate degree nursing programs*. Sudbury, MA: Jones and Bartlett.

Ooten, C., & Moore, K. (2009). *Managing the mean math blues: Math study skills for student success* (2nd ed.). Boston: Pearson.

Salamonson, Y., & Andrew, S. (2006). Academic performance in nursing students: Influence of part-time employment, age and ethnicity. *Journal of Advanced Nursing*, 55(3), 342–349.

Santrock, J. W., & Halonen, J. S. (2010). *Your guide to college success: Strategies for achieving your goals*. Boston: Wadsworth Cengage Learning.

Shane, D. L. (1983). *Returning to school: A guide for nurses*. Englewood Cliffs, NJ: Prentice-Hall.

Simon, L. (2009). *New beginnings: A reference guide for adult learners*. (4th ed.). Upper Saddle River, NJ: Prentice-Hall.

Steele, R., Lauder, W., Caperchione, C., & Anastasi, J. (2005). An exploratory study of the concerns of mature access to nursing students and the coping strategies used to manage these adverse experiences. *Nurse Education Today*, 25(7), 573–581.

Suggested Reading

Atkins, R. (2009). *Getting the most from nursing school: A guide to becoming a nurse*. Boston: Jones and Bartlett.

Carter, C., Bishop, J., & Kravits, S. L. (2001). *Keys to success: How to achieve your goals* (2nd ed.). Upper Saddle River, NJ: Prentice-Hall.

Dembo, M. H. (2000). *Motivation and learning strategies for college success: A self-management approach*. Mahwah, NJ: Erlbaum.

Ferguson, V. D. (Ed.). (1997). *Educating the 21st century nurse: Challenges and opportunities*. New York: NLN Press.

Gardner, J. N., & Jewler, A. J. (2000). *Your college experience: Strategies for success*. Belmont, CA: Wadsworth.

Griggs, S., & Dunn, R. (Eds.). (1999). *Learning styles and the nursing profession*. Boston: Jones and Bartlett.

Kramer, G. L., and Associates. (2007). *Fostering student success in the campus community*. San Francisco: Jossey-Bass.

Thibeault, S. (2001). *Stressed out about nursing school: An insider's guide to success*. Orlando, FL: Bandido Books.

Thorkildsen, T. A. (2002). *Motivation and the struggle to learn: Responding to fractured experience*. Boston: Allyn & Bacon.

VanBlerkom, D. L. (2002). *Orientation to college learning* (3rd ed.). Belmont, CA: Wadsworth Group.

Resources for Writing Professional Papers and Support for English Language Learners

Brians, P. (2003). *Common errors in English usage*. Wilsonville, OR: William James and Company.

Ellis, D. (2006). *Becoming a master student* (11th ed.). Boston: Houghton Mifflin

Lane, J., & Lange, E. (1999). *Writing clearly: An editing guide* (2nd ed.). Boston: Heinle and Heinle.

Raimes, A. (2004). *Grammar troublespots: A guide for student writers* (3rd ed.). England: Cambridge University Press.

http://owl.english.purdue.edu: Purdue University's Online Writing Lab. (Last accessed 7.6.2011).

www.back2college.com/library/faq.htm: Answers to frequently asked questions for adult students returning to school. (Last accessed 7.6.2011).

www.m-w.com: Merriam-Webster On-Line (dictionary, thesaurus, and Encyclopaedia Britannica). (Last accessed 7.6.2011).

www.aamn.org: The American Assembly for Men in Nursing. (Last accessed 7.6.2011).

www.nurselookup.com: A Web site promoting men in the nursing profession. (Last accessed 7.6.2011).

www.malenursemagazine.com: Male Nurse Magazine. (Last accessed 7.6.2011).

www.minoritynurse.com: A Web site for minority nurses. (Last accessed 7.6.2011).

www.ncbi.nlm.nih.gov/sites/entrez: A service of the U.S. National Library of Medicine and the National Institutes of Health. Serves as a search engine for locating publications and articles. (Last accessed 7.6.2011).

www.ncbi.nlm.nih.gov: National Center for Biotechnology Information. (Last accessed 7.6.2011).

www2.liu.edu/cwis/cwp/library/workshop/citation.htm: A guide to the citation styles for research papers, including APA, MLA, AMA, Turabian, and Chicago. (Last accessed 7.6.2011).

2

Role Development and Transition

By the end of this chapter, the student will be able to:

1 Differentiate between change and transition.

2 Differentiate between ascribed and acquired roles.

3 Describe the process of role choice in personal development.

4 Compare and contrast the stages of personal and adult development of selected theorists.

5 Describe family developmental stages and the effects of individual issues on family development.

6 Apply stage development theories.

7 Outline the stages of professional role development.

8 Describe the phases of role socialization.

9 Summarize the phases of role transition.

10 Differentiate between intrapersonal and interpersonal aspects of role conflict.

11 Discuss methods for conflict management.

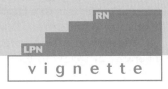

vignette

Juan Martinez, LVN, is a 23-year-old bachelor who works in an outpatient clinic for the Veterans Administration. Although he has been practicing only for 2 years, Juan has become bored with his role and does not feel it offers him the challenges it did when he first started. Some of his discontentedness stems from the fact that although he helps with basic assessment of clients and implementing care, he really wants to further develop his assessment skills and acquire management skills. Although no one in his family has ever attended college, he believes he could be successful in a college degree program. After visiting with a college counselor, Juan enrolls in college to pursue registered nursing and attain his ADN. As he progresses through the program he finds he is in fact successful and finds his course work challenging and fulfilling. Once again he is excited about nursing and his emerging new role as an RN. He is enjoying being a student, learning, and applying new theories to client care.

The notion of role development and transition is typically not part of the decision-making process of returning to school. These terms imply a very formal mode of thinking, when the actual reasons for returning to school may be much more pragmatic. However, in making the decision to pursue a degree in professional nursing, you already realize that a major life change is going to take place. This is the reality of role development and role transition.

● DEFINITIONS

ROLE is often defined as a person's particular function as it relates to others' functions. Certain behaviors must be learned so roles and functions become part of a whole. For example, one of your roles may be that of the oldest sibling. This role is defined by the fact that there are younger siblings. Behaviors for this role are learned; there are expectations of helping with the care of the younger children or having more responsibilities because you are the oldest. When a person is placed into a new situation, it often feels awkward and unfamiliar because of the uncertainty regarding the role and its obligate behaviors. You may recall how you felt as a new LPN/LVN in your first job, or how you are now feeling on your return to school. For each role, expected behaviors are learned for survival and success.

35

ROLE DEVELOPMENT Development in a role refers to the growth that occurs as a person learns the functions, expectations, and behaviors for a particular role. In your practical/vocational nursing education, you were taught specific tasks and behaviors to function within that role. You developed the skills that were necessary to perform a specific job, and as a result, you grew and expanded your knowledge and abilities. Once employed as an LPN/LVN, you continued to expand your knowledge and skills, adding experiential knowledge.

Each person develops roles that relate to the roles of others. Shane (1983) referred to these as role clusters. For example, you will develop as a student nurse in relation to nursing instructors, staff nurses, and other student nurses.

You may also be a parent, spouse, daughter or son, sibling, and employee. There are expectations for each of these roles. These behaviors are learned as part of the role development process. In your return to school, you will learn the role expectations and behaviors needed to be an RN. This process will be influenced by your other roles and experiences.

Role development is not always a voluntary process. Later in this chapter, the concepts related to role development are discussed in more detail.

ROLE CHANGE Throughout a person's life, there are many role changes. Role change consists of adding a new role, dropping an old role, or modifying the behaviors associated with an existing role (Shane, 1983). Experiences, expected behaviors, and personal values influence development in each new change.

ROLE TRANSITION Transition refers to a passage or shift from one place to another or from one role to another. Role transition indicates a period of change, often major change. It may involve letting go of some functions while adding others. You may have experienced the necessity of being a caregiver for a parent or grandparent. In this transition, you recognize that you have lost some of the functions of being a child and added those of parenting. In essence, you made the shift to your parents' shoes. The LPN/LVN role has involved certain role expectations and behaviors. In the process of acquiring the skills and knowledge needed to be an RN, you will experience changes in the way you think, act, and are. The process of role transition is individual and will not only affect you but may also have a profound effect on others. In the transition process, it is common for a person to experience role strain or stress. These concepts are examined later in this chapter.

Refer to Display 2.1 for definitions of role terms.

---

display 2.1   Definitions of Role Terms

Role: a particular function that is defined by its relationship with other functions; expected behaviors for a role are learned

Role development: growth within a particular role as a person learns the functions, expectations, and behaviors for that role

Role change: addition or subtraction of a role or the modification of behaviors associated with a particular role

Role transition: passage or shift from one role to another; involves changing the way one thinks and acts

---

thinking critically

Consider your current role change to that of student nurse. Analyze the behavior changes and expectations that you anticipate for this role. What is similar to your previous student experiences? What is different?

• TYPES OF ROLES
Ascribed Roles

Adults are given or acquire many roles. Ascribed roles are roles that are not chosen.

GENETIC ROLES

Many ascribed roles are genetic, such as those related to gender, age, and skin color. Previously in this chapter, the example of being the oldest sibling was used to demonstrate the necessity to learn behaviors for each role. It is also an example of an ascribed role.

SOCIAL MILIEU

Ascribed roles can also relate to the social milieu. This includes ethnic, religious, or familial roles, which have certain functions and expectations. For example, if you are born into a family with a particular religious affiliation, you are expected to learn the particular aspects of the religion, which may include the way you dress or eat, where you go to school, or who you marry. The ascribed roles related to social milieu carry with them expectations of certain behaviors and values. Ascribed and acquired roles are differentiated in Display 2.2.

Acquired Roles

Acquired roles are roles a person receives or takes on during a lifetime. These range from roles of choice, such as being a parent, to those over which there is little control, such as being an invalid. In your work as an LPN/LVN, you may have cared for clients who must adjust to a new role of being ill or disabled. It is not a role of choice, but it is an acquired role that involves similar issues of learning behaviors, expectations, and functions. Acquired roles can be personal, societal, or professional.

PERSONAL ROLES

Personal roles are those you assume as an individual. They can include marital status, parenting, or choice of friends. There are learned behaviors and expectations for each of these roles. The manner in which we behave depends on the relationship. Your role functions and expectations vary on any given day from being a parent to a spouse to a close friend.

display 2.2	Differentiation Between Ascribed and Acquired Roles

ASCRIBED ROLES

Genetic	**Social Milieu**	
Gender	Ethnicity	
Age	Religion	
Position in a family	Family role	
Skin color		

ACQUIRED ROLES

Personal	**Societal**	**Professional**
Marital status	Religious organizations	Job role
Parenting	Community organizations	Member of professional
Choice of friends	Political organizations	organization
Illness		Professional appointment

SOCIETAL ROLES

Societal roles are those you assume as a member of a group. These may involve affiliations with religious, community, or political organizations. For example, you may have certain positions within a social organization: secretary of a church committee, school board member, or member of a political candidate's campaign organization. You are obligated to learn the expectations for each of these roles.

PROFESSIONAL ROLES

Professional roles are those you assume related to your career or vocation. They may include job role, membership in a professional organization, or possibly a professional appointment to a committee or board. One of your reasons for returning to school is to acquire new knowledge and skills that will enhance your ability to take on new job roles and to join other professional organizations and boards. These roles require that certain expectations defined by a group and accepted by an individual are met.

thinking critically

Consider the many roles in your life. Differentiate between your ascribed and acquired roles. In what ways do the ascribed roles influence the acquired roles? Determine whether any of your acquired roles will be changed or modified as you return to school. Will any of your ascribed roles pose additional challenges for you? If so, how might you cope with these challenges?

● ROLE DEVELOPMENT

Role development is discussed briefly in the beginning of this chapter in the Definitions section. At this point, it is essential to examine this process more closely.

The following text reviews concepts of role choice and personal, family, and professional development. These concepts will assist you in understanding your own role development and transition as you move from the role of an LPN/LVN to that of a professional nurse.

Role Choice

Your decision to become an RN was not one that you made on a whim. It has been a careful process of weighing the advantages and disadvantages, as well as determining the priorities in your life. Although you may have had some help with this decision, it can be a lonely and agonizing time. You may have had to overcome some personal issues related to finances or child care, or perhaps your family did not support your decision to return to school. The educational road for some will be more difficult than for others. Your colleagues have different experiences and expectations. You may have noticed that strangers, some who are very different from you, who have more or less LPN/LVN experience, or who seem more or less knowledgeable, surround you. These factors may influence you in some way, but it is hoped that they will not deter you.

---

thinking critically

Review your list of ascribed roles. Consider what these roles mean to you. For example, is your age at this time beneficial? How might you use these ascribed roles to your advantage as you enter the nursing program?

Acquired roles may involve choices. Your decision to continue your education has involved an active process on your part. Generally, you have not been able to sit back and let someone else make the choice for you. It is impossible to predict the implications that returning to school can have on you and your life. You have undoubtedly experienced a variety of emotional states in your decision-making process. Now that you are actually pursuing further education by returning to school, it is necessary for you to examine two aspects of this choice: commitment and balance.

COMMITMENT

Commitment is the process of pledging to assume a role, perform a job, or accomplish a goal. Your decision to return to school initiated this process. However, you also have commitments to other ongoing roles that demand your attention. You have often heard that one must be able to set priorities. As you examine the commitment you have to your various roles (eg, worker, parent, spouse), you will need to maintain a commitment to the highest priorities of each role and maintain balance in your life.

BALANCE

As you make a commitment to your new role as a returning student and adjust priorities among other roles, achieving overall balance in your life will again become a challenge. Stephen R. Covey (1989, 2004) identified the seven habits of highly effective people. His seventh habit, called "Sharpen the Saw," focuses on renewal and keeping ourselves in balance. Covey (2004) stated, "Sharpening the saw is about constantly renewing ourselves in the four basic areas of life: physical, social/ emotional, mental, and spiritual. It's the habit that increases our capacity to live all other habits of effectiveness" (p. 153).

The need for balance in life transcends time and culture. As Sylvia Lee noted,

> The Native American Medicine Wheel, in which life is only in balance when its physical, mental, emotional, and spiritual components are in balance, offers an old-world model for a new-world environment. Many other ancient models echo this theme— Taoist principles among them (Longworth, 2003, p. vii).

thinking critically

You have already made some changes when you decided to return to school. What are those changes? How are these changes affecting your life's balance? What strategies can you use to restore balance to your life?

Barriers

You may experience some barriers in your educational journey. Some of these barriers are internal, and some are external. The following are examples of internal barriers to role development:

- Fear of failure
- Lack of confidence
- Confusion regarding new expectations
- Feelings of being overwhelmed

Palmer (2007) described fears common to college students, including fear of failing, not understanding, being drawn into issues they would rather avoid, having their ignorance exposed or their prejudices challenged, or looking foolish in front of peers. Such fears may serve as internal barriers to you being an active participant in class discussions, seeking clinical experience, and experiencing success in the ADN program.

Other barriers to role development are external. They may include issues surrounding family needs, child care, financial concerns, job demands, and personal needs. These barriers have a tremendous impact on your ability to succeed. Barriers and fears of the re-entry process are discussed in Chapter 1. Subsequent chapters provide you with some strategies to assist in overcoming barriers by adapting to change and developing an individualized plan for role transition.

thinking critically

Identify internal and external barriers as you embrace role transition. Design a plan of action to deal with these barriers.

• PERSONAL AND ADULT DEVELOPMENT

This section is an overview of adult developmental theory. Researchers such as Erikson, Piaget, and others have proposed theories that provide an explanation for adult development. You may recall these theorists from your LPN/LVN education. A review of these theories will assist you in more objectively examining your own development and personal journey. It will also provide you with a perspective to evaluate the development of your clients and to recognize the effects of illness on their development.

Erikson

Erik Erikson is one of the earliest theorists to delineate development in terms of phases or stages. He views these stages in terms of psychosocial development throughout the life span. Personal development occurs with passage through each stage. Erikson theorizes that a person develops by proceeding through developmental tasks or crises at each stage. Success or failure in resolving a crisis will influence a person's ability to deal with the next stage and may affect how he or she is as an adult.

Table 2.1 outlines Erikson's eight stages of psychosocial development, the time in a person's life when each stage occurs, the developmental task or crisis for each stage, and the possible consequences for success or failure in resolving each task or crisis.

Piaget

Jean Piaget is another early theorist who examined cognitive development, which is the process of understanding and knowing. He identified four stages related to intellectual development: sensorimotor (manipulation), preoperational (egocentric thought), concrete operations, and formal operations (abstract thought). Table 2.2 summarizes these four stages of cognitive development, the approximate age that each stage takes place, and what cognitive process is involved. Piaget theorizes that cognitive development occurs in a continuum from infancy on; it is an additive process in which new experiences are understood as a result of previous knowledge.

Piaget considered formal operational thought to be the highest level. To achieve this level, one must progress through the stages of manipulation and concrete thinking to consider all variables and solve problems. In his theory, this occurs in adolescence. Other theorists do not agree; they believe that abstract thinking or formal operations develop later in life with the appropriate experiences (Stevens-Long, 1988). These concepts are important for you for two reasons. First, your thought processes are more concrete as a result of your previous educational experiences. Shane (1983) attributed this to the rigid style used in nursing schools, where formal operations may not be encouraged. These concepts are also important when considering the learning needs of your clients. Your approach for teaching a specific procedure will differ, depending on the age of the client and the ability of that individual to use formal or concrete operations. You may also find that some of your clients will revert to previous modes of thinking when they are faced with stress.

table
.... STAGES OF PSYCHOSOCIAL DEVELOPMENT—ERIKSON
2-1

Stage	Approximate Age	Developmental Task or Crisis	Consequences of Success or Failure
Trust vs. mistrust	Birth–18 mo	Learn to trust others and self	Success: sense of predictability and certainty Failure: sense of abandonment and distrust
Autonomy vs. shame and doubt	18 mo–3 y	Learn to develop sense of choice and self-restraint	Success: sense of self-control without loss of self-esteem Failure: defiance, willfulness, sense of loss of control with shame and doubt
Initiative vs. guilt	3–5 y	Learn to have goals, develop judgment, and perceive self-behavior	Success: sense of responsibility and cooperation; ability to use positive judgment Failure: lack of self-confidence; fear of doing the wrong thing
Industry vs. inferiority	6–12 y	Develop skills and knowledge to complete tasks: use motor and cognitive skills	Success: sense of success and competence Failure: sense of inadequacy and hopelessness
Identity vs. role confusion	12–20 y	Develop a sense of self and abilities and an inner sense of commitment, morality, and ethics	Success: a positive sense of self and a knowledge that one has abilities and values Failure: doubt about sexual and vocational identity; confusion about individual identity; can lead to identification with heroes and cliques
Intimacy vs. isolation— early adulthood	20–40 y	Develop intimate relationships and make commitments to work and to others	Success: intimate relationship and positive commitments to work and to others Failure: avoidance of intimacy; problems with commitment
Generativity vs. stagnation— middle adulthood	41–60 y	Establish family and assist in the guidance of the next generation; be creative and productive	Success: feeling needed by family and helping the future generation; feeling productive and valuable Failure: concerned more with self; feeling useless and without value; stagnated
Integrity vs. despair—late adulthood	61 y–death	Resolve that life has meaning and worth	Success: accept one's life as meaningful and fulfilling; that something has been left for the next generation Failure: fear death; cannot see that life has had meaning

table
....
2-2
STAGES OF COGNITIVE DEVELOPMENT—PIAGET

Stage	Age	Cognitive Process
Sensorimotor	Birth–2 y	Senses and motor activity give information about the world and its objects; infant relies on totally direct experience; at the end of this stage, language skills increase, and the sense of object permanence is recognized apart from self.
Preoperational	2–7 y	Time of exploration and curiosity: child is very interested in the world; explains the world so that it makes sense to self; increased language skills and imagination help child use mental images and symbolic play.
Concrete operations	7–12 y	Child uses systematic thought and is able to apply universal rules: reversibility of thought (add and subtract); classification of objects by size or mass; and consistency of quantities when physical appearance changes (ie, pour liquid from narrow to wide container—amount remains the same). Child is able to learn in a procedural or sequential method.
Formal operations	12 y–adulthood	Child is now able to think in abstract terms and to use reasoning and scientific processes; also can conceptualize the future.

This theory provides you with a framework to assess the learning needs of your clients and to then devise a realistic plan for teaching new information.

Kohlberg

The development of moral reasoning was researched extensively by Lawrence Kohlberg. He determined that an integral part of socialization of a child from any culture is to teach the child the difference between right and wrong. This, in essence, gives the child a sense of values. Kohlberg's concept of moral development is similar to the concepts of Erikson and Piaget. As a child identifies with parents or other caregivers, she or he is either positively or negatively reinforced for particular behaviors. If the reinforcement is consistent, a child's personal sense of values will be greatly influenced by the value system of the caregivers.

Kohlberg's stages of moral development are presented in Table 2.3. The first stage of preconventional moral thought signifies the beginning of value development in early childhood. The child is dependent on adults for survival and learns to view moral behavior as the avoidance of disapproval or punishment from adults. Conventional moral thought develops in the preteen years. At this time, the child is able to define the rules and expectations of society and better understands the consequences if the rules are broken. The last stage is called postconventional or principled moral thought. As the teenager moves into adulthood, she or he develops an abstract moral sense that enables her or him to determine what is just or unjust.

table
2-3
STAGES OF MORAL DEVELOPMENT—KOHLBERG

Stage	Definition	Characteristics
Preconventional moral thought—early childhood	Obedience and punishment Action for personal satisfaction Interpersonal agreement	Believes action is right if not punished: wrong if punished Responds to bribery; will comply for personal gain Acts to please others and maintain relationships
Conventional moral thought—preteen	Law and order Personal values/standards	Understands and responds to authority; maintains social order Has sense of morality; protects rights of all
Principled moral thought—teenager to adult	Universal ethical standards	Has a conscience; respects other humans and believes in mutual trust

Nurses develop a professional value system in much the same way (Taylor, Lillis, LeMone, & Lynn, 2011). Depending on your own stage of personal development and experiences, you may have some difficulty assimilating these factors. You are also faced with teachers, clients, and colleagues whose value systems may differ from yours. As you grow and develop in your professional role, you will be more sensitive to various beliefs. Later in this text, ethical decision making is addressed. It will be helpful to apply Kohlberg's theory of moral development as you study ethical decision making.

Gilligan

Carol Gilligan (1982) developed a theory of moral development from a woman's perspective. As a student of Kohlberg and later as a colleague, she objected to the generalization of his theory to women because his theory was based on work done with males and then applied to females. The similarities in their theories are that they both identify three stages of moral development. However, Kohlberg's theory is based more on rules and justice and the development of abstract thinking, whereas Gilligan asserts that women's development is seen more in terms of relationships, caring, and connectivity. In Kohlberg's research with girls and women, he concluded that women were not able to reach the higher level of moral development, and that women were in some way deficient. Gilligan based her research on the stories or "voices" of girls and women, finding that their sense of moral reasoning is based on relationships, responsibility, and caring. This countered Kohlberg's earlier work.

Gilligan's three stages of moral development are as follows:

1. Orientation to individual survival: The individual views the moral decision as one that is necessary for her own survival in terms of herself only. There is a sense of obligation to one's own needs.

2. Goodness as self-sacrifice: The individual makes a moral decision based on meeting the needs and expectations of others and not hurting others. The obligation is to others and not self in this process.
3. Morality of nonviolence: The individual determines that the moral choice must be responsible to self and others and must involve caring and not hurting. The individual remains obligated to nonviolence.

As the individual progresses through these stages, there is an emphasis on the relationships within a particular situation and the importance of caring, attachments, and connectedness. Table 2.4 provides a brief comparison of the theories of Kohlberg and Gilligan.

Levinson

Another theorist who advocates a stage theory approach is Daniel Levinson. He has identified various stages and phases through which a person proceeds in the developmental process. Within each phase are periods of stability and transition and certain tasks that have to be completed. Table 2.5 shows the five stages that have been identified for adulthood, with the approximate ages involved and the tasks to be completed.

Levinson describes three phases within each of the five stages. The first phase is referred to as the novice phase, during which the individual begins to focus on new tasks that soon become the most significant. The second phase is called the culminating phase. This is a period of stability wherein tasks are achieved and maintained. The last phase is the transition phase, in which the present tasks lose their importance and other tasks begin to take precedence. The greatest turmoil, according to Levinson, occurs in the transitional phase. He theorizes that each phase can be as long as 5 to 7 years and may involve another 5 years of modification. As a result, adults spend many years in uncertainty.

Levinson's theory again poses interesting ways to examine your personal development. Consider the tasks with which you are absorbed as you return to school.

table 2-4   COMPARISON OF STAGES OF MORAL DEVELOPMENT—KOHLBERG AND GILLIGAN

Stage	Kohlberg	Gilligan
First	*Preconventional moral thought:* Child connects wrong acts with punishments; obedience through avoidance of punishment.	*Orientation to individual survival:* Child's moral decisions are based on survival of self, self-protection
Second	*Conventional moral thought:* Child responds to authority to maintain law and order.	*Goodness as self-sacrifice:* Child bases moral decisions on meeting the needs of others and not causing hurt to anyone.
Third	*Principled moral thought:* Individual develops standards and values that determine his or her sense of morality and ethics.	*Morality of nonviolence:* The individual determines that moral choices involve responsibility to self and others and involve an ethic of caring and nonviolence.

table
·················· STAGES OF ADULT DEVELOPMENT—LEVINSON
2-5

Stage	Age	Task
Early adult transition	18–20 y	The young adult begins the process of entering the adult world and leaving the security of childhood; independence is strongly desired.
Entrance into the adult world	21–27 y	The young adult begins adult career paths and adapts to an adult lifestyle that involves a variety of choices.
Transition	28–32 y	At this stage, the adult may choose to maintain the chosen path or to modify current life structures.
Settling down	33–39 y	The adult settles in at this stage and experiences stability within work, family, and social structures; views self as an expert in many ways.
The payoff	45–65 y	Within this stage, the individual is self-directed and is able to use influence with others and assess what life has been and needs to be.

It is a time of change and transition, and so it can be expected that it will be a time of turmoil, according to Levinson. You can also apply these concepts to your adult clients and determine what effect changes in health, pregnancy, or illness might have on a person's development. Does this alter or prolong the transition phase, or deter a person from completing essential tasks? Levinson's theory provides another framework to assess a client's developmental progress.

Sheehy

Thus far, most of the theorists presented have based their work on research studies of males, with the exception of Carol Gilligan. Other theorists view personal and adult development differently for females and males. A prominent person in this area is Gail Sheehy. In closely examining the work of stage theorists, she has noted that the developmental stages for men and women are different, and that there is more development in the adult stages than some theorists have presented. Women have traditionally been faced with more restrictions in the first half of their life cycle than have men. They have been the primary caregivers of children and elderly parents and the chief keepers of the home, as well as caring for almost anything else that needs care. Although women increasingly work outside the home, many caregiving tasks continue to be their responsibility, and frequently women choose work that complements the caregiver responsibilities. During the second half of their life cycle, women begin to look at self-development and at this time may choose to return to school and begin, advance, or change careers. Men have typically been more active in their careers and education during the first half of their life cycle and in the older adult years are more ready to think about leisure activities and retirement.

Traditional female and male roles are becoming more similar in the 21st century. Work and leisure roles that used to distinguish men and women are no longer as clearly defined. Gender stereotypes may not be as different as they once were, but life experiences do affect individual development, and any of the theories presented is limited to the population that has been studied.

Sheehy has identified stages or predictable crises of adulthood. On the basis of research of both men and women, she indicates the ages when one would generally go through each stage and points out gender differences if they are obvious. She is not so concerned with age as she is with the sequence of the stages. Table 2.6 outlines the stages, or crises, identified by Sheehy and their particular defining characteristics.

Sheehy believes that adult development needs to be better described in terms of men's and women's experiences. She also recognizes that adulthood does not represent easy work. Instead, it can be difficult and at times painful. Sheehy (1976) stated,

> The work of adult life is not easy. As in childhood, each step presents not only new tasks of development but requires letting go of the techniques that worked before. With each passage some magic must be given up, some cherished illusion of safety and comfortably familiar sense of self must be cast off, to allow for greater expansion of our own distinctiveness. (p. 21)

Sheehy's work provides a means to continue to examine your own development. Each of us progresses or develops at his or her own pace. Sheehy noted that the tasks for each stage are never completely done or eliminated, but we move on to the next step out of necessity or because other issues take precedence. Consider these aspects as you review the information given in Table 2.6. It is also a means to assess your clients and better understand the needs of each.

Stevenson

Joanne Sabol Stevenson is another author who has studied adult development, particularly the middle years of the life cycle. She referred to this as middlescence. "'Middlescence' is a term that originated in a facetious comment about the age group in the middle. Someone considered adolescence on the one side and senescence on the other and quipped that middlescence is in the center" (Stevenson, 1977, p. 1). She delineates four stages of adult development:

- Youth or young adulthood: 18 to 30 years
- Middlescence I (the core): 30 to 50 years
- Middlescence II (the new middle years): 50 to 70 years
- Late adult years: 70 years to death

Within each stage are tasks that have to be accomplished. She recognizes that some tasks are in process and may overlap into a subsequent stage, secondary to individual experiences and idiosyncrasies. Stevenson uses the suffix "-ing" to denote that the tasks are in operation but not necessarily complete, representing a dynamic process of development. Table 2.7 presents each of Stevenson's stages and the tasks for each stage. Again, review the material with your own development in mind but also consider the impact that changes in health, pregnancy, or illness might have as you think about your clients.

table
.... STAGES OF ADULT DEVELOPMENT—SHEEHY
2-6

Stage	Approximate Ages	Defining Characteristics
Pulling up roots	18–20 y	The young adult experiences the need to have autonomy and also to be taken care of. At this time, the struggle is to establish an adult identity separate from parents. "The tasks of this passage are to locate ourselves in a peer group role, a sex role, an anticipated occupation, an ideology or world view. As a result, we gather the impetus to leave home physically and the identity to begin leaving home emotionally" (Sheehy, 1976, p. 27).
The trying 20s	The 20s	Within this stage, the adult begins to settle into life work and to attempt intimacy while continuing the process of self-identity. Sheehy refers to the establishment of life patterns in this stage, such as *locked-in*, *wunderkind*, or *caregiver*.
Catch-30	Late 20s–early 30s	During this stage, adults question the wisdom of the choices made in their 20s. They may feel the need to change jobs or careers or to settle into marriage and start a family. Or, they may commit to extending their lives in the same direction they took in their 20s.
Rooting and extending	Early 30s	Settling in truly begins in this stage. The focus usually is on putting down roots and raising young children.
The deadline decade	Middle 30s–middle 40s	This stage marks a turning point in which adults recognize that they are halfway through the cycle of life. It is a time to reevaluate where one is, what one is doing, and what one should be doing. Many adults return to school or change careers at this stage.
Renewal or resignation	Mid-40s on	Adults accept their lives as they are and accept that no one will ever fully understand oneself and that blame cannot be placed on one's parents. Friends are important, but this adult also values privacy.

Stevenson is a nurse and has presented some implications in this process. She differentiates maturational crises from situational crises. Maturational crises are the turmoils or stresses that occur in developmental transitions, such as leaving home or making the decision to have children. These crises are similar for many people. Situational crises are the remarkable events that occur only to some of us. Personal illness, a catastrophic accident, the untimely death of a parent or spouse, or divorce are examples of situational crises. The stage at which these events occur influences a person's ability to cope. For example, an acute illness at the age of 45 years has great

table 2-7	STAGES OF ADULT DEVELOPMENT—STEVENSON	
Stage	Approximate Age	Tasks
Youth or young adulthood	18–30 y	Achieving relative independence from parental figures: attaining a sense of responsibility; developing roles and positions; achieving intimate relationships; beginning parenting; making personal values integral with work and social values
Middlescence I	30–50 y	Assuming responsibility for self-development and for growth of associated organizations; assessing one's work roles; assisting the younger generations: and older generations; involving oneself in a variety of organizations; optimizing responsibilities
Middlescence II	50–70 y	Achieving ways to maintain survival; taking interest in societal changes; maintaining mutually supportive relationships with family members; enjoying increased leisure time; adapting to aging
Late adult years	70 y–death	Assuming the need to share experience and wisdom; putting affairs in order; pursuing new interests; learning new skills; assessing one's life; adapting loss of significant other

implications for that individual in terms of lost income, lack of support for dependent family members, and inability to meet community and work-related obligations. Continue to consider these aspects as you study this material.

thinking critically

Select one of the theories outlined in the preceding material. What stage best describes your present status? Why? With what tasks are you most concerned? Do any issues remain unresolved or problematic? How is this stage impacted by your role transition to student and then to RN?

NCLEX–RN *Might Ask*   2.1

The student nurse is monitoring the progress of a client with juvenile diabetes in a community clinic setting. The client is a 15-year-old girl who is having problems with her diet that stem mainly from having to eat in the high school cafeteria with others of her age. According to Erikson, this child's stage of development is

    A. Trust vs. mistrust.
    B. Industry vs. inferiority.
    C. Identity vs. role confusion.
    D. Intimacy vs. isolation.

• See Appendix A for correct answer and rationale.

Family Development

In addition to personal development, individuals also grow and develop within the context of human relationships, which generally involve a family unit. Evelyn Duvall and Murray Bowen have studied family development.

DUVALL

Family development is perceived by some theorists in the context of a life cycle, with developmental stages and tasks similar to personal development. Duvall (1977) theorized that if a person understands who the family members are (including age, gender, and position in the family); what their status is in terms of race, ethnicity, and social standing; and what stage they are in the family life cycle, much can be predicted about what is happening with the family at a particular time. Duvall describes eight stages of family development within the framework of a family life cycle (Table 2.8).

With each stage, she delineates specific tasks that require adaptation and acquisition of new responsibilities and challenges. For example, a family with young children has the task of adapting to members of the next generation. The parents must acquire parenting skills, adapt their own relationship to make room for

table
2-8   STAGES OF FAMILY DEVELOPMENT—DUVALL

Stage	Developmental Tasks
Marriage of young couple; no children	Growth in marital relationship; adjustment to in-laws; decision regarding having children
Birth of children	Growth in parenting roles; adjustment in marital relationship; resolution of conflicting roles: spouse, parent, daughter/son, sibling, employee
Family with preschool children	Adaptation to children who are very involved with their environment; adjustment in marital relationship; involvement of children in socialization activities, such as church and nursery school, and other activities
Family with school-age children	Encouragement of achievements of children in school and other activities; adjustment in marital relationship; coordination of child and adult activities
Family with adolescents	Promotion of teenagers' responsible independence; maintenance of communication with all family members; adjustment in marital relationship
Family with offspring who have left home	Adaptation to empty nest; adjustment in marital relationship; growth of relationships with married offspring and grandchildren
Family in early retirement	Adaptation to retirement and increased leisure activities; strengthening of marital ties; adjustment to being older
Family in old age	Maintenance of marital relationship; adjustment to widowhood and loss of friends; adaptation to aging

children, and adjust relationships with other family members, such as aunts, uncles, and grandparents.

It is obvious that not all individuals and families fit into such predictable stages. There are many variations of family units. Brief examples include the following:

- Couples without children
- Families who have children early in a marriage and then much later
- Homosexual couples
- Children raised by grandparents or other caregivers
- Single-parent families
- Families with a member who is chronically ill or who has a disability

However, Duvall's theory provides a means to begin examining family relationships and roles and the impact of individual needs on family needs. For example, if there is a sick family member during the school-age stage, it may prevent the family from participating in community and educational activities. It is not always possible to mesh individual and family needs. If a family does not quite conform to the expectations of the community, pressure may be placed on them. A young child with HIV may be isolated, along with the family. A biracial or homosexual couple may be shunned. These factors will interfere with the developmental tasks of the family. In addition, a parent or caregiver with substance abuse may place a heavy burden on other family members financially, socially, and developmentally.

BOWEN

Murray Bowen proposes that the family is an interrelated and interdependent system that is influenced by each of its members and by external factors, such as the community, the environment, and life events. The interrelationships that exist between and among family members are so great that when one individual is changed, the whole family system will be affected. For instance, if a child becomes chronically ill, the parents will be focused on that child and may parent the siblings differently than they did before the child's illness. The siblings may begin to have behavior problems in school or vague physical ailments as a result of the first child's illness and the changed parenting. All family members are affected by the condition of one member. Bowen's approach to family therapy consists of treating the individual not as an entity separate from the family, but rather as part of a family unit, all of whom should be involved in the counseling. In this way, family members are able to face issues and deal with them together, instead of making one member responsible.

In your work as an LPN/LVN, you have already included family members when caring for an individual. As you move into the RN role, there will be an increased emphasis on the family unit. As health care delivery continues to evolve, the family plays a critical role. Not only must you assess a person, but you must also assess the family because the health status of individual members is affected by the function of the family. The family assessment will provide you with a clearer picture of the person's primary social context, family stressors, risk factors within the family, and the family's adaptation and coping mechanisms.

thinking critically

Review Duvall's stages of family development. Is there a stage that describes your current status? What is the same? What is different? What impact will your return to school have on your family's development? What impact will the situations of other family members have on your development as you return to school?

● PROFESSIONAL ROLE DEVELOPMENT

Role development is defined in the beginning of this chapter. The addition of the word "professional" requires a brief definition. To be a member of a profession, one must have special preparation and education to acquire knowledge and skills to perform a certain role. Professional role development implies acquiring the skills and knowledge that are needed to function within a particular role. Growth and development within the role are influenced by previous experiences and the expectations for that role by members of the profession and those who interface with such individuals.

Cohen

Professional role development may also evolve in stages. Cohen (1981) identified four stages that relate to Erikson's developmental stages (Table 2.9). The first stage is called unilateral dependence, in which a student professional begins to learn theoretical content and to practice in a limited way under the supervision of an instructor. The second stage is negative independence, which provides the student professional more opportunities to apply theory to practice and to internalize some of the professional role behaviors that fit with her or his own values and self-concepts. Cohen identifies the third stage as dependence/mutuality, in which the student professional begins to recognize role limitations to be acceptable to other

table 2-9 PROFESSIONAL ROLE DEVELOPMENT—COHEN

Stage I	Unilateral dependence	Inexperienced student learns theoretical concepts for role development; applies theory to practice in a limited and supervised way.
Stage II	Negative independence	Student has increased opportunities to apply theory to practice and assumes more responsibility; develops confidence and takes on some of the role values; also is more willing to question traditional patterns and ways of knowing.
Stage III	Dependence/mutuality	Student is able to be more realistic about role expectations, and questions reflect a higher understanding of theoretical concepts; recognizes role limitations.
Stage IV	Interdependence	Student is able to make independent judgments and to take on the professional role; student's professional identity is more secure and not in opposition with other roles.

professionals and to society in general. The last stage is called interdependence, in which the professional role seems more real. The individual is able to accept more responsibility and to believe that the professional role is part of her or his identity. The comfort level is much higher because the person generally believes that the professional role is not in conflict with other roles.

Your professional role development has already begun. Your decision to become an RN initiated the process. As you progress in your academic program, you will acquire the knowledge, skills, and abilities needed to be a professional nurse.

> **thinking critically**
>
> How has your role as an LPN/LVN affected your professional role development? Explore positive and negative effects and your present stage of professional role development. What will help or hinder you in reaching Cohen's fourth stage?

Professional Role Socialization

Professional role socialization is a complicated process during which an individual not only learns the necessary cognitive and motor skills for a particular role but also gains an identity with an occupation and adopts the values and norms of that occupational group. According to Cohen (1981), four goals are associated with role socialization. The student will

1. acquire technical and theoretical skills
2. take on the values of the profession
3. modify the professional role to one that is personally and professionally acceptable
4. balance the professional role with other roles

Several models have been developed to define the process of professional role socialization. The model developed by Hinshaw (1986) depicts three stages for socialization or resocialization for a professional role (Table 2.10). In the first stage, students change their concepts of role expectations from those they had anticipated to those being taught by professional role models. The second stage is a time of attachment to role models within the educational and clinical settings. It is also a time when students have conflicts about incongruences of role behaviors that were not anticipated or expected. During this time, it is essential that role models assist students to cope with these incongruences. The last stage is the internalization of the values and standards of the new role.

In your socialization to the RN role, you will take on the values and standards for that role. As an LPN/LVN, you may not recognize all the differences that exist between the two roles, except in terms of tasks. In the mid-1900s, Kelman (1958) identified three processes of attitude change:

1. Compliance: An individual demonstrates appropriate behaviors to receive positive feedback but has not internalized the values.
2. Identification: The individual is selective about the particular behaviors that are personally acceptable; this often depends on particular role models.
3. Internalization: The individual believes and accepts the new standards of behavior as part of her or his own value system.

table
············
2-10   MODEL OF PROFESSIONAL ROLE SOCIALIZATION—HINSHAW

Stage I	Transition from anticipated role expectations to those that are taught	Adults who are new to a profession are committed to learning the expected role behaviors.
Stage II	Attachment to important role models; identification of inconsistencies	Attachments are made with significant faculty or staff members. Role models are important and essential. At this time, questions also arise regarding situations that are incongruent with those presented by role models.
Stage III	Internalization of role values and standards	The individual takes on the values and standards of the professional role. If the incongruencies have been significant in the second stage, the internalization of values may be affected.

These processes of attitude change still remain present today as an LVN/LPN transitions to the RN role. Your education to become an RN will not only provide you with new skills but also change the way you think and who you are. Moving to the professional role of the RN will cause you to develop deeper analytical and critical thinking skills. Chandler (2010) describes the world entered by new Registered Nursing graduates as one of staff shortages and greater patient acuity, "demanding sophisticated assessment skills, initiating clinical interventions, using management skills, and demonstrating leadership capabilities" (pp. 22–23). Socialization into this new professional role will require new knowledge and skills beyond the directed level of nursing practice experienced at the LPN/LVN level as you assume these autonomous responsibilities in a leadership role as an RN.

• ROLE TRANSITION

Role transition means the passage or shifts from one role to another and involves changing the way one thinks and acts. William Bridges (1980, 1991, 2001, 2003) differentiated between change and transition. He defined change as a "situational shift" (getting a new boss, having a child, or returning to school). Bridges (2001) described transition as "the process of letting go of the way things used to be and then taking hold of the way they subsequently become" (p. 2). He noted that transition is the way we come to terms with change. Bridges (2001, 2003, 2009) further divided transition into three phases: endings, neutral zone, and beginnings.

Endings

Every transition begins with an ending. We have to let go of the old before we can pick up the new—not just outwardly, but inwardly, where we keep our connections to the people and places that act as definitions of who we are. Bridges designates four aspects of endings:

1. Disengagement: separation from a familiar place within the social order. At various times, a person voluntarily or involuntarily is disengaged from activities, relationships, places, or roles that have been important.

2. Disidentification: loss of self-definition; a process of not being quite sure of who you are. Often, the old identity can interfere with transition because it is hard to let go of what you were.

3. Disenchantment: the realization that the beliefs and views in the past are no longer real. Life is a series of disenchantments in the many transitions; disenchantment may be related to the loss of a relationship or a change in career. The disenchanted person recognizes the old view as sufficient in its time but insufficient now.

4. Disorientation: the lost and confused feeling that a person experiences when in transition. There is a sense of unreality about even ordinary events; nothing feels the same.

Neutral Zone

The second phase of role transition described by Bridges is called the neutral zone. During this phase, a person is "in limbo," a temporary state of emptiness or loss or an in-between state of affairs. It is a time when a person appears to be in a void but is actually contemplating important inner thoughts. The first function of this phase is one of surrender, in which a person gives in to the emptiness and does not try to escape it. A second function is one of renewal, recharging, and possibly redirecting. The last function is a change in perspective about what a person has always known and learning how to view it differently.

Beginnings

The last phase of transition identified by Bridges is called beginnings. There is no clear path that can tell a person that a new beginning is at hand. Instead, there is just an initial hint that something is different. It occurs within the person, although the transition may be the result of changing jobs, changing relationships, or continuing an education. The beginning in the transition process is part of a continuum; it is a new chapter of one's life that is beginning. As the beginning becomes part of the whole, the person reintegrates the new identity with the old identity. None of us are the same as a result of a transition; rather, we are changed in many ways. Bridges' phases of transition are shown in Display 2.3.

thinking critically

As you read through role socialization and transition, where do you see yourself? Assess the stage or phase that you are currently experiencing. What will define your new beginning?

ROLE CONFLICT

Role conflict develops when an individual is faced with expectations that are incompatible with each other. This can be intrapersonal or interpersonal. Intrapersonal role conflict occurs within one's self when an individual struggles with multiple personal role expectations. For example, in your role as a student nurse, you may

---

| display **2.3** | **Bridge's Phases of Transition** |

PHASE I: ENDINGS

Four types of endings:
1. Disengagement   3. Disenchantment
2. Disidentification   4. Disorientation

PHASE II: NEUTRAL ZONE

Three functions:
1. Surrender
2. Renewal and recharging; redirection
3. Change in perspective

PHASE III: MAKING A BEGINNING

- A "loop in the life-journey"
- Reintegration of new identity with old identity

---

face conflict with the necessity of having to study as opposed to spending time with significant others in your life. Interpersonal role conflict occurs between two individuals when each has different expectations about the same role. An example of this type of conflict might occur in relation to others' expectations of you in your role as a nurse. You may think that your role is to spend time with a client with newly diagnosed diabetes so that you can begin teaching the process of self-care, whereas your supervisor may think that it is more important that you complete your written documentation. Role conflict is a component of role stress, in which a person realizes that role obligations are conflicting or that role demands are too difficult or impossible to fulfill. Feelings of discomfort, frustration, and anxiety can occur; this is referred to as role strain.

Many women who are trying to balance motherhood with returning to school or work experience role strain and role overload (Garey, 1999; Granrose & Kaplan, 1996; Holcomb, 1998). This phenomenon also occurs in men who are single parents or who have assumed more care-giving and parenting responsibilities in the home.

Bolton (2000) described role overload for many women as they engage in what she called "the third shift." In addition to dealing with concerns about work while at home and those of home while at work, many women invest mental energy into reflecting on these two roles. They are continually assessing how well they are balancing home and work roles, which one is being compromised, and whether they are exercising good judgment in the choices they make each day. This role overload is often particularly present in Latino, Asian, and other cultures where the family plays an important role, and women in particular are expected to care for family first. Gandara and Contreras (2009) describe such barriers for Latino students, where role overload can be particularly challenging. Federal and community-based programs available at most colleges can be especially helpful in assisting students in overcoming role conflict and balancing the multiple role expectations of one's culture.

Role overload has been exacerbated during the current recession in the United States. The economic downturn has caused families to experience increased financial constraints, and family members assuming multiple roles to "make ends meet." Assuming additional employment and caretaking roles has become common, as extended family members rely on limited family workers for income, housing, and caretaking. The unemployed and those displaced from business and home foreclosures place additional burdens and role expectations on remaining family members.

Lastly, those who are veterans, returning from the war, may be experiencing a greater than normal anxiety in transitioning both to civilian life and to the student role. One veteran stated, "I am more terrified of going to college than I was going to war." Such challenges in role transition require additional services, which can be found through your college advisor, student services personnel, and veteran's affairs staff.

As a returning student, you may be experiencing a greater than normal amount of role overload and/or challenges in role transition. It is imperative that you seek assistance from your nursing advisor, or college counselor to access resources that can assist you.

Unfortunately, role conflict cannot be avoided, and so it is important to develop methods of coping with conflict constructively. Five methods can be used to resolve conflict (Display 2.4):

1. **Avoidance:** This is also called withdrawing from or denying conflict. When this method is used, conflict is generally not resolved and may actually be perpetuated. Example: You checked a book out of the library and then loaned it to a fellow student. She returned it to the library late, and you were billed for the fine. You decide to pay it rather than asking the student to do so.

2. **Compromise:** This approach uses the techniques of bargaining or negotiating. It is recognized that there must be a give and take for the solution to be determined. Generally, compromise works well, although the conflict issue may recur. Example: You and your spouse arrange to accomplish household chores based on time limitations and abilities. Both of you agree that it is a good plan that will satisfy the need for a clean house and mutual responsibilities.

3. **Accommodation:** In this method, a person attempts to smooth over the conflict or to suppress the problems. Often, a peaceful environment will be maintained, but one person may feel as though she or he has made a tremendous sacrifice and is inwardly angry and frustrated. Example: In Example 2, one partner may not follow through on the predetermined tasks, and so the

---

display 2.4   **Five Methods of Resolving Role Conflict**

1. Avoidance
2. Compromise
3. Accommodation
4. Competition
5. Collaboration

other partner says that she or he understands and helps the partner finish the undone household chores.

4. **Competition:** In this strategy, one person decides to force the issue and to place personal goals or desires over those of others. This sets up a conflict of power. Example: A group of students meet to plan for an end-of-the-year banquet and select a leader. One student spends 10 minutes describing her experience in her LPN program chairing the banquet committee, the success of the banquet, and how grateful her classmates were for her leadership. The group agrees to let this student have primary responsibility for planning this banquet.

5. **Collaboration:** This strategy requires participants to be willing to problem solve and confront the issues with the intent of setting mutual goals. All participants are involved in the decision-making process. Example: A group of student nurses is concerned about the volume of paperwork required by clinical instructors. The instructors recognize that there is a lot of work, but they believe it is necessary to ensure that each student is prepared for each clinical assignment. The chairperson arranges a meeting with the students and instructors to develop methods that validate student preparation without being overly burdensome.

---

thinking critically

Consider each method of conflict resolution. Think of an example of your own for each method. Would another method have been more satisfactory? Why?

NCLEX–RN *Might Ask*   2.2

A client asks a nursing student what the changes to her role have been as she has gone from LPN to RN. The nurse would be *incorrect* by stating the following:

 A. "I have acquired more advanced technical and theoretical skills."
 B. "I have learned to balance my roles as wife and mother with my professional ones."
 C. "I have interwoven new professional values into my existing ones."
 D. "I have changed my professional roles to only what is acceptable to me personally."

· *See Appendix A for correct answer and rationale.*

● CONCLUSION

Role development and transition are complex processes that have individual and universal concepts. In this chapter, personal development is presented in relation to the work of stage theorists who perceive development in terms of stages and critical tasks that occur in a sequential pattern. Adult development is described as an ongoing and dynamic process. Family and professional role development is presented in terms of stages of development.

Concepts related to role socialization, role transition, and role conflict are presented with an emphasis on the meanings these concepts have for the LPN/LVN role transition process. Understanding the theories and concepts of role development and transition enhances a person's ability to examine her or his own experiences and to better assess client experiences. The impacts of role changes and health status changes are varied and yet more predictable when all concepts are considered. You will find many opportunities to apply this information in your personal and work experiences, including your transition to the RN role.

student exercises

1. Interview a student in your class.

2. Identify the various roles for this student.

3. Differentiate the individual's ascribed and acquired roles.

4. Select a theorist or theorists to determine the tasks with which this individual is concerned.

5. Ask the student to describe the role of her or his family and what her or his role is within that family.

6. Explore with the student what role changes are forthcoming.

7. Determine whether there are role conflicts involved and what methods are used for coping.

References

Bolton, M. E. (2000). *The third shift: Managing hard choices in our careers, homes, and lives as women*. San Francisco, CA: Jossey-Bass.

Bridges, W. (1980). *Transitions: Making sense of life's changes*. Menlo Park, CA: Addison-Wesley.

Bridges, W. (1991). *Managing transitions: Making the most of change*. New York, NY: William Bridges and Associates, Perseus Books.

Bridges, W. (2001). *The way of transitions: Embracing life's most difficult moments*. New York, NY: William Bridges and Associates, Perseus Books.

Bridges, W. (2003). *Managing transitions: Making the most of change* (2nd ed.) Cambridge, MA: DaCapo Press.

Bridges, W. (2009). *Managing transitions: Making the most of change* (3rd ed.). Philadelphia, PA: Perseus Books Group.

Chandler, G. E. (2010). *New nurse's survival guide*. New York, NY: McGraw-Hill.

Cohen, H. A. (1981). *The nurse's quest for a professional identity*. Menlo Park, CA: Addison-Wesley.

Covey, S. (1989). *The seven habits of highly effective people*. New York, NY: Simon & Schuster.

Covey, S. R. (2004). *The 8th habit: From effectiveness to greatness*. New York, NY: Free Press.

Duvall, E. M. (1977). *Marriage and family development* (5th ed.). Philadelphia, PA: JB Lippincott.

Gandara, P., & Contreras, F. (2009). *The Latino education crisis: The consequences of failed social policies*. Cambridge, MA: Harvard University Press.

Garey, A. I. (1999). *Weaving work and motherhood*. Philadelphia, PA: Temple University Press.

Gilligan, C. (1982). *In a different voice: Psychological theory and women's development*. Cambridge, MA: Harvard University Press.

Granrose, C. S., & Kaplan, E. E. (1996). *Work-family role choices for women in their 20's and 30's: From college plans to life experiences*. Westport, CT: Praeger.

Hinshaw, A. S. (1986). Socialization and resocialization of nurses for professional nursing practice. In E. C. Hein & M. J. Nicholson (Eds.), *Contemporary leadership behavior: Selected readings* (2nd ed.). Boston, MA: Little, Brown and Company.

Holcomb, B. (1998). *Not guilty: The good news about working mothers*. New York, NY: Scribner, Simon & Schuster.

Kelman, H. C. (1958). Compliance, identification, and internalization: Three processes of attitude change. *The Journal of Conflict Resolution, 2*(1), 51–60.

Longworth, N. (2003). *Lifelong learning in action: Transforming education in the 21st century*. New York, NY: Routledge/Falmer.

Palmer, P. J. (2007). *The courage to teach: Exploring the inner landscape of a teacher's life* (10th Anniversary ed.). San Francisco, CA: Wiley and Sons.

Shane, D. L. (1983). *Returning to school: A guide for nurses*. Englewood Cliffs, NJ: Prentice-Hall.

Sheehy, G. (1976). *Passages: Predictable crises of adult life*. New York, NY: Dutton and Company.

Stevens-Long, J. (1988). *Adult life* (3rd ed.). Mountain View, CA: Mayfield.

Stevenson, J. S. (1977). *Issues and crises during middlescence*. New York, NY: Appleton-Century-Crofts.

Taylor, C., Lillis, C., LeMone, P., & Lynn, P. (2011). *Fundamentals of nursing: The art and science of nursing care* (7th ed.). Philadelphia, PA: Lippincott Williams & Wilkins.

Suggested Reading

Alexander, C. N., & Langer, E. J. (1990) (Eds.). *Higher stages of human development*. New York, NY: Oxford University Press.

Ellis, J. R., & Hartley, C. L. (2009). *Managing and coordinating nursing care* (5th ed.). Philadelphia, PA: Lippincott Williams & Wilkins.

Leddy, S., & Pepper, J. M. (2010). *Conceptual bases of professional nursing* (7th ed.). Philadelphia, PA: Lippincott Williams & Wilkins.

Rossi, A. S. (Ed.). (1985). *Gender and the life course*. New York, NY: Aldine.

Sheehy, G. (1981). *Pathfinders*. New York: Morrow and Company.

Valentine, P. (2001). A gender perspective on conflict management strategies of nurses. *Journal of Nursing Scholarship, 33*(1), 69–74.

On the (WEB) *http://www.piaget.org:* The Jean Piaget Society. (Last accessed 7.6.2011).

http://www.gailsheehy.com (Gail Sheehy's Web site). (Last accessed 7.6.2011).

http://www.webster.edu/~woolflm/gilligan.html (Information about Carol Gilligan). (Last accessed 7.6.2011).

For more information on Adult Development Theory, go to *www.google.com* and enter "Adult Development Theorists" or the specific theorist you wish to learn more about.

3

Adapting to Change

● LEARNING OUTCOMES

By the end of this chapter, the student will be able to:

1 Explore the paradoxes of change.

2 Differentiate individual and organizational change.

3 Summarize factors that motivate change.

4 Compare and contrast types of change.

5 Describe the process of planned change.

6 Outline Lewin's process of change.

7 Discuss the effects of change on individuals and systems.

8 Apply theoretical effects of change.

9 Describe methods for adjusting to change.

10 Give examples of positive outcomes of change.

adaptation
ambivalence
autonomy
biotechnology
change agent
change paradox
conflict
crisis
distress

driving forces
eustress
flexibility
general adaptation
   syndrome
individual change
loss
organizational change
resistance

resonance
restraining forces
self-actualization
stakeholders
transactional change
transformational
   change

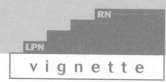

v i g n e t t e

Deborah Pogwist is a 54-year-old LPN who has worked in the mental health unit of a state hospital for the past 25 years. She is taking her first clinical nursing course in the ADN program. After having difficulty with the clinical component in a hospital setting, she is meeting with her nursing adviser, John Tercha, to discuss her problems adjusting to change.

DEBORAH: I feel so inadequate! I remember being in the hospital setting years ago, but why do I need to go through this again when there is a job opening where I have worked for 25 years? I just feel that I'm jumping through hoops!

ADVISOR: I hear what you're saying, and I understand. It is often very uncomfortable for adults to be in a new environment. It sounds as if you feel frustrated and are not sure whether the concepts you are learning are applicable to your professional work.

DEBORAH: Exactly! Do I really have to do all of this?

ADVISOR: Yes, you will have to complete the clinical objectives for the courses. However, I can assure you that the newness will wear off, and even though you cannot see the relevance of what you are learning, it is part of the bigger picture. This picture includes helping you become more flexible, more well rounded, more educated, and more of a critical thinker. Change is a difficult process, but it is necessary. Let's review what specific difficulties you are having and use change theory to help you through this first clinical course transition.

● CHANGE DEFINED

William Bridges (2001), a leading author on change and transitions, identified several change paradoxes that define its dynamic state (Display 3.1). A paradox is a statement that seems absurd or contradictory but is based on fact.

Change is ever present in our daily lives. With change, each person, group, or organization has the opportunity to develop, grow, and adapt. Change is inevitable and dynamic. Each of us copes with change in unique ways. Our responses to change are affected by what is occurring in our lives, our needs, and our experiences.

---

display 3.1   **Paradoxes of Change**

- To achieve continuity, we have to be willing to change.
- Change is the only way to protect whatever exists; without continuous readjustments, the present cannot continue.
- The very things we now wish that we could hold onto and keep safe from change were themselves originally produced by change.

● PROCESS OF CHANGE

Examining the process of change is particularly important for student nurses for several reasons. First, you are experiencing personal change by returning to school. Second, you will be presented with many aspects of change within the nursing curriculum. For instance, in issues related to trends in health care, the faculty may present you with current methods of delivering care and have you explore how the future in health care delivery will be affected by biotechnology or economic concerns. Third, as you prepare for your own role transition, you will learn about the new roles nurses have today and will have in the future. It is essential to understand that change is inevitable. Change occurs even when you think societal and work roles and values are stable or resistant to change. As Lapp (2002) noted, change is inevitable in today's world and the challenge for each individual is to learn to be more comfortable outside his or her "comfort zone."

● INDIVIDUAL AND ORGANIZATIONAL CHANGE

When differentiating individual change from organizational change, remember that change always implies the alteration or modification of behaviors or functions. Within the individual, change may occur without any plan at all, or it may be the result of much planning. Later in this chapter, types of change are described. Organizational change also results in behavior or function alterations but has the potential to have a greater impact on parts of an organization and its individuals. Display 3.2 compares individual and organizational change. Change within an organization involves modifying working practices and procedures, causing individuals to work in different ways. This can produce a great deal of fear among employees. Carter and Alfred (1999) noted that "Change, by its very nature, represents breaking with the past. Ironically, it is most successful when the process honors and respects institutional history and tradition" (p. 28).

● FACTORS THAT MOTIVATE CHANGE

Many factors motivate change. If you were to examine your reasons for desiring a change from your role as an LPN/LVN to that of an RN, you may identify some aspects that are described in the following text. You may also recognize some factors that have played a part in other life changes.

Crisis

One factor that can precipitate change is a crisis—a turning point or a critical time in the course of an event. As discussed in Chapter 2, a situational crisis involves an unexpected event, such as a natural disaster, loss of a loved one, illness, or divorce. This type of crisis can motivate an individual to make other changes. For example, a 40-year-old nurse who had recently been through a divorce recognized a need to further her education and develop a professional career. This may not have happened if she had remained in the marriage.

Conflict

Another factor that can influence the process of change is conflict. There is always an implied sense of battle or opposition when the term conflict is used. In relation to change, it also denotes a struggle or variance with a particular situation or person. Conflict may result in change because an individual is frustrated with the current circumstances. An example is that of a man who has not been happy in his position as a nurse at a local hospital. He wants to practice nursing in a more holistic way and believes that the fragmented care system is not adequate. Although he has spoken to his boss many times, he has been unable to make any changes in the health care delivery system. Finally, he decides that he can no longer deal with the conflict, and so he resigns. He is subsequently hired by a community health agency that practices a more holistic approach. Conflict motivated him to make a change.

Disappointment

Everyone has experienced disappointment at some point. Disappointment is related to a sense of failure at not meeting expectations or fulfilling certain plans and can be another motivator for change. A nursing student who has done poorly in math has avoided working on math problems. After failing her first quiz, she meets with her advisor, spends time with a college tutor, and purchases a step-by-step nursing math review text. This student nurse has vowed to change her practice habits, so that she will pass the next quiz and improve her clinical performance.

Lack of Rewards

Another stimulus for change is lack of rewards in the current circumstances. An individual may be in a position that affords little recognition or reward. This situation can motivate the person to take courses or advanced training or to change jobs to gain more rewards and prestige.

Desire for Autonomy and Self-Improvement

The last factor that can activate change is the desire for autonomy and self-improvement. A person may feel stagnated and powerless in a particular position and thus may take appropriate steps to change the situation. For instance, a certified nursing assistant may enjoy her or his work but not feel able to influence policy or procedures. She or he may also want to learn more and take on additional responsibility. This sense of powerlessness and need for self-improvement is a potent factor for change.

---

thinking critically

Identify factors that have caused you to make a change in your life. Give examples of changes that you have made. Analyze the results of these changes and how certain behaviors or functions were affected.

● TYPES OF CHANGE

There are various types of change—some are developmental, some are unplanned, and some are planned—that an individual or organization can face. From your own experiences, you can probably identify some of these. The following sections define three types of change that are generally encountered.

Developmental Change

Developmental change is change in which a person proceeds through stages in a fairly predictable order. Tasks are identified for each stage that must be accomplished to complete a stage. Examples of this type of change are described in the previous chapter.

Unplanned Change

Unplanned change can refer to positive or negative, desired or undesired change that was not planned. An example of positive unplanned change would be an unexpected promotion within an organization, whereas a negative unplanned stage might be unannounced layoffs at a place of employment. Two types of unplanned change are forced change and spontaneous change.

FORCED CHANGE

Forced change is a type of change that is imposed on an individual or organization that requires action, often of an immediate or emergent nature. An example would be a fire in a person's home, in which the entire home and its contents are lost. Family members are forced to consider rebuilding the home and replacing lost items, as well as realizing that everything is forever different.

SPONTANEOUS CHANGE

Spontaneous change refers to change that is impulsive or effortless and is often random or unpredictable. For example, when a person begins a new job, she or he may take on the characteristics of other coworkers. This may involve buying the same types of clothes or becoming interested in similar activities. In retrospect, it may seem like a planned response, but in reality it occurred spontaneously and without forethought.

Planned Change

Planned change involves advanced strategy by a change agent. Ellis and Hartley (2009) described a change agent as a "champion" who is responsible for leading the group to change. Members who are affected by the change are referred to as stakeholders. In an organization, anyone can become the change agent and present ideas to the stakeholders. For example, a planned change is your return to school; you probably made careful plans to achieve your goals. These plans may have included child care or other personal issues, revision of work schedules, or a change in daily activities. Other planned changes may have occurred in your workplace. Schedule changes are an example. Some health care settings have opted to have their employees work 12-hour shifts. To establish that schedule, an implementation plan is developed, so that the transition to the new schedule is as smooth as possible. This is the process of planned change. There are several types of planned change.

INCREMENTAL CHANGE

Incremental change involves a planned change that occurs gradually in steps or stages. This type of planning is often applied to long-term projects, such as hospital mergers or curriculum changes. You may have planned your return to school in increments. You may have taken your general education courses first at the initial stage of your education. The second part of the process involves completing the nursing courses. By doing this, you are able to continue working or have greater ability to care for a family or remain involved in other interests.

RAPID CHANGE

Change that is planned quickly may or may not be successful. For instance, rapid plans may need to be developed in rescue situations to assist people quickly in precarious situations. Rapid change can also mean the implementation of an organizational plan without considering the ramifications. As an example, a nursing organization recognizes that staff positions need to be eliminated fairly quickly because of reduced census or revenue shortfalls. The plans are made to eliminate positions based on seniority, without considering what units have the highest staffing needs and how staff might need to be transferred and oriented. The plan is implemented quickly but without considering the fallout.

TRANSACTIONAL CHANGE

Transactional change occurs for mutual benefit. For example, nursing faculty and students determine that a change is needed in clinical experiences so that all seniors have the opportunity for a leadership experience. Representatives of both groups meet to plan the best method to accomplish this goal. The plan is formed so that all parties are able to transact an appropriate and mutually agreeable plan.

TRANSFORMATIONAL CHANGE

Transformational change occurs within the process of planned change. In your return to school, a change will occur as you progress through your ADN course work. With this process of change will come not only new knowledge and skills but also a new way of thinking and being. Transformation implies that there is a radical difference in an individual or a group as a result of change.

---

thinking critically

Review the types of change that have been described. Think of experiences that have involved change in your life. Categorize these changes according to the previous descriptions. Consider these changes in terms of individual, group, and organizational changes. Are any of them transformational in nature? Why? What has been the impact of these changes?

NCLEX–RN *Might Ask*   3.1

The nurse is taking care of a large group of clients in a community care setting. Because of the high influx of new clients, the nurse manager independently decides to make a radical change in the way clients are assessed and processed. This type of radical change would be most consistent with

  A. Transactional change.
  B. Transformational change.
  C. Unplanned change.
  D. Spontaneous change.

· *See Appendix A for correct answer and rationale.*

● STAGES OF PLANNED CHANGE

The process of change is complex because it involves the modification of behaviors. Unplanned change is, obviously, less structured and more haphazard than planned change. When change is planned, there will be a more systematic approach that entails problem solving, decision making, and deliberate steps. Kurt Lewin is a

---

display 3.3   **Lewin's Stages of Planned Change**

Unfreezing: An individual, group, or organization identifies the need for change and the need to change behaviors. It is necessary to identify restraining and driving forces for the planned change.

Moving: Strategies for the planned change are developed. The individual, group, or organization gathers data, formulates plans, and enlists the support of all those involved with the change.

Refreezing: The process of change is completed. The individual, group, or organization internalizes the behavior changes and attitudes that were identified as necessary for the change process.

---

social scientist credited with doing the first work in change theory. The following text outlines his theory of planned change. Display 3.3 summarizes Lewin's (1951) three stages of planned change, which are still in use today.

Unfreezing

The first stage that Lewin (1951) identified is referred to as the unfreezing stage, in which a person, group, or organization is motivated to bring about change. There is a need to learn new behaviors. This stage is one of imbalance and disequilibrium; it is very unsettling. During this stage, two types of forces are present: those against and those in support of the change.

RESTRAINING FORCES

Restraining forces are those that inhibit change. For example, as you have become motivated to return to school, you undoubtedly have encountered some restraining forces. For example, some of the restraining forces may have been related to family concerns, loss of income while in school, lack of confidence in your ability to succeed, or coworkers who fear you will be leaving.

DRIVING FORCES

Opposing such restraining forces are driving forces. These are the forces that encourage and sustain change. For example, your motivation to return to school may have been supported by such forces as your desire for more decision making, increased clinical skills, more recognition, or the encouragement and support of a family member, mentor, or friend.

Moving

The second stage that Lewin (1951) identified is called moving. During this stage, plans are detailed and initiated. It is important to collect data and supplemental information from as many sources as possible. In addition, it is helpful if most, if not all, people involved are in agreement that change is desirable. For example, you entered the moving stage after you began making plans to return to school. At this time, you formulated plans for child care or alternative work schedules. You may also have obtained information about financial aid and scholarships. You gathered as much information as possible to assist you in your plans. You may have enlisted the advice of a colleague who had been through this process. It may have been necessary for you to persuade those around you that this was an important move for you and that you needed their support and understanding. Use of "win/win agreements" as discussed in Chapter 1 can be helpful during this stage.

It is during this second stage of change that transitions occur, as described in Chapter 2. Letting go of the past (ie, accomplishing endings) becomes essential to make room for new beginnings. Role conflict may increase as both you and others around you work to put old roles behind you to prepare for new ones. Often, there is a sense of loss for the role left behind.

Refreezing

Lewin's (1951) last stage is called refreezing. The change has occurred and is now part of the individual, group, or organization. Refreezing requires a commitment to change and the stabilization of restraining and driving forces. There is a change of behaviors and attitudes within the change process. In continuing with the same example, as you re-enter school, one change has already occurred: You are a student nurse again. You have internalized the value of continuing your education and have made the commitment to become an RN. This change is part of who you are. Your family, friends, and coworkers have also made adjustments to this change.

---

thinking critically

Recall a planned change with which you were recently involved. Critique your change as viewed through the three stages of planned change described by Lewin. What steps were taken to initiate the change? What were the restraining and driving forces? What was your role in the planned change? What role conflict did you experience? When did you become aware that you had made a transition and were prepared for the refreezing stage? What was the impact on those around you?

• EFFECTS OF CHANGE

Change can have many effects. Some are expected, and some are not. As previously stated, individuals cope with and adapt to change in unique ways.

Stress, Distress, and Eustress

Stress, distress, and eustress are terms defined by Hans Selye (1976) to describe various conditions that humans experience. Stress is a universal response to any situation or factor that disturbs a person's equilibrium. It has become a familiar term to all of us and may be a term that you will use frequently while in nursing school. Selye called the side effects of stress distress and eustress. Distress is the negative or maladaptive effects of change or stress, whereas eustress represents the more beneficial effects.

With any stress or change, nonspecific bodily changes occur. If a person is able to cope effectively with change, the side effects will be kept to a minimum, but poor adaptation to stress or change results in damaging side effects, or distress. Physical signs of distress can include prolonged elevated blood pressure, increased gastric acid secretions, and decreased urine output. Emotional signs may include insomnia and hyperexcitability. There also may be behavioral changes such as depression or anger. Selye (1976) believed that some conditions (eg, hypertension, ulcers, certain emotional disturbances) represent diseases of adaptation. Although many researchers and physicians argue differently, the concepts of distress and eustress provide a means for you to evaluate the typical coping patterns of your clients.

General Adaptation Syndrome

As the previous paragraphs indicate, a common effect of any change, planned or unplanned, is stress, which disturbs an individual's equilibrium. Selye (1976) was the first to describe a nonspecific general response to stress, which he called general adaptation syndrome. He differentiated stress as a condition of the body that is characterized by the changes that occur within the body. A stressor is defined as any factor that upsets the equilibrium and results in stress. For example, a student may experience nausea before making a class presentation. The stressor is the impending presentation; the stress is the condition of nausea.

Selye (1976) delineated three stages that occur in the general adaptation syndrome: alarm reaction, resistance, and recovery or exhaustion. Table 3.1 shows these stages.

table
3-1   STAGES OF THE GENERAL ADAPTATION SYNDROME

Stage	Body Responses
Alarm reaction (fight or flight)	Increased release of hormones by the autonomic nervous system: • Increased heart rate • Increased oxygen intake • Increased blood sugar • Increased mental acuity • Increased blood flow to muscles • Increased blood pressure • Decreased flow to the kidneys • Decreased urine output
Resistance	Stabilization: • Hormone levels return to normal • Cardiac functions return to previous levels • Adaptation to stressor(s)
Recovery or exhaustion	Defense mechanisms described in the alarm reaction stage are exhausted Decreased energy levels Fatigue Decreased ability for adaptation Death

ALARM REACTION

The first stage of the general adaptation syndrome is the alarm reaction. The body responds to a particular stressor, such as an extreme in temperature, infection, verbal abuse, or other conscious and unconscious factors. With this process, the defense mechanisms of the mind and body are activated. The autonomic nervous system releases large amounts of hormones into the body. Blood volume is increased, and blood glucose levels rise to meet energy needs. Increased epinephrine results in a higher heart rate, more blood flow to muscles, better oxygen intake, and greater mental alertness. Norepinephrine is released in greater quantities to decrease blood flow to the kidneys. Increased rennin secretion will result in more angiotensin production, thus elevating blood pressure. This process initiates the fight-or-flight response and may last for a short period to many hours. A person is ready for action during this phase.

RESISTANCE

The second stage is called the resistance stage. During this stage, the alarm reactions stabilize. The hormone levels and cardiac functions return to previous levels. The person attempts to adapt to the stressor or to cope more effectively with its effects. For example, if a person has sustained a fracture, the body responds by beginning the process of healing at the site of the fracture. This would be considered recovery. If the stressor is more difficult, such as hemorrhage, adaptation may be impossible, and the outcome is exhaustion. In both cases, the individuals enter the next stage.

RECOVERY OR EXHAUSTION

The third stage is referred to as the stage of recovery or exhaustion. The body will either recover or find it can no longer cope with the stressor, having exhausted its ability to defend itself. The effects of stress may involve the entire body. A person who experiences psychological trauma will enter a state of exhaustion and demonstrate physical and emotional symptoms, such as abdominal pain, insomnia, or depression. If the state of exhaustion is severe, such as the state that follows unchecked hemorrhage, death may occur.

The concepts of stress and adaptation should be familiar to you from your LPN/LVN program. One's ability to adapt to stress also describes the ability to adapt to change. Adaptation involves a person's capacity for change as she or he is faced with new experiences. Understanding how you adapt to change can assist you with some of the stress you may encounter as you return to the student role.

---

thinking critically

Recall a situation that has created stress for you. Review the stages of the general adaptation syndrome. Determine what physical, emotional, or behavioral changes occurred. What was the outcome of the change that took place? What is your general response to stressful situations? How do you adapt? What resources are available to you if you experience stress during the nursing program? What are some positive mechanisms you can employ to adapt to change?

NCLEX–RN *Might Ask*

(3.2)

The nurse is caring for a client in the emergency room after an automobile accident. Although there are no visible signs of injury, the client's heart rate, blood pressure, and respirations are elevated. The client's peripheral oxygenation level is 100%, the blood glucose level is slightly elevated, and the client is answering questions appropriately. The nurse knows that this stage of the general adaptation syndrome is

    A. Normal.
    B. Alarm reaction.
    C. Resistance.
    D. Exhaustion.

· *See Appendix A for correct answer and rationale.*

Ambivalence

Another effect of change is ambivalence. This term pertains to opposing views an individual may have for a particular situation, person, or other factor. For instance, some claim to have experienced a love–hate relationship with a particular person. This means that within one's self are conflicting emotions of love and hate.

Feelings of ambivalence can occur when a person is experiencing change. During the change process, a person may have mixed feelings about what the change will involve. At some point, you may have decided to change your hairstyle or facial hair. Halfway into the change, you may have been tentatively pleased, yet also appalled about this new look. This is ambivalence.

thinking critically

Consider changes that you have experienced, for example, a marriage, divorce, birth of a child, loss of a job, economic pressures, or change in a partner or living arrangements. Analyze ambivalent feelings you had about these changes. How did you resolve the ambivalence?

Resistance

Resistance has been defined as conduct that tries to preserve the status quo. Ellis and Hartley (2008) noted that most people are initially resistant to change, especially if the change requires news skills and new patterns of behavior, or will take additional time to learn. There is always comfort in the way things are. Fear of the unknown or a lack of self-confidence can hinder a person's ability to welcome change. Other factors that may be involved include the following:

* Past experiences with change may not have been positive. Example: An employee who resists change states that previous job changes always meant loss of job, pay, or informal seniority standing with coworkers.
* Resistance to change is higher if an individual or group has not participated in the decision to make the change. Example: The head nurse in an intensive care unit decides to implement the use of computerized standard care

plans. The equipment that is purchased is labor intensive to learn and not nurse friendly. Many of the staff nurses are irate and refuse to comply with the change.

- Lack of communication throughout the change process increases resistance. Example: Employees of a medical clinic are informed that there will be a change in the management structure to make the organization more efficient and less costly. They are told that more information will be coming soon. After several weeks of hearing nothing, some of the employees are disgruntled. Rumors are rampant, and many of the employees are now vehemently opposed to any change that may occur, although they initially recognized a need.
- Passive resistance may be manifested as inefficiency, lethargy, failure to complete tasks, increased errors in job performance, or poor attitudes. Example: A nurse at a small hospital is unhappy about being floated to a similar medical–surgical unit. Although she goes to the assigned unit, she barely speaks to the other staff nurses and displays a sullen attitude when she sees the supervisor.

Resistance to change is important to consider not only from a personal or organizational point of view but also from the perspective of clients. Many of your clients will experience change, much of which may be undesirable and unwanted. These clients may resist the efforts of the health care system to accomplish the needed changes.

CULTURAL RESISTANCE FACTORS

Predictability and linearity of change is basically a Western phenomenon. Looking at change from the Eastern perspective can help us learn much. Taoist and Confucian philosophies view change as cyclic and ongoing, rather than as having an end point. Life is a quest for balance and harmony within an ever-changing environment. Resistance may occur when needed changes are incompatible with cultural beliefs. For example, some people of Hispanic background believe that illness is caused by diet imbalance and that certain foods in combination restore balance, even though some foods may be contraindicated in some medical conditions.

SOCIAL RESISTANCE FACTORS

Resistance may also occur when needed changes are not seen as normal within a social group. For example, a woman with chronic bronchitis does not change from her weekly social routine of playing bingo, even though the game is played in a smoke-filled room, which aggravates her bronchitis.

PSYCHOLOGICAL RESISTANCE FACTORS

Finally, resistance to change may occur when needed changes produce anxiety secondary to fear of the unknown, lack of confidence, loss of control, and fear of being a burden. For example, a client with newly diagnosed diabetes is afraid to give himself injections because he is afraid that poor technique will make the disease worse.

(Display 3.4)

---

thinking critically

Consider a change that has occurred in your workplace or within another organization. Review the factors that increase resistance to change. What types of resistance did you observe? What strategies were used to overcome the resistance? Was the change a success or a failure? Why?

You must assess your clients' feelings and attitudes about a particular change. You must also not impose change without regard to a person's cultural, social, and psychological beliefs. According to Creasia and Parker (2007), change is better perceived if a client/stakeholder is actively involved in the change process (Display 3.4).

Loss

Change frequently involves some type of loss. The death of a spouse is an obvious example of loss. However, other changes can induce a sense of loss. Many recent graduates report a sadness or grief when they complete a program of study. This is often related to leaving school, being separated from friends, and beginning something new and unknown.

INDIVIDUAL LOSS AND CHANGE

Elisabeth Kübler-Ross (1969) developed a model of death and dying that describes stages when dealing with loss and change. You likely are familiar with this model from your LPN/LVN training. The first stage is denial, in which an individual refuses to believe that anything has happened or is different. Others may believe that everything is under control. In the second stage, the person experiences anger; she or he is mad at everyone and everything. The third stage is the bargaining stage, in which a person attempts to barter or deal to make things better or to delay reality. Depression is the fourth stage; it occurs when the person fully recognizes the impact of the loss. She or he frequently withdraws and is mournful and lonely. The last stage is acceptance, in which the individual is more at peace with the loss and has come to terms with the situation.

ORGANIZATIONAL LOSS AND CHANGE

Perlman and Takacs (1990) developed a model based on Kübler-Ross' model to describe the phases that are seen within an organization that is involved with

---

display 3.4   **Improving Reception to Change**

Change will be better received if a person perceives a need for change, is open to change, has the ability to have choices regarding the change, and commits to the change process.

change. These phases can be used to depict the emotions that one may experience with any change. The following is a brief description of each stage:

Phase 1: Equilibrium—A person is happy with the current conditions, believes that everything is in balance, and experiences anxiety if the status quo is threatened.

Phase 2: Denial—When change becomes apparent, the person attempts to act as if nothing has changed or will change; the person may choose to ignore what is happening or not participate in activities that help prepare for change.

Phase 3: Anger—Within this stage, the individual actively resists change by being visibly angry, disgruntled, and uncooperative. The person typically blames others and wants everything fixed.

Phase 4: Bargaining—A person tries to negotiate to keep things from changing. The person is willing to make some concessions in an attempt to maintain as much of the status quo as possible.

Phase 5: Chaos—The person feels powerless to stop the change or to make it better. She or he feels insecure and disoriented because the change does not make sense.

Phase 6: Depression—The individual grieves and feels tremendous sorrow for the loss or change. She or he also experiences self-pity and emptiness.

Phase 7: Resignation—The individual is lethargic and mechanical; the change is passively accepted.

Phase 8: Openness—Within this stage, the individual becomes more engaged with the change and is more willing to be involved in the activities needed to complete the change.

Phase 9: Readiness—The individual continues to be more engaged and enthusiastic about the change; she or he is more willing to participate in necessary activities.

Phase 10: Re-emergence—The person now values the change and is willing to make a personal investment in the change process.

The models by Kübler-Ross and Perlman and Takacs are compared in Table 3.2. These models will assist you in contemplating what change can mean for an individual or a group. It is helpful to consider these aspects when you are experiencing personal changes or when your clients are forced to adapt to a new situation. As with any stage theory, the phases may not be as clear or sequential as outlined, but the emotions that can accompany any change will be similar. The following critical thinking activity requires that you role play the part of a client and imagine the stages of change that this client will experience.

thinking critically

Mr. Fleming is 40 years old. He is a lawyer in a prominent law firm. He is married and has two young sons. Last weekend he was on a long bicycle ride and was hit by a truck. His injuries included a severe traumatic injury to his left foot, resulting in a below-the-knee amputation. His other injuries were not as severe. Consider the stages or phases of change shown in Table 3.2 and explain in each stage or phase what you might observe in terms of his behavior and emotions.

table
3-2
COMPARISON OF MODELS OF STAGES OF INDIVIDUAL LOSS AND CHANGE
(KÜBLER-ROSS) AND PHASES OF ORGANIZATIONAL CHANGE (PERLMAN AND
TAKACS)

Stages of Individual Loss and Change (Kübler-Ross)	Phases of Organizational Change (Perlman and Takacs)
	Phase 1: Equilibrium
Stage 1: Denial	Phase 2: Denial
Stage 2: Anger	Phase 3: Anger
Stage 3: Bargaining	Phase 4: Bargaining
	Phase 5: Chaos
Stage 4: Depression	Phase 6: Depression
	Phase 7: Resignation
Stage 5: Acceptance	Phase 8: Openness
	Phase 9: Readiness
	Phase 10: Re-emergence

NCLEX–RN *Might Ask*   3.3

The nurse is caring for a client who has had a radical mastectomy. The client refuses to look at her operative site and be involved in dressing changes. This client's behavior best describes which stage of grieving?

   A. Depression
   B. Denial
   C. Bargaining
   D. Acceptance

· *See Appendix A for correct answer and rationale.*

Resonance

The term resonance is generally used to define the reflection or reverberation of sound. However, it also describes the response of a system to changes from inside or outside the system. For example, if an individual has a cold, not only are the nasal passages affected, but malaise, fever, and general discomfort also occur. Likewise, the individual who is depressed will also be fatigued and disengaged from day-to-day activities. An entire system is affected by what is happening to a part or parts.

General systems theory is often used to explain the interrelatedness of parts of a system and the resonance response. When one part of a system experiences change, the whole system responds. The system can be a human, a family, an organization, or a community. Although the parts may be defined as separate, each part has a function that contributes to the total function of the system. A change in one part resonates throughout the system.

The nursing profession has always held a holistic view of wellness and illness. Within this holistic view, change within one part affects the entire system. The whole is considered greater than and different from its parts. In using the holistic perspective, a person constantly experiences change internally and externally. These changes resonate within the entire system. An open system must be maintained for the exchange of energy, information, and matter to occur.

Following are examples of changes that occur to a part in which the entire system responds.

EXAMPLE 1

Alice dives into a cold pool. She experiences a sense of shock as she hits the cold water. She also feels other sensations related to internal changes, such as blood vessel constriction, an inability to focus on anything except the immediate sensations, and a feeling of discomfort. Alice will also experience other changes, depending on how long she remains in the pool. Her internal environment responds to the changing external environment.

EXAMPLE 2

There are four members of the Allen family. The parents both work outside the home. Their two teenage daughters go to the local high school. The father has not been home from work on time for many weeks. When he arrives home, it is obvious that he has been drinking. The parents frequently fight about this situation. The oldest daughter is frequently having headaches and stomachaches. Her grades at school have dropped. Her teachers are concerned about the change in her demeanor—she is withdrawn, quiet, and inattentive.

EXAMPLE 3

A respected resident of a small town dies suddenly as the result of a heart attack. Members of the community experience shock, dismay, and grief after this event.

In these examples, part of the system is affected by a change in the internal or external environment; the change resonates within the system, and the entire system responds in some way to the change that has occurred. The concepts related to general systems theory present a holistic approach to the effects of change. Nurses are able to intervene more effectively and holistically if they recognize how change in one part affects change of the whole.

thinking critically

Reflect on your own examples of resonance following change that have happened to you, within your family, work setting, or community. Consider how change to one part affected the whole. What changes did you note resonated throughout the whole system? How did the whole system also resonate refreezing, as Lewin described, after the change? Discuss this with another person in that system. How do the observations and perceptions of resonance by that individual compare with yours?

● ADJUSTING TO CHANGE

In the process of adjusting to change, turmoil exists. Heath and Heath (2010) describe human beings as having two separate, and sometimes competing "systems" in our brains —a rational system that plans and thinks logically, and an emotional system that reacts intuitively and with instincts. When these two systems are in conflict during the change process, change can be quite arduous. Adjusting to change is not always an easy task. Emotions vary widely, from despair to joy, with much tension and doubt in between. Porter-O'Grady (2003) noted that even experienced nurses can become overwhelmed by large amounts of change unless they approach it in an organized way and keep the ultimate goal in mind. This requires aligning the rational and emotional systems toward a greater goal.

You have probably learned through experience how to adjust more readily to change. Senge et al. (2011) note that we must confront fear and anxiety. They describe the conflict that can exist between those who embrace and believe in the change and those who either do not believe in the change or resist it. As you embark on the registered nursing program of study, you may find yourself confronted at times with such challenges. Sometimes it helps to read about others coping with change processes in order to view ourselves more objectively and thereby better cope and reach resolution. Two fun and easy-to-read books on change that describe how different people react and adjust to change may be helpful to you. In *Who Moved My Cheese?*, author Spencer Johnson (1998) used the analogy of a maze. Two mice, Sniff and Scurry, and two "little people," Hem and Haw, demonstrate differing reactions to change when a new cheese is introduced into the maze. In *Our Iceberg Is Melting: Changing and Succeeding Under Any Conditions*, author John Kotter (2006) used the analogy of penguins who live on an Antarctic iceberg and described their approaches in adjusting to change. On reading these two light but informative texts, you will likely see yourself and those close to you in various reactions and adjustments as you experience role transition and change in entering the registered nursing program.

---

thinking critically

Read the texts by Johnson and Kotter presented above. With which characters do you identify? What can you learn from other characters to help you adjust to the change you are experiencing in your role transition to a student nurse, and then an RN?

Attitude

The primary method for adjusting to change is often related to the attitude one has about the change. The manner in which one approaches change can have a major effect on the ability to adapt. For instance, an employer informs a nurse who has been employed full time by a community health agency for 7 years that only full-time nurses will be taking emergency calls in the future. The nurse can approach this change in several ways. The first is to endorse the change as positive for continuity of care for the clients who are seen by the agency. The second approach would be to lament to the employer that this is not a fair system and that everyone should have to take calls. This nurse has some control over her or his adjustment to change, depending on which attitude she or he adopts.

In other changes that are more sudden, or in which an individual has less control, it may be more difficult to have the appropriate attitude. If a loved one dies suddenly, a positive attitude will assist a person to adjust, but other strategies are generally used. For instance, one person may solicit the support of other family members and friends. Others may benefit from joining a support group consisting of people who are experiencing a similar situation. Some people plunge into work or other activities so that they can get on with the business of living and avoid dwelling on the loss.

Flexibility

Maintaining an approach that incorporates flexibility also assists with successful adaptation to change. Katz, Carter, Kravits, Bishop, and Block (2009) noted that especially during rapid change or unplanned change, flexibility can help you shift priorities quickly to minimize negative results and move ahead. Flexibility allows you to discover unforeseen opportunities and to grow. In *The Reflective Life*, Tiberius (2008) advocates that one acquire self-knowledge in order to be more successful at what one attempts, and to set future goals. She notes the need to know our values, but to have the wisdom to be reflective, to question these values, and to be flexible to change as needed.

Coping Strategies

Coping strategies vary and often depend on the circumstances and previous coping methods used. When faced with change, one person may try to avoid it, whereas another faces it directly. A third person may try to enlist the support of others or gather more information to deal with the change more effectively. All these methods may be effective in the adjustment to change.

In your return to school, you must identify what strategies will assist you in being successful. Obviously, a positive attitude is extremely beneficial, not only for you but also for your student colleagues. It is often useful to develop a support system within the student nurse group. A small group of colleagues will provide support and guidance for many issues that you encounter while in school. Some find that it helps to study together or to socialize away from school to adjust more effectively to the changes caused by returning to school.

---

thinking critically

In your return to school, consider the strategies that are useful for you as you adjust to the changes that school necessitates. Summarize methods that help you cope with change. Compare these methods with those of another nursing student and assess alternative methods you each could use.

McKenry and Price (1994) emphasized that successful coping depends on both our perception of change (ie, how we approach it will determine the amount of stress it poses) and our ability to adapt to change. They noted that families under stress rely on both internal family system resources and external community resources. Reynolds (2009) provides examples of essential support skills for student affairs practice that help college students adjust to the changes they are experiencing. The significant rise in serious mental health issues, such as depression, anxiety, and substance abuse, is described. Reynolds emphasizes that students need to let their advisors know if they are experiencing serious stress because resources are available that can assist you.

William Bridges (2009) describes how individuals manage transitions as they move through three stages. In the first stage, that of "ending, losing, and letting go," one lets go of the old ways and the old identity. In the second stage, which he describes as the "neutral zone," "critical psychological realignments and repatternings take place." In the third and final stage, "the new beginning" is established. He states, "This is when people develop the new identity, experience the new energy, and discover the new sense of purpose that make the change begin to work" (pp. 4–5). It is at this time that you will experience positive outcomes of change.

● POSITIVE OUTCOMES OF CHANGE

Change has the possibility of many positive outcomes. Within any change process, the positive aspects of the change should be visualized as you embrace the change process. This will assist you in aligning rational and emotional systems toward common goals. In examining positive outcomes of change, the following relates to your process of returning to school and the changes that will occur.

The possible positive outcomes are as follows:

1. You will acquire more education and knowledge. Although the educational process can be overwhelming or frustrating at times, the benefit will be an increased ability to integrate theory with practice and to be more informed regarding client care and health care issues.
2. One of the reasons that you returned to school may have been related to a desire to increase responsibilities and scope of practice. The RN role will provide more opportunities for career mobility, flexibility, and professional development.
3. Another positive outcome of change will be monetary rewards. Salaries for RNs have improved in the last decade. The potential for financial growth continues to be greater within the professional roles, even with the uncertainty of future healthcare reform.
4. With any additional education, there is a greater potential for increased prestige. Although such recognition may not seem important or may seem to have elitist overtones, being recognized for increased knowledge and abilities and associated achievements reaps the reward of educational changes. The ADN and the title of RN bestow a distinct and honorable recognition and provide opportunities for increased decision making.
5. Along with increased prestige comes increased self-confidence and self-esteem. Maslow identified a hierarchy of basic needs. According to his theory, after physiological, safety and security, and love and belonging needs are met, an individual has needs of esteem and self-esteem. Esteem needs include respect from others, recognition, prestige, and importance. Self-esteem needs encompass those related to achievement, competence and independence, and

self-worth. Advanced education provides a greater means to achieve a belief in your own abilities and thus to have self-confidence and self-esteem.

6. A final positive outcome of change is self-actualization. Maslow theorized that the highest level of needs occurs when the other basic needs have been met. Self-actualization is the need to be all that you can be through self-fulfillment and reaching your potential. In your return to school, you are fulfilling a dream or a goal. You are also increasing your ability to solve problems, broadening your means to deal with various situations, and developing greater power to cope with stress. The positive outcomes of change are varied. Each change with which you are faced provides the opportunity for positive outcomes. In the following Critical Thinking activity, you are asked to consider some positive outcomes of change.

thinking critically

Critique an organizational change that has occurred in your workplace or within a community organization with which you are involved. Compare the positive outcomes experienced with that change, both for the organization and for yourself. Examine similarities and differences.

● CONCLUSION

Change is a dynamic and ongoing process. Many of the changes that we face are not of our choosing. However, we also have the ability to affect our own change and to plan for and deal with the results. Nurses must understand the dynamics of the change process. Not only do nurses face the challenges of personal changes, but they also encounter the changes that their clients face. The processes of stress and adaptation are important to understand the coping strategies that individuals may use. Nurses are also involved with organizational changes, which can involve complex processes personally and collectively. The effects of change are varied and often depend on individual and group coping mechanisms.

Nursing and health care in general is ever changing. Although it is impossible to predict what changes will occur in the future, it is certain that change will be continuous. You must recognize these dynamics and determine how your experience will assist you to adapt and be part of the change process.

student exercises

Recruit another student, peer, or friend to assist you with the following exercises:

1. Create a change situation that involves role playing a client who is faced with a new diagnosis of heart disease.

2. Determine what factors may motivate this client to change her or his lifestyle.

3. Develop a plan that will assist the client to make changes.

4. Discuss the possible effects of change related to the impact of the diagnosis and the need for a change in lifestyle.

5. What are the possible negative and positive effects?

6. While role playing, follow Perlman and Takacs's phases of change.

References

Bridges, W. (2009). *Managing transitions: Making the most of change* (3rd ed.). Philadelphia, PA: Perseus.

Bridges, W. (2001). *The way of transition: Embracing life's most difficult moments*. Cambridge, MA: Perseus.

Carter, P., & Alfred, R. (1999). *Making change happen*. Ann Arbor, MI: Consortium for Community College Development, University of Michigan.

Creasia, J., & Parker, B. (2007). *Conceptual foundations: The bridge to professional nursing practice* (4th ed.). St. Louis, MO: Mosby.

Ellis, J., & Hartley, C. (2008). *Nursing in today's world: Trends, issues, & management* (9th ed.). Philadelphia, PA: Lippincott Williams & Wilkins.

Ellis, J., & Hartley, C. (2009). *Managing and coordinating nursing care* (5th ed.). Philadelphia, PA: Lippincott Williams & Wilkins.

Heath, C., & Heath, D. (2010). *Switch: How to change things when change is hard*. New York, NY: Crown Publishing, Broadway Books.

Johnson, S. (1998). *Who moved my cheese?* New York, NY: G.P. Putnam's Sons.

Katz, J. R., Carter, C., Kravits, S., Bishop, J., & Block, J. (2009). *Keys to nursing success* (3rd ed.). Upper Saddle River, NJ: Prentice-Hall.

Kotter, J. (2006). *Our iceberg is melting: Changing and succeeding under any conditions*. New York, NY: St. Martin's Press.

Kübler-Ross, E. (1969). *On death and dying*. New York, NY: Macmillan.

Lapp, J. (2002). Thriving on change. *Caring Magazine, May*, 40–43.

Lewin, K. (1951). *Field theory in social science*. New York, NY: Harper & Row.

McKenry, P. C., & Price, S. J. (1994). *Families and change: Coping with stressful events*. Thousand Oaks, CA: Sage.

Perlman, D., & Takacs, G. (1990). The ten stages of change. *Nursing Management, 21*(4), 33–38.

Porter-O'Grady, T. (2003). A different age for leadership, part 1. *Journal of Nursing Administration, 33*(2), 105–110.

Reynolds, A. L. (2009). Helping college students: Developing essential support skills for student affairs practice. San Francisco, CA: Jossey-Bass.

Selye, H. (1976). *The stress of life* (Rev. ed.). New York, NY: McGraw-Hill.

Senge, P., Kleiner, A., Roberts, C., Rose, R., Roth, G., & Smith, B. (2011). *The dance of change: The challenges of sustaining momentum in a learning organization*. London, UK: Nicholas Bradley Publishing.

Tiberius, V. (2008). *The reflective life*. Oxford, UK: Oxford University Press.

Suggested Reading

Friedman, T. (2006). *The world is flat*. New York, NY: Farrar, Straws & Giroux.

Harvard Business Review. (2011). *HBR's 10 must reads on change*. Boston, MA: Harvard Business School Publishing.

Kübler-Ross, E., & Kessler D. (2005). *On grief and grieving*. New York, NY: Scriber.

Lancaster, K. (1999). *Nursing issues in leading and managing change*. St. Louis, MO: Mosby.

Mauksch, J. G., & Miller, M. H. (1981). *Implementing change in nursing*. St. Louis, MO: Mosby.

Morrison, M. (1993). *Professional skills for leadership: Foundations of a successful career*. St. Louis, MO: Mosby.

Peters, T. (1998). *Thriving on chaos*. New York, NY: Alfred Knopf.

Porter-O'Grady, T., & Malloch, K. (2003). *Quantum leadership: A text book of new leadership*. Sudbury, MA: Jones and Bartlett.

Redman, G., Riggleman, J., Sorrel, J., & Zervil, L. (1999). Creative winds of change: Nursing collaborating for quality outcomes. *Nursing Administrative Quarterly, 23*(2), 55–64.

Salmond, S. (1998). Managing the human side of change. *Orthopaedic Nursing, 17*(5), 38–51.

Tiffany, C. R., & Lutjens, L. R. J. (1998). *Planned change theories for nursing: Review, analysis, and implications*. Thousand Oaks, CA: Sage.

 On the **WEB** For more information on change theory, go to *www.google.com* and enter "Lewin's change theory" or "change management." (Last accessed 7.6.2011). *www.elisabethkublerross.com* (Kübler-Ross's Web site). (Last accessed 7.6.2011).

4

Transitions Throughout Nursing's History

- **LEARNING OUTCOMES**

By the end of this chapter, the student will be able to:

1 Define professionalism and describe characteristics of nursing that qualify it as a profession.

2 Discuss the significant historic events in nursing that influenced its development.

3 Describe benchmarks of the evolution of nursing as a profession.

4 Summarize the various educational programs in nursing.

5 Describe the expanded roles that exist within the nursing profession.

6 Discuss the effects of societal trends on the profession and practice of nursing.

7 Give examples of the impact of changes in health care on the nursing profession.

● KEY TERMS

advocacy
alternative lifestyles
articulation
assisted living
assistive personnel
autonomy
baby boomers
bioethics
biomedical
    technology
bioterrorism
career mobility
cloning
cost containment
continuous quality
    improvement (CQI)
cryogenics
cultural proficiency
diversity
diagnostic-related
    groups (DRGs)
ecological
    intelligence
emotional intelligence
entrepreneurism

evidence-based
    practice (EBP)
experiential wisdom
external degree
flexible spending
    accounts (FSAs)
gender equity
genetic engineering
globalism
Health Insurance
    Portability and
    Accountability Act
    (HIPAA)
HIV/AIDS
health maintenance
    organizations
    (HMOs)
holistic nursing
health savings
    accounts (HSAs)
informatics
managed care
metaparadigm
mutual recognition of
    licensure

Nurse Licensure
    Compact
nursing informatics
outcomes assessment
palliative care
pandemic flu
political advocacy
post-traumatic stress
    disorder (PTSD)
preferred provider
    organizations (PPOs)
profession
professional code
professionalism
quality assurance (QA)
robotics
service learning
social policy
spiritual care
spiritual nursing
student learning
    outcomes (SLOs)
total quality
    management (TQM)
transition

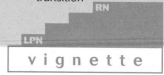

vignette

Joan Chin and Lucy Braveheart are two students who have formed a study group. They are meeting over coffee in the student center to discuss the upcoming lecture.

JOAN: Today we are supposed to discuss the history of nursing. History is something I've never been really good at. I think it's because I find it boring.

LUCY: I think it all depends on how it is presented. Rumor has it the professor has a unique way of presenting this topic. The fourth semester students say that she dresses up like Florence Nightingale and helps students learn her thinking through a monologue. Some say you can imagine what it was like back then.

JOAN: I guess I remember those history lessons in school where we were lectured to about historical battles and such.

LUCY: Being a Native American, I have always been interested in history. My people say, "You can never tell what it was like until you walk in someone's moccasins." I guess we'll be walking in Florence's today.

JOAN: Yes, my folks are third-generation Chinese. They value what the elders say. I guess it's so we won't repeat the same mistakes.

The history of nursing is rich and tumultuous. In many respects, the history of nursing is a reflection of society in general, women in particular, and the blurring of gender stereotypes. Although it may not seem important to know and appreciate nursing history, it is crucial to understanding and appreciating the world of nursing today. Depending on your perspective, nurses have existed in some form since there have been people on this earth. However, nursing as it is known today is a relatively young profession.

The workplace for nurses has changed radically in the past three decades, and significant changes continue. There is no doubt that nurses will always be challenged by changes in society, technology, and the health care industry. There will continue to be both new challenges and greater opportunities and rewards in nursing. The issues that confront nurses today are the foundation for the profession and practice of nursing tomorrow, just as those that came before us brought us to where we are today.

● DEVELOPMENT OF NURSING

The history and origins of nursing are rich and multifaceted. The evolution of nursing from ancient times through the ages was particularly influenced by Christianity. The Nightingale reform had a significant impact on the development of nursing in the United States, as did the evolution of nursing as a profession, the formation of professional nursing organizations, the women's movement, the acceptance of men in caregiving roles, and the more recent movement toward opening traditionally single-gender professions to both genders.

Ancient Origins

There have always been humans who have required care when they were sick, injured, with child, elderly, or dying. Women, as demonstrated by cave drawings of women caring for sick children or preparing a brew of herbs and bark to aid an ill person, have generally done this work. Although little is known about nursing as a specific entity in ancient times, both male and female caregivers can be found in early cultures. A return to holistic nursing and better acceptance of Eastern methods of health and healing today continue to shape and reshape nursing.

In ancient Egypt, there were identified physicians or healers. They were usually priests who were responsible for healing diseases. The priests acted as the link between humans and the gods. It was believed that people had to keep the gods happy to have good health and peace of mind. The priests or physicians did not interfere with the process of childbirth and infant care; they left that work to midwives and wet nurses. These women had developed special skills and abilities to assist friends and neighbors.

The ancient Israelites were important in the development of modern medicine in that they formulated strict codes for personal hygiene and cleanliness. They instituted careful handwashing techniques, boiling of water, meat inspection, and other sanitation measures. Some of their practices are still followed by Orthodox Jews today.

Hindu Indians had a team concept approach to the care of the sick. The team consisted of a patient, a healer (physician), and a nurse, who was male. Each person had identified duties and functions. The Hindus described the use of various instruments and surgical techniques that were used during ancient times. Many of the treatments that used herbs, plants, or animal parts were discovered by accident or trial and error.

Ancient China is known for the use of acupuncture, drug therapy, massage, hydrotherapy, and exercise to treat and prevent illness. Many of these same procedures and techniques are used today. The Chinese believed that a balance between Yang (the male elements of light, life, and optimism) and Yin (the female elements of dark, lifelessness, and cold) kept the body in harmony and health.

In other ancient cultures, such as those in South America, there is evidence that hygiene, diet, and herbal medicine practices were important. Not much is known about nursing care specifically, although it appears that women were esteemed for their knowledge of medicines. As with other ancient cultures, the emphasis was usually on the balance between good and evil spirits and the appeasement of the gods.

Christian Origins

With the advent of Christianity came a renewed focus on the value and dignity of human life. Bishops of the church were charged with caring for those in need, but the services were actually rendered by deacons and deaconesses. Men and women committed themselves to the care of the poor and sick. Women—in particular, deaconesses, matrons, widows, and virgins—took care of the sick in their homes. Phoebe, the first deaconess, is cited by Paul in the New Testament as providing nursing care. She is also called the first visiting nurse (Ellis & Hartley, 2004).

The deaconesses of the early Eastern Christian Church were required to be unmarried or widowed only once to serve in that capacity. They were often wealthy women of culture and education who were from fine homes and backgrounds, were ordained, and worked on an equal basis with the deacon. "These dedicated young women practiced 'works of mercy' that included feeding the hungry, clothing the naked, visiting the imprisoned, sheltering the homeless, and burying the dead" (Ellis & Harley, 2004, p. 117). They carried medicine and food in baskets to people's homes. The deaconesses were the early counterparts to the community health nurses of today. Display 4.1 highlights several women credited for their contributions to nursing in the early years of Christianity.

---

display 4.1   Early Nursing Leaders

Phoebe: First deaconess; carried letters for Paul; credited with being the first visiting nurse

St. Marcella: Established the first convent for women in her own palatial home; interested in the care of the sick; known as "mother of nuns"

Fabiola: After converting to Christianity, she established the first public hospital in Rome and devoted herself to the care of the sick and poor; she personally nursed many of them and was revered in Rome

St. Paula: A student of St. Marcella; traveled to Jerusalem and used her money to found hospitals and inns for pilgrims traveling to the Holy Land, in Bethlehem; she also established a convent and built hospitals for the sick and hospices for the pilgrims; the first to teach nursing as an art

As Christian churches were established, orders were formed that provided care for the sick, injured, poor, orphaned, widowed, and elderly. In early Christian times, men and women were considered equal, and there were more opportunities for single women to serve within these orders than had ever been available before. Within the religious orders, there was an established hierarchy of rank. This hierarchy demanded that there be absolute discipline and adherence to maintaining the rank and order. Some of the doctrines of faith, charity, servitude, and discipline of the early religious orders have continued to be part of modern nursing, serving to influence today's health care arena.

During the rise of Christianity, there was tremendous turmoil and chaos as battles and wars raged. Many men were killed, leaving many widows. Survival of widows during these troubled times was not a priority of society in general. For this reason, many of these women became interested in the various religious orders as a means of survival. Eventually, the Order of the Widows was formed. These women no longer had home responsibilities and were able to devote themselves to the care of the poor. As the church placed more value on purity of the body, the Order of the Virgins evolved. They were later called nuns nonnuptaeor, meaning "not married" (Zerwekh & Claborn, 1997). Convents were built to provide safe shelter for these women. However, they continued to care for the poor and the sick within these shelters. Deaconesses also existed in Western Europe, where they were called "matrons," but the Western church suppressed the deaconess movement, which became nearly extinct.

The Middle Ages (c. 500–1500 AD) occurred after the fall of the Roman Empire. The development of medical science and nursing care halted as the Christian Church advocated little concern for its growth and instead focused on preparing for the afterlife. Europe was divided into many kingdoms, which were continually at war with each other; poverty, illness, and starvation were widespread. Religious orders grew even stronger, particularly as deaconesses lost favor and decreased in great numbers. Monks and nuns of various religious orders assumed control of hospitals. However, they were more concerned with spiritual, rather than physical, care of the ill.

Military Origins

In the late Middle Ages, the Crusades occurred, lasting for about 200 years (c. 1090–1290 AD). The Crusaders were generally men of religious and military orders: priests, brothers, and knights. Their mission was to reclaim the Holy Land for the Christian faithful. As they traveled throughout Europe and the Near East, they gathered new information, learned new ways of doing things, and obtained different products and goods. The Crusaders were interested in the organized facilities for the sick that the Moslems used. As a result, similar hospitals were built near battlefields; the men were sometimes assigned to fighting and sometimes to caring for the sick and the injured. Eventually, military nursing orders evolved.

An example of a military nursing order was the Knights Hospitalers of St. John, located outside Jerusalem. These men staffed two hospitals and, in addition to caring for patients, frequently had to defend the hospital and the patients. They wore habits with a suit of armor underneath and the Maltese cross on top. Many nurses today wear pins that designate the school from which they graduated. One of the symbols used by some schools, such as the Nightingale School, is the Maltese cross, whereas other schools use another form of a cross. Additional symbols are also used, with many representing the military origins of earlier centuries. Military nursing orders advocated strict discipline and hierarchical lines of authority that emphasized devotion and obedience. These characteristics have extended to modern nursing and can be problematic in some settings.

As the Crusaders returned to their homes, they brought with them a vision of improvement. Religious and secular groups organized hospitals and clinics that were better able to meet the needs of the sick and the injured. The organizations became structured and ordered. The caregivers, or nurses, wore white robes and were given a hood on completion of a novitiate period. They remained responsible to a director or maitresse. During this time, nursing care was valued, although advances in medical science were not. Nursing care generally involved providing comfort measures and hygiene. There was no scientific basis for the nursing care. Toward the end of the Middle Ages, many countries were faced with rampant diseases and plague. The need for advancements in medicine was acute.

Protestant Reformation

Various Protestant churches were created as church leaders took issue with the Roman Catholic Church. In countries where the reformation was widespread, the care of the sick suffered because there were not enough nuns to provide that care. Deaconesses were urged to take on this work. However, the standards that had marked military and nursing orders were not maintained; thus, the quality of care greatly diminished. In addition, Protestant women had religious freedom, but they did not have other freedoms, such as being able to work outside the home. Society expected them to remain at home to provide care for children and the elderly and to assume other domestic responsibilities. As a result, the caliber of nurses was diminished. In countries such as England, nurses in the 1800s were generally considered to be drunkards or thieves because many women chose to do their jail time serving within a hospital setting. Conditions in hospitals were deplorable, and the mortality rates greatly escalated.

In the 15th to 19th centuries, medical progress was more profound. Many advances were made in the knowledge of anatomy and physiology, as well as in the use of pharmaceutical agents and surgical techniques. For example, the vaccination for smallpox was developed, the microscope was invented, and pasteurization was developed. However, the practice of nursing did not advance until after the mid-1800s.

The Nightingale Reform

In 1836, in Kaiserwerth, Germany, a young Protestant minister named Theodore Fliedner strove to revitalize the deaconess movement by starting a training institute for deaconesses. As part of this institute, he and his wife started a nursing course that included hands-on training and some lectures by physicians. Fliedner's work and the formation of other secular and religious groups once again laid the foundation for the growth of nursing.

Florence Nightingale was born in 1820 to a family of wealth and social standing. With her culture and education, she was expected to marry and continue the traditions of English society women. However, she had a strong desire to be a nurse. Her family considered this ambition absurd, but she nonetheless managed to learn about hospital reforms and public health issues and became an expert in these areas. In her travels and through information from friends, she learned about the institute at Kaiserwerth. Because this was a church-sponsored institution, she was allowed to attend the nursing program. She spent 3 months there learning as much as she could about nursing.

After she returned to England, she continued her own studies and served on a committee that oversaw the Establishment for Gentlewomen During Illness. Although her family was not happy about her continued interest in nursing and in hospitals, she was later appointed superintendent of this organization. Her work in that capacity resulted in general acknowledgment of her expertise about hospitals and the need for educated nurses. She was asked to take a group of nurses to the Crimean War battlefields to improve the conditions there. Thirty-eight nurses who met Nightingale's standards accompanied her to Scutari. The work that was accomplished there was nothing short of miraculous. When they arrived, the conditions were filthy and unsafe. Through Nightingale's extraordinary efforts and with the assistance of powerful English friends, the situation improved dramatically. Sanitary and hygienic measures were instituted and maintained, nutritious food was provided, and conditions radically improved. She was especially concerned about the welfare of the soldiers and was able to obtain sick pay benefits for them, along with other benefits that improved their health and well-being. The mortality rate was reduced from 50% to 60% to approximately 1% to 2%. Nightingale became known as the "lady with the lamp" and the ministering angel because of her late night rounds to ensure that all was well.

Improving conditions at the battlefields was not without its own conflicts. The physicians and military officers resented Nightingale's intrusion, and some of the nurses who were involved argued with each other and disagreed with Nightingale. She tended to be controlling to accomplish her mission and was known to be stubborn, obstinate, and strong-willed (Barritt, 1973). During her service in the Crimean War, she became ill with what was called the Crimean fever and came close to death. However, she recovered and remained in service until the end of the war.

When Nightingale returned to England, she essentially became a recluse due to her health problems. However, she still was able to exert a powerful influence on the development of nursing because of the widespread fame that she attained as a result of her accomplishments in the Crimean War. She wrote many books and reports that demonstrated her ability to use research and statistics. Many refer to her as the first nurse researcher, drawing conclusions that today would be termed "evidence-based nursing research." Nightingale also continued to work to develop nursing education and improve the conditions for soldiers, particularly those in foreign lands. She established the Nightingale Fund, which was later used to establish a training school for nurses, and was awarded the Cross of St. George by Queen Victoria.

---

display 4.2   **Nightingale's Principles for the Education of Nurses**

1. Nursing is an art and a science.
2. The student must be taught to treat the patient as a human, not a disease, and there must be compassion and empathy for each individual.
3. The emphasis must be on education, not service. For this reason, a school of nursing should be independent from the hospital.
4. Graduate nurses should always continue their education.
5. Nurses must be taught to take care of the sick and must not do the laundry, clean, run errands, and other such chores that take them away from their nursing responsibilities.
6. Education for nurses should be a combination of theory and practice.

NIGHTINGALE SYSTEM OF EDUCATION

Nightingale established a training school for nurses in 1860. It was founded at St. Thomas' Hospital as a 1-year program. Women between the ages of 25 and 35 years were selected based on qualifications relating to their character, conduct, and desire to be a nurse. The nursing program was highly structured and rigorous. Nightingale also recognized the need for both theory and practice in training nurses and saw that the educational program must stand alone, where students could focus on their training apart from hospital service. See Display 4.2 for Nightingale's principles for the education of nurses.

The Nightingale system of education is considered to be the beginning of modern nursing education and the start of professional nursing. Nightingale's insistence on discipline and high moral character had a profound effect on the growth of modern nursing and the education of nurses, effects that continue to influence nursing education today. Within the first two decades after the Nightingale Training School opened, there were graduates that became superintendents in hospitals throughout Europe, Asia, and the United States. A whole new system of professional nursing was introduced throughout the world.

thinking critically

Consider the following statement from Nightingale's (1992, a commemorative edition of the first edition published in 1859.) *Notes on Nursing: What It Is and What It Is Not:*

> I use the word nursing for want of a better. It has been limited to signify little more than the administration of medicines and the application of poultices. It ought to signify the proper use of fresh air, light, warmth, cleanliness, quiet, and the proper selection and administration of diet—all at the least expense of vital power to the patient. (p. 6)

What is the relevance of this statement to nursing as you know it today? How does this philosophy relate to the expansion of holistic nursing and spiritual nursing today? What would you add to this statement to reflect the broader, more comprehensive scope of professional nursing today?

Nursing in the United States

The growth of nursing in the United States was stimulated in particular by the Civil War. Prior to that, there was no organized method for caring for the sick, especially during times of war. Women were the primary caregivers in the home or in the homes of neighbors. There were few formal educational programs available, except those that were within Catholic sisterhoods, and nursing education was relatively unavailable to men and other religions and ethnicities.

The Civil War began in 1861. The obvious need for nurses prompted many women to volunteer to care for the wounded soldiers. Although they were not trained as nurses, they demonstrated great compassion and concern. The Union Army appointed Dorothea Dix, a woman who had championed causes for the mentally ill, to be the superintendent for these nurses and to provide some training for them. Women from religious orders also volunteered in the North and the South, and other women who were not trained nurses also assisted. In the South, fewer women volunteered because it was not socially acceptable. Many hospitals were built during the Civil War to house the large numbers of wounded soldiers. The nurses of this time experienced multiple difficulties: The working conditions were deplorable, the Army medical staff did not always think highly of them, and they were generally poorly treated. However, they persevered, and in some areas, their work was well received and respected.

After the Civil War, there was a recognized need for educated nurses. The popularity of Florence Nightingale in England and the proliferation of educated Nightingale nurses also helped promote the growth of nursing in the United States. In 1869, the American Medical Society proposed that the issue of trained nurses should be investigated. As a result of that study, three schools for the training of nurses opened in 1873: the Bellevue Training School in New York City, the Connecticut Training School, and the Boston Training School. Although these training programs were theoretically modeled after the Nightingale system, the major thrust was service, as opposed to education. Eventually, many schools of nursing opened. Hospitals realized that there was economic value in having student nurses deliver the bulk of patient care and other tasks. Essentially, the student nurses provided a free labor force for the hospitals. Despite the hardships, these programs were popular because they provided young women with the eventual means to earn a living. The choices for young women during these times were limited. Nursing was considered an acceptable alternative to traditional female roles and provided a slightly higher income than any other occupation available to women.

Uniforms and caps were not originally a traditional characteristic of training schools. In 1875, the first cap was used to cover long hair and particularly long, dirty hair. Its function was practical, not decorative. Later, a student at Bellevue Training School designed a student uniform. Eventually, caps, uniforms, and school pins came to signify a certain school or particular accomplishments within the school and have continued to be part of nursing heritage.

In the early 1900s, nurses were expected to be submissive within a hospital organization and to the dominance of physicians. As reported by Zerwekh and Claborn (1997), there was a similar expectation for women in the male-dominated society. The woman was esteemed by her husband and had limited power within the confines of the home and society. She was expected to be hard working and able to maintain harmony, while also being submissive to the demands of her husband. However, some women of this time worked hard for reform and laid the foundation for societal changes for women in general and nurses in particular. These issues are examined later in this chapter.

The first licensure laws for nursing did not exist until 1903, and even with the first law's passage, licensure was not mandatory or enforced. Hospitals continued to promote their own needs and not those of nurses or students. A few nursing programs moved to an educational setting, but the education continued to be practice driven and involved many long hours. There were many objections to nurses being overeducated and overtrained. Physicians in particular did not perceive a need for nurses to have increased education. Two important factors in the development of nursing in the United States were the upgrading of The Johns Hopkins School of Nursing in 1918 and the opening of the Yale School of Nursing in 1924. The first stressed the need for improved education of public health nurses, and the second was the first to be a separate university department with its own dean.

From the early 20th century emerged many of nursing's important leaders. Several notable ones are listed as follows:

- Linda Richards: Called American's first trained nurse, she moved from one hospital to another to establish new training programs and to upgrade the quality of nursing services.
- Isabelle Hampton Robb: She graduated from Bellevue Training School after having been a teacher. She was instrumental in improving conditions for student nurses and founded the program at Johns Hopkins. When she married and resigned her position, she still maintained an active interest in nursing. She authored nursing textbooks, helped in the formation of the first nursing organization, and was one of the founders of the *American Journal of Nursing*.
- Adelaide Nutting: She was a graduate of the Johns Hopkins program and later a principal of that school. She obtained the funding to improve the education for public health nurses and was a strong advocate for reform in nursing education. Nutting later developed the nursing department at Teachers College, Columbia University. She was able to establish a 3-year nursing program and to reduce a student nurse's workday to 8 hours.
- Lavinia Dock: She was an early graduate of Bellevue Training School and later an assistant to Isabelle Hampton Robb. She was an early organizer of what is now known as the National League for Nursing (NLN). She wrote *History of Nursing*, which remains a classic on that subject.
- Lillian Wald: She founded the Henry Street Settlement in New York in 1893. This marked the beginning of public health nursing in the United States. She was particularly interested in the ability of nursing graduates to provide high-quality care to people within their homes.

These are only a few of the individuals who helped change the course of nursing. The changes that occurred in the 20th century reflect the hard work and dedication of women who were compelled to advocate reform in nursing. Although the women's movement has often ignored their work, their accomplishments did affect the changes women have experienced in general.

The presence of African Americans and men in nursing is not well documented. The first African American graduate of a training program was Mary Mahoney in 1879. She was dedicated to the promotion of excellence in the care of private duty patients and the acceptance of African Americans within the nursing profession. Although African American nurses were not accepted for military service until World War II, Adah Thomas fought for the acceptance of African American nurses in World War I and was effective in getting African American nurses to work for the American Red Cross. The prejudice against men in nursing also was high, and essentially, men were not influential in nursing until after World War II. Today, however, nurses of both genders and many ethnicities are common, mirroring patients/clients in their care. This has strengthened the profession of nursing, as multiple perspectives yield an enriched database upon which evidence-based practice (EBP) can be built.

NCLEX–RN *Might Ask* (4.1)

A nurse is explaining the relevance of various changes in the history of nursing. The nurse is aware that symbols, organization, strict discipline, and hierarchical lines of authority have

  A. Ancient origins.
  B. Christian origins.
  C. Military origins.
  D. Protestant origins.

· See Appendix A for correct answer and rationale.

● PROFESSIONAL NURSING ORGANIZATIONS

The formation of nursing organizations initiated the process of using cooperative efforts to achieve common goals and missions. Nurses found that a collective voice was much more likely to have an impact on the development of nursing.

National League for Nursing

The first nursing organization in the United States was established in 1893. The group was initially called the American Society of Superintendents of Training Schools for Nurses in the United States and Canada. These nurses gathered for the purpose of improving and standardizing the education of nurses. In 1912, they changed the organization's name to the National League of Nursing Education. Membership was originally limited to nurses, but in 1943, the league decided to open membership to lay members. There continues to be two levels of membership: individual and agency. Schools of nursing and other agencies that provide nursing services are eligible for membership as agency members.

In 1952, a major reorganization took place, along with another name change. The league became the NLN and actually merged seven organizations into one. These groups were the National League of Nursing Education (1893), the National

Organization for Public Health Nursing (1912), the Association of Collegiate Schools of Nursing (1933), the Joint Committee on Practical Nurses and Auxiliary Workers in Nursing Services (1945), the Joint Committee on Careers in Nursing (1948), the National Committee for the Improvement of Nursing Services (1949), and the National Nursing Accrediting Service (1949). Although in some respects these were very diverse groups, they were able to formulate a common mission of promoting and providing for quality health care through effective nursing practice and education.

The National League for Nursing Accreditation Commission (NLNAC) of the NLN provides accreditation processes to schools that choose to participate. Accreditation by the NLNAC is a voluntary process for schools of nursing, involving the writing of a self-study report according to established criteria. Representatives of NLNAC then visit the school to evaluate and assess the nursing program according to the established standards. These visitors make recommendations regarding accreditation of the program. Graduation from an NLN-accredited program provides for national recognition and the acceptance of credits from another NLN-accredited program if a graduate chooses to continue her or his education. Not all schools participate in the process, which is labor intensive and costly. However, all schools participate in the accreditation/approval process conducted by their state board of nursing. That process is mandatory in most states.

Two other important contributions the NLN makes to nursing are high-quality publications and research studies on the practice of nursing and nursing education. The official journal of the NLN is *Nursing Education Perspectives.* This journal presents many current issues related to education, practice, administration, changes in health care delivery, research, and other relevant topics. The NLN also produces *NLN Position Statements* and the *Reflection & Dialogue* series to address important issues in nursing and nursing education. In addition, NLN produces many books, publications, and multimedia, and maintains a Web site www.nln.org. Last, in an effort to make available vital statistics on nursing and nursing education, the NLN in 2008 began publishing all its data on the Web at NLN DataView™.

Since its inception in 1893 for the purpose of improving and standardizing the education of nurses, the NLN has maintained as its central theme a commitment to nursing education and has continued to be the leading professional association for nursing education. (For more historical information on the NLN, visit the Web site www.nln.org.) The NLN mission states, "The National League for Nursing promotes excellence in nursing education to build a strong and diverse nursing workforce." The NLN implements its mission guided by four dynamic and integrated core values that permeate the organization and are reflected in its work:

CARING: promoting health, healing, and hope in response to the human condition

INTEGRITY: respecting the dignity and moral wholeness of every person without conditions or limitation

DIVERSITY: affirming the uniqueness of and differences among persons, ideas, values, and ethnicities

EXCELLENCE: creating and implementing transformative strategies with daring ingenuity

The NLN maintains a comprehensive database of nursing education programs, as well as surveys about nursing education. The NLN (2006) released its Excellence in Nursing Education Model comprising eight core elements:

- Clear program standards and hallmarks that raise expectations
- Well-prepared faculty
- Qualified students
- Well-prepared educational administrators
- Evidence-based programs and teaching/evaluation methods
- Quality and adequate resources
- Student-centered, interactive, and innovative programs and curricula
- Recognition of expertise

Studies on the competencies of associate degree and practical nurses conducted by the NLN have helped guide curriculum development in nursing education programs.

Last, the NLN embarked on an excellence initiative that culminated in a document highlighting 30 hallmarks of excellence in nursing education, with corresponding suggestions of indicators or questions to determine the extent to which a nursing program is achieving each "hallmark of excellence." An extensive glossary of terms is also included in the document. Three "hallmarks" were identified specifically for students:

1. Students are excited about learning, exhibit a spirit of inquiry and a sense of wonderment, and commit to lifelong learning
2. Students are committed to innovation, continuous quality/performance improvement, and excellence
3. Students are committed to a career in nursing

The full text of the hallmarks, indicators, glossary, and references can be viewed online at www.nln.org/Excellence/hallmarks_indicators.htm.

American Nurses Association

The Nurses' Associated Alumnae of the United States and Canada was organized in 1896 by a group of nurses who believed that group action by nurses would be beneficial. In 1903, Canada's name had to be removed from the name of the organization to be able to incorporate, according to the laws of New York. The name of this organization was changed to the American Nurses Association (ANA) in 1911, and Canadian nurses formed their own national organization. The ANA is known as the professional organization for RNs and limits its membership to RNs. There have been numerous changes throughout ANA's history, but it has always maintained a commitment to individual nurses, and in turn to the public, as recipients of the work nurses do. The ANA's mission statement is "Nurses advancing our profession to improve health for all." A significant change occurred in 1982, when the ANA adopted a federation model of membership. With this model, individual members join state nurses associations (SNAs), and the SNAs are members of the ANA. This was done in hopes of strengthening the state organizations and possibly increasing membership. Unfortunately, only a small percentage of employed nurses belong to their state organization. However, despite the relatively low membership, the ANA has been a powerful voice in nursing issues. The official journal of the ANA is *The American Nurse*. As a fresh, evidence-based voice of nursing, *American Nurse Today* covers cutting-edge issues in nursing practice and keeps nurses abreast of the ANA's advocacy on behalf of the profession. The journal also provides practical, clinical, and career management information that nurses can use to stay up to date on best practices, enhance patient outcomes, and advance their professional careers. ANA's Web site is www.ana.org, and the organization also publishes *The Online Journal of Issues in Nursing*, a peer-reviewed publication that provides a forum for discussion of the issues inherent in current topics of interest to nurses and other health care professionals. The intent of this journal is to present different views on issues that affect nursing research, education, and practice, thus enabling readers to understand the full complexity of a topic. The interactive format of the journal encourages a dynamic dialogue resulting in a comprehensive discussion of the topic, thereby building up the body of nursing knowledge and suggesting policy implications that enhance the health of the public.

The ANA comprises a number of councils that represent specialty areas. Standards of practice have been developed by each council, whose function is to be a forum for discourse related to continuing education, consultation, and other issues that pertain to that council's interests. There are also two congresses, one for nursing practice and the other for nursing economics, whose function consists of setting policies, standards, new programs, and other related responsibilities. Other activities of the ANA include the following:

- Advanced certification of RNs
- Accreditation of continuing education programs
- Participation in public policy issues
- Development of an economic and general welfare program
- Promotion and support of research activities
- Publication of journals, pamphlets, and multimedia

Several areas of controversy have been prevalent throughout ANA's history and may account for some of the reasons that nurses choose not to belong to this organization. One issue is ANA's position on entry into practice. In 1965, an ANA position paper advocated that the entry level for professional nursing should be the baccalaureate nurse. This issue has caused and continues to cause a great deal of conflict within nursing. Another area of conflict began in 1974 with the passage of the Taft–Hartley Act. This act legislated that professional nursing organizations could also be labor unions. Nurses in management positions or nurses who disagree with nurse professionals being represented by a bargaining unit frequently choose not to support the ANA. Other areas of conflict have related to ANA's legislative activities, in which it is rare to find consensus in dealing with various issues proposed for legislation. The ANA's active involvement in national and state health policy issues, although important, contributes to controversy over the positions and direction of the ANA by professional nurses. ANA's position statements on a wide array of issues can be found on its Web site. Several other organizations that are related to the ANA include the following:

- American Nurses Foundation: This organization is a tax-exempt, nonprofit organization committed to supporting research related to nursing. It provides analysis and research related to public policy, supports a group of nurse scholars who are involved with public policy and journalism endeavors, and funds research activities.
- American Academy of Nursing: The ANA established an honorary association to recognize nurses who have made a meaningful contribution to the nursing profession. Nurses so honored are called fellows and use the title Fellow of the American Academy of Nursing.
- International Council of Nurses (ICN): This is the international organization for professional nurses. The ANA is one of the many national nursing organizations with membership in the council. There are 98 national members. The council's headquarters are in Geneva, Switzerland.
- National Student Nurses Association (NSNA): Founded in 1952, this organization comprises students enrolled in associate, baccalaureate, diploma, and generic graduate nursing programs. Although affiliated with ANA, NSNA is its own organization. Two nonvoting consultants are appointed by ANA and NLN to assist the all-student 10-member board of directors. NSNA's official journal is titled *Imprint*. In 2005, NSNA also began publishing *Imprint en Espanol*.

National Council of State Boards of Nursing

The National Council of State Boards of Nursing (NCSBN) comprises the boards of nursing from all 50 states in the United States and its five territories: American Samoa, Guam, Northern Mariana Islands, Puerto Rico, and the Virgin Islands. The mission of the NCSBN is to provide leadership to advance regulatory excellence for public protection. To that end, the NCSBN conducts studies of nursing practice to develop current, relevant test plans for the NCLEX for RNs and LPN/LVNs. These test plans are revised every 3 years, following a comprehensive workplace analysis, to ensure that they are up to date with current practice. In conjunction with the revision of the test plan, the NCSBN also reviews and updates the passing score of the NCLEX. More information is available on testing in Chapter 1, and on the NCSBN Web site www.ncsbn.org.

Another effort by the NCSBN is the study of continued competence in nursing for post–entry-level RNs and LPN/LVNs to ensure that nurses maintain continued competence in the profession following initial entry. The NCSBN has also recently taken a lead role in examining certification requirements for advanced practice registered nurses (APRNs). Each state's Nurse Practice Act outlines the scope of practice for APRNs. Similar to RN and LPN/LVN licensure, this often presents a barrier to nurses practicing in multiple states, and/or moving from one state to another, when the scope of practice for APRNs differ between states. In order to support licensure, certification, and practice portability, the NCSBN recommends APRN certification examinations as a basis for licensure decisions, advocates the APRN compact for mutual recognition of licensure to promote quality advanced practice nursing care within states and across state lines, and endorses the 2008 *Consensus Model for APRN Regulation: Licensure, Accreditation, Certification & Education*. The ANA's new *Nursing: Scope and Standards of Practice for Nursing* (2010) outlines standards also for APRNs. However, since practice is regulated at the state level under each state's Nurse Practice Act, efforts have been ongoing to gain support for this Consensus Model for APRNs. More than 40 Nursing Organizations thus far have endorsed the model. More information on the NCSBN and its activities can be found on the organization's Web site www.ncsbn.org.

Other Nursing Organizations

There are more than 50 organizations for and about nursing, including Sigma Theta Tau, nursing's professional honor society. Many clinical nursing specialties have their own organizations, and some organizations are international. There are also organizations for nurses that are related to educational, religious, ethnic, and other special interests. The National Organization for Associate Degree Nursing was founded in 1984 to be the voice for associate degree nursing (ADN). This organization serves to protect and strengthen ADN. The official publication of this organization is *Teaching and Learning in Nursing*. All of these groups have recognized the importance and value of sharing ideas, research, and experiential knowledge, as well as collective effort and advocacy.

---

thinking critically

As an LPN/LVN, do you currently belong to any nursing organization? As you enter professional nursing practice, your role will include advancing the profession. What areas of nursing do you feel need collective effort for redesigning or advancing the profession of nursing? Which nursing organization do you believe has an interest in this area or similar areas? What are the advantages of collective effort?

NCLEX–RN *Might Ask*   4.2

A nursing student is discussing information on nursing organizations with her clinical preceptor. The nurse is aware that the agency that endows nursing schools with accreditation is the

    A. American Nurses Association (ANA).
    B. American Medical Association (AMA).
    C. National League for Nursing (NLN).
    D. National Student Nurses Association (NSNA).

· See Appendix A for correct answer and rationale.

● EVOLUTION OF NURSING AS A PROFESSION

In the development of nursing as a profession and nurses as professionals, it is necessary to assure the public that the title of nurse represents a defined scope of responsibility and obligation to professional criteria and standards of practice. Joel (2002) described nursing as a profession with a unique, distinct role and autonomy. He argued that nurses as independent thinkers who work with autonomy will contribute more to the health care delivery system. Grossman and Valiga (2005) noted that professionalism also involves belonging to organizations, participating in projects, and being involved politically to advance nursing and help create the preferred future for the profession.

● QUALITIES OF A PROFESSIONAL

Leddy and Pepper (Hood, 2005) described certain qualities necessary to be considered a professional:

1. Intellectual characteristics: Professional practice is based on a body of knowledge gained from research and experience. The education is a combination of general and specialized courses.
2. Service to society: Professional service entails ethical commitment and legal responsibility to the public. Within this service, the public must be guaranteed the competence of professional nurses by a licensure or credentialing system. Ethical obligations are defined by a code of ethics. The *Code of Ethics for Nurses with Interpretive Statements* (ANA, 2008) is discussed later in this chapter.
3. Autonomy: By definition, autonomy means that the individual has self-determination over functions within the workplace. A professional must be responsible and accountable for her or his actions. Nurses have had more difficulty achieving autonomy because of the hierarchal nature of nursing organizations and the continued dependence on the medical profession.
4. Shared personal values: Many values are important to the growth and development of a professional, just as characteristics of commitment, accountability, responsibility, ethical and moral standards, and caring are important to the maturation of the profession as a whole.

thinking critically

Which of the qualities described by Leddy and Pepper (1998) have contributed to your motivation and desire to become an RN? Why are these qualities important? How do you see your nursing practice changing in these four areas as you transition from LPN/ LVN to the RN role?

The move toward mandatory licensure; the development of nursing diagnoses, separate from medical diagnoses; the development of a social policy statement and a code of ethics for nurses; the growth of nursing theory and nursing conceptual models, and the establishment of doctoral degrees in nursing; the advances in nursing science and nursing research; and the formalization of evidence-based practice have all promoted nursing as an independent profession. Leddy and Pepper (Hood, 2010) describe the profession of nursing as one that has gained many of the characteristics of a profession, but is still an "emerging profession" since it has yet to adopt a standardized education for entry into the profession. Currently, there are three levels of education that qualify persons to take the licensing exam for professional nurse registration: diploma, associate degree, and baccalaureate degree nursing programs. These will be discussed later in this chapter.

● LICENSURE

In the late 1800s, there was a move in the United States to license nurses. Nursing leaders of that time believed that a mechanism should exist to assure the public that nurses were competent to practice nursing according to defined standards. Licensed nurses would be titled RNs. These early leaders recognized that the great variance in nursing education programs did not guarantee adherence to any standards. The organizations that preceded the NLN and the ANA supported the licensure of nurses. Although it was a difficult battle, licensure was eventually achieved, and a national examination called the NCLEX-RN was instituted. It is interesting to note that Florence Nightingale did not support nursing licensure. She advocated instead for ongoing education for nurses. Today, we call this "lifelong learning," and RNs participate in continuing education after initial licensure. See Display 4.3 for more information about the history of nursing licensure.

The early licensure laws granted permissive licensure, which means that the person was "permitted" to be licensed if requirements were met. Licensure was

---

display 4.3 | The History of Nursing Licensure

1867 Dr. Henry Wentworth Acland first suggests licensure for nurses in England.
1892 American Society of Superintendents of Training Schools for Nurses formed in the United States.
1901 New Zealand initiates first nursing licensure in the world.
1903 United States initiates nursing licensure (NC, NJ, NY, and VA—in that order).
1915 ANA drafts its first model nurse practice act.
1919 England initiates nursing licensure.
1923 United States completes nursing licensure in all 48 states.
1935 First mandatory licensure act in the United States: New York (effective 1947).
1946 Ten states include definitions of nursing in the licensing act.
1950 State Board Test Pool Examination in use in all states and US territories.
1965 Twenty-one states include definitions of nursing in the licensing act.
1971 Idaho recognizes expanded practice in its nursing practice act.
1976 California institutes mandatory continuing education for relicensure.
1982 NCLEX-RN initiates use of nursing process as its organizing framework.
1987 North Dakota requires baccalaureate degree for RN licensure (rescinded 2003).
1994 Computer-adapted testing (CAT) adopted nationwide for licensure.
1998 Mutual Recognition Nurse Licensure Compact (NLC) finalized; Utah first to adopt.
2000 Nursing Licensure Compact Administrators (NLCA) formed; NURSYS completed, housing licensure and disciplinary data on nurses from more than 30 states.
2003 NCLEX-RN introduces computerized multiple option and short answer questions.
2006 Twenty-three states complete adopted legislation to implement the NLC.
2007 NCLEX-RN begins new "integrated client needs" format; interactive CAT individualizes testing for each candidate.
2008 NCSBN adopts *Advanced Practice Registered Nurse (APRN) Model Act/Rules and Regulations* for licensure/certification of APRNs.
2010 Most recent test plan for NCLEX-RN implemented; new passing scores established.
2011 Twenty-four States have adopted NLC.
2011 APRN Compact: Utah, Iowa, and Texas have passed laws authorizing joining the APRN Compact.

Adapted in part from Ellis, J. R., & Hartley, C. L. (2008). *Nursing in today's world: Trends, issues, and management* (9th ed.). Philadelphia, PA: Wolters Kluwer/Lippincott Williams & Wilkins; and NCSBN, retrieved July 6, 2011 from www.ncsbn.org/nlc

not required for a person to practice nursing. For that reason, employers made a distinction between RNs and nurses. North Carolina, New Jersey, New York, and Virginia first granted permissive licensure in 1903. Mandatory licensure was later advocated as an additional assurance to the public that all nurses were registered and thus met specific criteria and standards. In 1938, the first mandatory licensure law was passed in New York, and today, all 50 states require nurses to pass the NCLEX-RN examination and to be licensed and registered as professional nurses. Some states distinguish between "active" and "inactive" licensure status, requiring continuing education to maintain active status.

Nurse practice acts evolved as licensure laws were enacted. Their purpose is to

- Define nursing
- Stipulate the qualifications to practice nursing
- Outline the methods of obtaining licensure, licensure renewal, and interstate endorsement or reciprocity
- Establish and maintain rules and regulations of nursing
- Delineate unlawful acts, misconduct, or disciplinary actions
- Name the state agency (and its functions) that will oversee the nurse practice act (usually the state board of nursing comprising nurses, other professionals, and consumers)

By 1923, all states had some form of a nurse practice act. Since then, nurse practice acts have changed to reflect changes in nursing, the advent of the national examination and mandatory licensure. Licensure of APRN is also covered in many states' nurse practice acts. It is imperative that licensed nurses are familiar with the nurse practice act for the state in which they practice, not only for current practice regulations but also to keep informed of changes and requirements for licensure renewal.

Approximately half of the 50 states have adopted the NLC for mutual recognition of licensure between and among states. In more recent years, many boards of nursing have adopted regulations for APRN in specialty areas, and many states are also considering the APRN Compact for mutual recognition of licensure for APRNs.

• AMERICAN NURSES ASSOCIATION'S SOCIAL POLICY STATEMENT

Defining nursing has historically been problematic for the nursing profession. There are many viewpoints related to philosophical and practice perspectives. To address this issue, the ANA formulated and published *Nursing's Social Policy Statement* (ANA, 1980). This document was developed to assist nurses in conceptualizing their practice; to provide direction to educators, administrators, and researchers within nursing; and to inform other health professionals, legislators, funding bodies, and the public about nursing's contribution to health care (ANA, 1980).

Within this policy statement, the ANA incorporated the use of the nursing process and the diagnosis and treatment of human responses. This defined the autonomous and unique practice of nursing. The statement also stipulated that nurses are responsible and accountable to society for their actions, which may be in a variety of settings for clients of all ages. The ANA asserts that nurses must include preventive health measures in their practice. The policy statement also included a section about specialization in nursing practice, spearheading the move toward advanced nursing practice.

The statement has been important to the development of the nursing profession in that responsibility and professional accountability are viewed as an essential element of professional nursing practice. Obviously, as knowledge and roles change, changes must also be made in the responsibilities. However, the accountability to the public remains unchanged; nurses accept defined responsibilities for providing care at a particular level. They are always accountable and must practice according to state rules and regulations, standards of practice, and the policy statement. The *Nursing's Social Policy Statement* has been revised three times since its adoption, with the most recent revision in 2010. *Nursing's Social Policy Statement*, and two other documents, *Nursing: Scope and Standards of Practice* (also last revised 2010) and *Guide to the Code of Ethics for Nurses: Interpretation and Application* (2008) serve as an ongoing core foundational trio for guiding the profession of nursing.

• AMERICAN NURSES ASSOCIATION'S CODE OF ETHICS FOR NURSES

A professional code of ethics is a guide for ethical behavior of practitioners in that professional field. A professional code does not have any legal authority, but it does advocate ethical and moral behavior for the profession's practitioners.

To address ethical issues in nursing, the ANA (1985) developed the *Code for Nurses with Interpretive Statements (Code for Nurses)*. The ANA began a process to review and revise the code in 1995, with extensive review and input from practicing nurses and nursing organizations, and culminating in the new *Code of Ethics for Nurses with Interpretive Statements (Code of Ethics)* in 2008. As shown in Display 4.4, the *Code of Ethics* clearly expresses nursing's own understanding of its ethical standards, commitment to society, and the ethical obligations and duties of every individual entering the profession. The full *Code of Ethics for Nurses with Interpretive Statements* can be viewed and purchased online via ANA's Web site.

There is also an international code of ethics for nurses, *The ICN Code of Ethics for Nurses*, which can be found on the ICN Web site at www.icn.ch/icncode.pdf. The preamble to *The ICN Code of Ethics for Nurses* states:

> Nurses have four fundamental responsibilities: to promote health, to prevent illness, to restore health and to alleviate suffering. The need for nursing is universal.
>
> Inherent in nursing is respect for human rights, including cultural rights, the right to life and choice, to dignity and to be treated with respect. Nursing care is respectful of and unrestricted by considerations of age, colour, creed, culture, disability or illness, gender, sexual orientation, nationality, politics, race, or social status.
>
> Nurses render health services to the individual, the family and the community and co-ordinate their services with those of related groups. (ICN, 2006)

| display **4.4** | **Nine Provisions of the ANA Code of Ethics for Nurses** |

1. The nurse, in all professional relationships, practices with compassion and respect for the inherent dignity, worth, and uniqueness of every individual, unrestricted by considerations of social or economic status, personal attributes, or the nature of health problems.
2. The nurse's primary commitment is to the patient, whether an individual, family, group, or community.
3. The nurse promotes, advocates for, and strives to protect the health, safety, and rights of the patient.
4. The nurse is responsible and accountable for individual nursing practice and determines the appropriate delegation of tasks consistent with the nurse's obligation to provide optimum patient care.
5. The nurse owes the same duties to self as to others, including the responsibility to preserve integrity and safety, to maintain competence, and to continue personal and professional growth.
6. The nurse participates in establishing, maintaining, and improving health care environments and conditions of employment conducive to the provision of quality health care and consistent with the values of the profession through individual and collective action.
7. The nurse participates in the advancement of the profession through contributions to practice, education, administration, and knowledge development.
8. The nurse collaborates with other health professionals and the public in promoting community, national, and international efforts to meet health needs.
9. The profession of nursing, as represented by associations and their members, is responsible for articulating nursing values, for maintaining the integrity of the profession and its practice, and for shaping social policy.

From American Nurses Association. (2001). *Code of ethics for nurses with interpretive statements* Washington, DC: Author. Retrieved August 15, 2010, from http://nursingworld.org/ethics/code/protected_nwcoe303.htm. Revised Edition, 2008.

● NORTH AMERICAN NURSING DIAGNOSIS ASSOCIATION INTERNATIONAL

Since the mid-1960s, the concepts related to the nursing process have become more common in the nursing world. In most educational and practice settings, some form of the nursing process is used. This involves assessing the client, making nursing diagnoses, formulating and implementing plans of care, and evaluating the client to determine the effectiveness of the care plan. Later in this text, in-depth information about this process is presented. It is mentioned here because one component of nursing as an independent profession has been the development of a nursing diagnostic taxonomy, separate from medical diagnoses and those of other professions. This means that diagnoses are classified and ordered based on a set of principles in the discipline of nursing. The North American Nursing Diagnosis Association International (NANDA-I) has guided the development of this process.

In 1976, NANDA-I was formed as an organization made up of individual and group RN members. Its purpose is to provide a forum to discuss information and issues related to nursing diagnoses and to develop uniform language for nursing diagnoses. Members may propose new problems or diagnoses by preparing appropriate research and documentation and submitting them to NANDA-I for consideration. Committees review the proposals and then present them to the membership at the national convention. The organization provides and promotes this taxonomy as a common language for nurses and the profession of nursing. The most current taxonomy of NANDA diagnoses can be viewed and purchased via the Web site at www.nanda.org. These diagnoses are used in the autonomous practice of professional RN in developing comprehensive individualized nursing care plans for patients, and directing the work of LPN/LVNs, Certified Nurse Assistants (CNAs), and nonlicensed assistive personnel.

• STANDARDS OF PRACTICE

Important to any profession is an understanding of the scope and standards of practice expected of practitioners in that profession. The ANA publishes not only the *Nursing: Scope and Standards of Practice* described earlier but also similar documents for clinical specialties (eg, pediatric nursing, psychiatric and mental health nursing) and other special functions of nurses (eg, nursing informatics [NI]).

• EVOLUTION OF NURSING SCIENCE

As nursing developed as a profession, with its Social Policy Statement, Code for Nurses, Taxonomy of Nursing Diagnoses, Licensure, Registration, and Standards of Practice, the science of nursing was also emerging. Doctoral degrees in nursing were initiated, and research was undertaken to identify nursing theory, construct conceptual models of nursing, and articulate the key constructs of nursing.

Masters (2005) described the metaparadigm of nursing as the four key phenomena, or concepts, with which the discipline of nursing concerns itself. These are man/person, environment, health, and nursing. Nurse theorists have studied each of these concepts to develop conceptual models of nursing on which curricula in nursing education programs are built.

The evolution of the science of nursing has resulted in an increasing emphasis on EBP, to be discussed later in this chapter. Theory guides practice, and practice informs theory. Three types of doctoral programs are in place for nursing: the doctor of philosophy (PhD), doctorate of nursing science (DNS), and the doctorate of nursing practice (DNP). The International Network for Doctoral Education in Nursing (INDEN) began out of efforts from the University of Michigan, when it hosted the 1995 Doctoral Forum in Nursing titled "Generating Nursing Science in a Global Community." There emerged a desire to create an international network for dialog and global collaboration among doctorally prepared nurses, resulting in the formation of INDEN in October 1999. The most current information on doctoral programs in nursing can be found on the organization's Web site at www.umich.edu/~inden.

• TRANSITIONS IN NURSING EDUCATION

You may be aware that nursing education has made many transitions since the late 1800s. Again, the history of nursing can often be told in part by the educational methods that are used. Florence Nightingale believed that the education of nurses should be a function separate from service to patients. However, in the United States, hospitals and physicians advocated to have nurses educated within a hospital setting to essentially provide an inexpensive labor force. It took many years and hard effort to change this mentality in order to support nursing education as a collegiate experience, where students attain theoretical knowledge as a foundation for not only technical skills but also client assessment and higher-order thinking and problem solving.

Educational Program Similarities

With the many educational options that are now available, nurse educators from the various programs recognize that there are almost as many similarities among programs as there are differences. For example, the student bodies generally have a large variance in age. The average age is often around 30 years. Many students are married or have partners. Many have children, and single parents and mixed families are common. More men are entering nursing, and the profession comprises a wide array of ethnicities. Students are often entering nursing as a second or third career. For some, it is the first time in higher education, and for others, it is a return to school after having earned other certificates or degrees. Most students work at least part time to pay the rising costs of tuition, fees, books, and uniforms and to support themselves and their families.

To meet the needs of older students and those with family and work responsibilities, evening, weekend, part-time, and distributive education (including online) programs are available. A challenge for nursing programs has been the increased cost of nursing education and how to provide quality education at a greatly reduced cost in nontraditional formats. Nursing education programs are among the most costly programs on college campuses and often struggle for adequate funding to provide high-quality, relevant, technologically advanced instruction.

Other similarities revolve around program essentials. The state board of nursing or other designated state agency must approve all programs. Some schools also seek NLN accreditation. All programs require that faculty possess or are seeking graduate degrees. Both theoretical and clinical components are required in registered nursing programs, and students participate in practicum assignments in a variety of clinical settings. Many programs also use practicing RN mentors in the more advanced clinical components of the program. The challenges to nursing students and faculty are many. There are five basic modes of entry to becoming an RN.

DIPLOMA PROGRAMS

The oldest form of nursing education is the diploma program. These programs began in 1873 and were initially similar to on-the-job training programs. Traditionally, they were strict and structured modes of instruction, practice, and conduct. Most diploma programs continue to be located in hospitals, require 3 years to complete, and include basic theory courses along with structured clinical experiences. Many diploma programs are now affiliated with local colleges, so students may receive college credit for general education courses. Graduates of diploma programs are prepared to function as primary caregivers in hospital and ambulatory care settings. They are not educationally prepared for administrative, school nursing, or public health positions. There has always been a fierce loyalty to diploma education; however, the number of diploma programs has declined since the 1980s, partly because of the increased costs for the programs and partly because of the growing number of ADN programs, which are of 2 years in duration and confer the associate degree on completion.

ASSOCIATE DEGREE NURSING PROGRAMS

ADN programs were instituted in the 1950s as a result of Mildred Montag's published doctoral dissertation in 1952 titled "*Education for Nursing Technicians.*" She proposed that technical nurses could be educated in 2 years within a community or technical college and work as RNs. Although there was much opposition to this mode of education, the postwar need for nurses was an impetus for the start of these programs as an additional mode of entry to registered nursing practice. Initially, seven programs were started. They were so successful that many community colleges started similar programs. This second mode of entry has become very popular, with nearly 900 ADN programs in place nationally today. ADN programs provide an accessible, affordable mode of entry into professional nursing, and research has shown that NCLEX-RN pass rates and job performance as an RN are comparable to other modes of entry into practice.

ADN education was designed to have a balance between general education and nursing courses, without affiliation to a particular hospital, but rather clinical nursing experiences in one or more agencies for "hands-on" practicums to accompany collegiate theoretical classes. These programs are generally 2 years in duration and are usually located in community and technical colleges. However, some programs are found in 4-year colleges or within hospitals. ADN graduates are prepared to be direct caregivers in hospitals, long-term care facilities, and ambulatory care settings. They are not prepared educationally for nursing administration, school nursing, public health nursing, or nurse educator positions, although some may work in these settings as part of a "tiered, team approach" to health care delivery.

BACCALAUREATE DEGREE NURSING PROGRAMS

Baccalaureate of science in nursing (BSN) programs were first established in 1909 at the University of Minnesota. They are the third mode of entry to registered nursing. Early programs were 5 years long; however, most programs are now 4 to 5 years. The early programs were greatly opposed by most nurses and physicians, who did not see the need for women and nurses to have higher education. BSN programs today generally begin with 2 years of liberal arts and science education. Nursing courses are concentrated into the last 2 years. Clinical education is similar to that of ADN programs but also includes the use of research in the practice setting. BSN graduates are prepared to care for clients in a variety of settings, including administrative, school, and public health settings.

MASTER'S DEGREE PROGRAMS

A fourth option available to prospective nursing students is the master's degree program that leads to an initial degree in nursing at the master's level. These programs are designed for students who already hold bachelor's degrees in other majors and decide to become RNs. Generally, the programs last 2 to 3 years and involve a combination of undergraduate- and graduate-level courses. Graduates of these programs can practice in settings similar to BSN graduates but have graduate course preparation to engage in research-related nursing activities, case management, and teaching in a nursing education program.

FOREIGN NURSES

The last mode of entry into registered nursing is designed for foreign nurses immigrating to the United States, many of whom are non-English or limited English–speaking adults who practiced nursing in their native country. Each state's board of nursing establishes requirements for foreign nurses who desire to become licensed RNs in the United States.

● CAREER MOBILITY OPTIONS

Career ladder programs provide several opportunities for nursing education. They are sometimes called multiple entry/exit programs. For example, a person who is already an LPN/LVN may enter the second year of an ADN program after completing prerequisite general education courses and a transition course. Alternatively, a person may enter a 2-year ADN program and exit at the end of the first year after completing a practical vocational nursing program option. These types of programs are popular because a student can better meet her or his needs in terms of education and work.

Other career mobility options are related to people who are already RNs but are seeking a higher degree. Many baccalaureate programs have direct "2 + 2" articulation agreements with local community colleges. Essentially, this means that units or credits from the community college freshmen and sophomore courses transfer directly to the 4-year program so that the student enters at the junior-year level and completes 2 more years to attain a BSN. Some ADN and BSN programs offer students the opportunity to take challenge examinations for credit in lieu of some of the courses.

A final option is the availability of external degree programs, in which courses that are required for a BSN may be taken at a local community college, online, or on a self-study basis. Often, a student must have a preceptor or advisor for this process. There are benefits in that the student has more flexibility and can eliminate some of the problems related to traveling and work schedules. Drawbacks are that students do not always have the benefit of learning from other students' experiences and must be able to discipline themselves to succeed in an independent study model.

The choice for initial entry to becoming an RN is important, regardless of which route is taken. However, the business of nursing education is not terminated with the initial process. Nursing must always include a dedication to lifelong learning. Continuing education units (CEUs) are now mandatory for relicensure in most states. Many CEU courses are available to nurses through work, professional organizations, or local community colleges. There are also options available for seeking higher degrees as a way to continue education. Advanced practice roles require a master's or doctoral degree, as do many jobs in specialty areas and nursing education. Many nurses also seek advanced certification in a specific practice area through the ANA or other professional organizations. Continuing education in nursing is essential for remaining current in the practice of nursing.

• FACTORS THAT HAVE INFLUENCED TRENDS AND TRANSITIONS IN NURSING

Throughout history and continuing today, influences outside the realm of nursing have had a major impact on the growth and development of nursing. Nursing does not exist in a vacuum. As technology and communication advance, so does the influence of society on the profession and practice of nursing. In the following section, a brief examination of some of the historic and societal trends that influence nursing is presented.

Impact of War

The impact of war has been mentioned several times in this chapter. In theory, nursing education was born in the United States as a result of the Civil War. When the Spanish-American War occurred in 1898, injured soldiers required the services of nurses from training schools, although the military physicians were greatly opposed. There was less opposition after the war, but it was 1901 before the Army Nurse Corps was created. The Navy Nurse Corps was founded in 1908.

World War I initiated a new dimension for military nurses; injuries caused by shrapnel and gas were now evident, and there were massive numbers of casualties. This war also created a great demand for nurses, which prompted quicker training programs to satisfy some of the demand. After this war, a nursing shortage continued, secondary to the return to longer training programs.

World War II created more demand for nurses and more need for them to be at the battlefront. Educational programs were not providing the necessary numbers, so the Cadet Nurse Corps was created, in which students received tuition and living costs in exchange for serving as a military or civilian nurse for the duration of the war. The curriculum for these programs was shortened, which prompted all nursing programs to reevaluate the duration of programs. Eventually, nurses in the military achieved officer status, but it took longer for male and African American nurses to gain equal status.

The Korean War initiated the use of mobile army surgical hospital units. Nurses were in greater demand than ever. The Vietnam War and the Persian Gulf War emphasized the important role that nurses continue to have in wartime. However, by this time, ADN programs were plentiful, providing a low-cost, high-quality educational program in a shortened time frame.

An additional impact of war on nursing is the challenge nurses face in meeting the needs of veterans suffering from post-traumatic stress disorder (PTSD) and difficulties encountered entering and adjusting to civilian life. The nature of war has changed in today's era of Middle Eastern war (Afghanistan, Iraq, etc.). Today's veterans have experienced not only the carnage of war itself, but also the use of suicide bombers, terrorism, and bombings injuring and killing women, children, and civilians in general. These have had lasting psychological impacts on veterans and an increase in PTSD.

Women's and Men's Roles in Society

Throughout time, nursing has been, and continues to be, a female-dominated profession, although both genders are now widely accepted in the nursing profession. Changes in both women's and men's roles in society, however, have had an impact on nursing.

Traditionally, the work that women did was undervalued. Raising children, housekeeping, and caregiving roles were expected and mostly unpaid. Research done predominantly by men, of men, yielded results incorrectly attributed to women. Various works such as Kohlberg stages of moral development did not portray the "different voice" of women. Although women were not included in his study, Kohlberg generalized his results to both genders, concluding that women were not able to reach the higher level of moral development and were in some way deficient (see Chapter 2). The women's movement, which began in the 1960s as a component of the "Sixties Revolution" (free love, antiestablishment, zero population growth, civil rights, gay rights, peace, and talk of the upcoming "Age of Aquarius"), brought with it a new emphasis on the role of women and equal rights. *The Second Sex* by Simone De Beauvoir and *The Feminine Mystique* by Betty Friedan were already in print, and bookstores carried dozens of books on women's roles. Reaching perhaps a peak in the late 1970s and early 1980s with Title IX (gender equity) and affirmative action legislation, researchers began to study the development of women, and nurse theorists began to study the profession of nursing.

Carol Gilligan, a student of Kohlberg, conducted research on women and produced the seminal text, *In a Different Voice* (1982), in which she contrasted men's ethos of "justice and rights" with women's ethos of "care and connectedness." She concluded that women's moral reasoning, based on the latter, was not inferior, just "different." Women's roles in general, and more specifically in nursing, began to be valued. The development of nursing as a profession, with advanced degrees, research, and an independent taxonomy of diagnoses, all contributed not only to the valuing of nursing but also to the value of women.

Concurrent with, and subsequent to, the women's movement, men were also questioning their traditional roles. With the onset of more "career moms" came more "stay-at-home dads." Men were no longer viewed as inadequate when choosing to assume caregiver roles, and such phrases as "the sensitive man," "it's okay to cry," and "you're okay, I'm okay" were coined. Gender equity began to apply to both genders, and nursing became a more acceptable, feasible career for men, as did other caregiver professions.

Over the past three decades, as Basow (2010) notes, there has been an explosion of research on the psychology of women, gender, and roles. Most notable is the recognition and appreciation of diversity, the impact of social context, and the influence of individual identity within gender: race, ethnicity, class, sexual orientation, and so forth. All these research findings continue to shape nursing, as a female-dominated profession, today. As more men enter the profession, and as men's and women's roles in society continue to evolve, so too will the profession of nursing.

Societal Trends and the Changing Role of Nursing

Societal trends have had, and continue to have, an impact on nursing. Several of these are described in the following sections and listed in Display 4.5.

AGING POPULATION

As the population ages, there are increasingly greater numbers of elderly people who require health care services. This is partly due to the baby boomers entering their sixties and partly due to advances in health care that detect disease early and thus prolong life. The inclusion of elder care and gerontologic concepts in nursing curricula increased in the 1990s. Emphasis began to be placed on individualizing care for three distinct groups of elderly—the old; the very old; and the very, very old. Emerging concepts in caring for the well but frail elderly, as well as concepts of family-centered care for four- and five-generational families, are now included in nursing curricula.

display **4.5**	Societal Trends That Have Influenced the Profession of Nursing
Aging population	Quality outcomes
Shortened lengths of stay	Medical benefits, social security, and reimbursement programs
Nursing shortage	Changes in family structures and alternative lifestyles
Diversity, multiculturalism, and emotional intelligence	Nursing informatics, telehealth, and Health Insurance Portability and Accountability Act (HIPAA)
Immigration issues and foreign nurses	Experiential wisdom and evidence-based practice
HIV/AIDS and pandemic flu	Holistic and spiritual care
Disaster preparedness, bioterrorism, and homeland security	Nursing entrepreneurism
Advancing technology, bioethics, and globalism	Health care advocacy and service learning
Health care reform	Social policy and political advocacy
Managed care and collaborative practice	

SHORTENED LENGTHS OF STAY IN HOSPITALS

Acute care settings have seen a shift to clients who are more critically ill than in the past, yet are staying in the hospital for shorter periods of time. Fewer hospitalized patients are ambulatory. There is also a greater need for high-tech and highly skilled care in long-term and home care settings. Many surgeries and procedures previously performed on clients as inpatients are now being shifted to the outpatient setting, creating a greater demand for outpatient nursing services and increased acuity in inpatient settings. For nurses working in inpatient settings, the ability to prioritize care to more acute patients, think critically, and watch for complications is imperative, as are increased technological skills. Nurse–patient ratios also need to be addressed because nurses can only safely care for a smaller number of patients than in the past. Many states are passing legislation to limit the nurse to patient ratio to ensure safety to the public. Nursing education has to continue to be vigilant and creative in preparing graduates for this new environment.

NURSING SHORTAGE

Throughout history, there have been numerous times when there was a nursing shortage, especially in times of war. However, today, several societal trends are contributing to an alarmingly increased nursing shortage.

First, as mentioned earlier, the population is aging due to the baby boomers entering retirement, and life expectancy is increasing due to advances in medical and nursing science. This means that many nurses in the current workforce are also retiring at a time when there is an increased need for care. These retirees include both nursing faculty and those in clinical practice. As La Rocco (2006) noted, the average age of graduates from nursing programs rose from 24 in 1984 to 31 in 2000. These new nurses will remain in active practice a shorter length of time than their earlier counterparts.

Increased patient acuity and shortened lengths of stay also mean that nurses cannot care safely for as many patients as in the past, thereby further increasing the demand for nurses. Nurses may experience more stress from this increased level of patient acuity, finding themselves working overtime and taking fewer rest breaks throughout the shift. Additionally, many facilities have designed the forty hour work week into shift schedules of "4 tens" or "3 twelves" which can lead to further fatigue. Erickson (2010) notes the importance of healthy work environments, and their relationship to quality outcomes in patient care. Such challenges in nursing may cause prospective students to choose other professions, further contributing to the nursing shortage.

Because the nursing shortage is of such grave concern, nurses and nursing organizations are joining to seek solutions. A significant event took place in 2001, when the ANA invited the NLN and other national nursing organizations to join together to address the nursing shortage. A summit was held with participants from 60 national nursing organizations, and the resulting document, *Nursing's Agenda for the Future: A Call to the Nation* (ANA, 2002), was published. A steering committee of 19 national nursing organizations including ANA, NLN, and NSNA identified 10 domains, or areas of focus, for their work, with the goal of achieving *Nursing's Agenda for the Future* by the year 2010. The 10 domains are listed in Display 4.6. These organizations have made some progress in moving the national agenda, but the challenges are great and such work continues today.

| display **4.6** | **Ten Domains for Achieving Nursing's Agenda for the Future** |

Leadership and planning	Economic value
Delivery systems	Work environment
Legislation/regulation/policy	Public relations/communication
Professional/nursing culture	Education
Recruitment/retention	Diversity

From American Nurses Association. (2003). *Nursing's agenda for the future: A call to the nation.* Washington, DC: Author. Retrieved June 28, 2007, from www.ana.org/naf

---

The nursing shortage continues, and is expected to grow as we approach 2020. Compounding this problem is the shortage of qualified and experienced nursing faculty. Economic pressures in the workplace are causing the health care industry to reduce costs, and therefore reduce RNs in preference to lower paid health care professionals. RNs also find nurse to patient ratios impeding their ability to provide comprehensive professional care to patients. Economic pressures in nursing education programs are causing increased teacher to student ratios, thereby minimizing critical thinking activities in the classroom and laboratory settings, and reducing overall annual nursing student cohorts as institutions contain costs through the reduction of costly programs such as nursing. Benner, Sutphen, Leonard, Day, and Schulman (2010) describe these increasing shortages of both nurses and nursing faculty and pose an agenda for educating nurses to address today's health care industry challenges. The authors suggest increased use of simulations and case studies to prepare tomorrow's nurses for client challenges they will face in the workplace, and an examination of other workforce issues.

DIVERSITY, MULTICULTURALISM, AND EMOTIONAL INTELLIGENCE

Ethnic diversity has increased greatly in the United States, resulting in a growing need for caregivers who are multiculturally sensitive and who value diverse perspectives, views, and values. In some areas of the country, two of three clients are of minority populations, and in a few states, the new majority is persons of color. Thus, the need for nurses who reflect this cultural diversity to better meet client needs is acute. Educators need to prepare nurses to think and act from a multicultural perspective, and nursing school recruitment, admission, and retention practices need to address this challenge of increasing the ethnic diversity of student and graduate nurses. Strategies to diversify faculty are also of value, to attract and retain both male and ethnically diverse nursing faculty.

Parvis (2003) stressed the need for effective leadership in our multicultural workplace. Lindsey and Roberts (2005) advocated the development of "cultural proficiency" across all levels of education. They describe the cultural proficiency continuum, as well as the six stages of development for individuals, leaders, and organizations to become culturally proficient (Table 4.1). As an RN, you will be expected to both model and provide leadership for the development of cultural proficiency in health care settings and among those you supervise.

table
4-1   LINDSEY AND ROBERTS' CULTURAL PROFICIENCY CONTINUUM

Stage of Social Competence	Behaviors
Cultural destructiveness	Any action that negates, disparages, or purges cultural practices or expressions of culture different from your own
Cultural incapacity	Any action that elevates the superiority of your own culture values and beliefs while suppressing cultures different from your own
Cultural blindness	Any policy, practice, or behavior that ignores existing cultural differences or that considers such differences inconsequential
Cultural precompetence	Recognizing that your skills and practices are limited when interacting with other cultural groups
Cultural competence	Any policy, practice, or behavior that uses the essential elements of cultural proficiency for the individual or the organization: assessing culture, valuing diversity, managing the dynamics of difference, adapting to diversity, institutionalizing cultural knowledge
Cultural proficiency	Knowing how to learn and teach about different groups in ways that acknowledge and honor all people and the groups they represent

Adapted from Lindsey, R. B., & Roberts, L. M. (2005). *The culturally proficient school: An implementation guide for school leaders.* Thousand Oaks, CA: Corwin Press, Sage.

Becoming culturally proficient also means being aware of one's own and others' emotions. Goleman (1998) stated that leaders must be attentive to emotional intelligence. He emphasized the need for those who want to be successful, especially as leaders, to learn more about their own and others' emotions and what motivates them in order to inspire, work collaboratively, and adapt to change. As our society becomes more diverse, nurses must develop emotional intelligence. Moss (2005) described the emotionally intelligent nurse as one who is better equipped to provide leadership in issues of day-to-day patient care and ethical dilemmas. Moss also pointed out that emotions become even more important in our ever-increasing technological world, and the emotionally intelligent nurse will be a stronger member of the collaborative health care team.

IMMIGRATION ISSUES AND FOREIGN NURSES

Another societal trend is the public debate over issues of immigration. The nursing shortage and the overall shrinking workforce compared to the overall population have placed an increased emphasis on immigration issues. Foreign nurses are being relied on by the health care industry in greater numbers, and state boards of nursing are challenged to adopt appropriate regulations for nurse licensure. This comes at a time when mutual recognition, through the NLC, is also being adopted, thereby complicating decisions on legislation and regulations.

The ANA has noted that creating a positive environment for all RNs, foreign or US educated, will result in better patient outcomes, improved retention of nursing staff, and optimal performance by the health care facility. Strategies that create a positive work environment and facilitate successful integration of internationally recruited nurses are the focus of several 2007 meetings cosponsored by ANA, ICN, and the Commission on Graduates of Foreign Nursing Schools. Federal legislation to relax nurse immigration standards in response to the US nursing shortage, however, is being met with opposition by the ANA and others who are concerned about decreasing standards and other ethical implications of the proposals. (For current information on this topic, refer to the ANA's Web site at www.ana.org.)

HEALTH CARE REFORM

Today's political agendas surrounding health care reform emphasize access, medical record portability, primary preventive care, cost containment, and choice in caregivers. There is also more emphasis on primary preventive care that is more community based. The primary care provider will serve as a gatekeeper in the continuum of health care needs. The role of acute care centers is changing to one of providing only acute, intensive care. Simple surgeries, procedures, and treatment of illness are provided in community-based settings whenever possible. Cost-containment efforts emphasize quality care in more reduced and efficient ways, and insurance carriers are funding only limited inpatient stays. Restorative and rehabilitative services are being required to be conducted in ambulatory care settings. Communities must ensure that services are integrated and consolidated so that costly duplication is eliminated. The work that nurses, especially advanced practice nurses, do now is held in high esteem because of nursing's holistic and preventive tradition. The quality of care and the reduced cost of that care will be greatly influenced by the work that nurses do.

Grossman and Valiga (2005) posed that the new leadership challenge for nursing is to create its future. They stated, "To continue to participate successfully in health care, nursing will need to persist in finding ways to use resources wisely, validate the effects of nursing interventions on patient outcomes, and develop new ways to provide high-quality and cost-effective care" (p. 28). This will require not only incremental change but also transformational change in health care reform. For a more in-depth exploration of transformative leadership, refer to Burns (2003).

MANAGED CARE AND COLLABORATIVE PRACTICE The expansion of health care systems and health maintenance organizations (HMOs) caused by mergers and cost-saving strategies is affecting nursing and how clients receive care. The use of preferred provider organizations (PPOs) and diagnostic-related groups (DRGs) in an effort to contain skyrocketing inflation in health care costs has had some impact. However, the use of unlicensed assistive personnel to defray costs is causing the profession of nursing to be concerned with the quality of care being given. Nurses are aware that many "tasks" they perform are also accompanied by skilled assessment and critical thinking skills for which unlicensed personnel are not trained. For example, while taking vital signs, the nurse may also notice early signs or symptoms of sepsis, which likely will not be noticed by unlicensed assistive personnel, who are merely taking vital signs.

The initiation and expansion of managed care approaches, compared to the traditional primary care approach, has raised concerns for nurses who want to ensure illness prevention and health promotion for their patients, in addition to medical treatment. In managed care settings, a patient often sees different physicians and other providers at each visit and/or each day during a hospitalization. This is not only confusing to patients but can also lead to missed secondary complications not passed on from one provider to another or not observed when subtleties are only seen with consistent observation over several days.

Two trends have developed in nursing as a result of managed care approaches and the increased use of electronic devices (rather than human senses) to monitor patients' conditions. First, nursing has returned to its "roots," focusing on "holistic health care," viewing the patient as a complex biological system, where all components interface and have an impact on each other: biological, psychological, sociological, emotional, and spiritual. Eastern healing philosophies are becoming more apparent, blended with Western medicine, and health care reimbursement is examining the cost-benefit of reimbursement of preventative medicine, which was previously excluded. Whole fields of holistic and spiritual nursing and nursing specialties are emerging. These are discussed in a later section in this chapter.

Second, a "team approach" has become critical in managed care settings, and today's RN must engage as a "collaborative practitioner." When nurses collaborate, they work with other members of the health care team to think critically, drawing on the expertise of various team members to analyze and solve complex problems in patient care. Wheatley (1999) argued that organizations are self-organizing and that collaboration by all members of the team is essential for creativity and developing the best strategies for quality outcomes. Laura Hendrix (2004) provided some practical tips on organizing information about the patient to provide a comprehensive picture of the patient before contacting a colleague health care provider. She emphasized that by presenting a comprehensive description of the patient's condition, nurses exercise and demonstrate critical thinking and judgment skills, learn more about the patient themselves, and strengthen collaboration among members of the health care team.

QUALITY OUTCOMES Efforts to incorporate quality assurance (QA), total quality management (TQM), and continuous quality improvement (CQI) practices are adding work to already overworked nurses. Although these initiatives are designed to ensure accountability for quality-based outcomes, the increased management of patient/client care is removing nurses from the "soft skill" side of promoting health, patient education, and meeting psychosocial needs.

Accrediting associations for nursing programs, higher education, and health care agencies are all monitoring for quality outcomes. Colleges and universities are being held accountable for student learning outcomes (SLOs) in order to be regionally accredited. Outcomes assessment, evaluation, performance indicators, organizational "scorecards," and accountability measures are prominent in society today as policy makers determine allocation of limited resources. This is impacting health care agencies, nursing programs, and nurses themselves. For nursing, such information not only drives finances but also, even more importantly, is necessary for nursing research, continuous improvement of quality patient care, and the expansion of EBP (discussed later in this chapter). In 2007, the ANA hosted its first annual National Database of Nursing Quality Indicators (NDNQI) data use conference. The conference focused on such topics as how hospitals use NDNQI reports to improve the quality of nursing care, how nurse staffing affects patient outcomes, mandates for public reporting initiatives, data collection practices, and cost savings achieved with quality improvement. This is consistent with the growing emphasis on the science of nursing and EBP.

MEDICAL BENEFITS, SOCIAL SECURITY, AND REIMBURSEMENT PROGRAMS Perhaps the greatest challenge for older persons today is the change in medical benefits, social security, and reimbursement programs. Not only are such changes confusing, they raise fears for both patients and health care providers. What costs will be covered by insurance providers, Medicare, and social security programs? How will noncovered costs be paid?

For nurses and other health care providers both employment and retirement planning must take into account such programs as Medicare health savings accounts (HSAs), flexible spending accounts (FSAs), prescription plans, long-term care insurance, and the emerging national health care agenda. As health care agencies struggle with rising costs and cost containment strategies, reductions in benefit packages can drive nurses to other professions, contributing to the nursing shortage and, ultimately, further compounding cost escalation. In addition, issues of guardianship and who is covered on benefit plans arise with the increase in same-sex couples, mixed families, and alternative lifestyles and living arrangements. These all impact the nurse's role both in planning care and legal compliance.

CHANGES IN FAMILY STRUCTURES AND ALTERNATIVE LIFESTYLES

Another societal trend effecting nursing is the diversification and change in family structures. As discussed previously, the aging population has resulted in multigenerational families. Also, alternative lifestyles have resulted in an increase in same-sex couples and public policy debate regarding same-sex marriage and individual rights. For nursing, this raises ethical dilemmas in issues of patient confidentiality; legal guardianship; and authorization for surgery, medical procedures, organ donation, and end-of-life decisions.

HIV/AIDS AND PANDEMIC FLU

The AIDS epidemic has greatly influenced the world of nursing. Implementation and maintenance of standard precautions can minimize the danger of AIDS and other bloodborne pathogens, but health care workers continue to have increased risks. This has prompted some nurses to leave the profession and has possibly deterred others from seeking a nursing education. In other ways, the workplace has become a safer environment for health care workers if the universal precautions are practiced. The concern over an impending pandemic flu is also of concern to nursing. Detailed plans for such a disaster are needed in all health care settings. Nurses will play a lead role in such an event and will need to be prepared for the challenges involved.

DISASTER PREPAREDNESS, BIOTERRORISM, AND HOMELAND SECURITY

The world in the 21st century differs greatly from earlier times. In just the first 5 years, the United States experienced the World Trade Center attack on September 11, 2001; subsequent acts of terrorism and bioterrorism; and disasters such as Hurricane Katrina on the Gulf Coast and the Asian Tsunami in the Pacific Ocean. These have caused the health care industry, and nursing in particular, to respond to the need for disaster preparedness. Wright and Vesala-Husemann (2006) examined the vulnerability of communities and countries facing disaster based on their coping ability and the nature and extent of the disaster. Addressing nutrition and other health care issues and building capacities in such settings are discussed.

Both the ANA and ICN have established Web pages devoted to terrorism, bioterrorism, and disaster response, with information for nurses on how to care for patients, how to cope and protect themselves, and how to prepare for disaster. Many articles have been written on these topics, health care agencies have adopted new policies and procedures in the event of such emergencies, and nursing programs have added curricula focused on preparing nurses adequately to face such challenges.

The NCSBN and individual state boards of nursing have also responded to issues of disaster preparedness and homeland security. Some states have implemented criminal background checks for nurse licensure applicants.

ADVANCING TECHNOLOGY, BIOETHICS, AND THE GLOBAL ECONOMY

Technological changes and the growing trend toward specialization have changed the educational needs and practice of nurses. In most settings, nurses must also be highly skilled technicians who are well trained to manage highly advanced technology. Computer-based documentation and high-tech caregiving equipment are now common, demanding new skills from all RNs. As advances continue in medical care, the need for highly specialized nurses will increase. Like technology advances in acute care settings, the technology in home care and long-term care settings has also escalated. This has an obvious impact on families and health care providers in those settings. Along with this "high-tech" environment, the "high-touch" skills of nurses will be of even greater importance as clients and their families require more patient teaching and communication to allay fears and care for themselves at home.

Bioethics and societal trends such as organ replacement, joint replacement, life-prolonging procedures, cryogenics, genetic reengineering, cloning, and stem cell research pose ethical dilemmas for health care professionals. Nurses, in collaboration with other health care professionals, must think critically about these issues to examine their secondary effects on patients, their families, and society as a whole. Nursing organizations must study and engage in critical dialogue about these controversial issues. The ANA announced its support for the Stem Cell Research Enactment Act of 2007, which promotes the ethical use of stem cells for research and therapeutic purposes that impact health. In a January 11, 2007, press release, ANA President Rebecca M. Patton, MSN, RN, CNOR, stated, "ANA supports participation in the ethical, legal, and social debate surrounding stem cell research by all communities. We are committed to working through a political action to improve the health of the nation." Today's nurses will need to be knowledgeable of these issues not only to be politically active but also to engage in patient education on a daily basis.

Technological advances in telecommunications have provided greater opportunities for medical consultation and the portability of medical records. However, this has placed patient confidentiality at greater risk, and it challenges today's nurse to be especially mindful of privacy issues. This is discussed in more depth later in this chapter.

Another challenge of the societal trend toward multimedia and advanced telecommunications is what Goleman (2007) calls "creeping disconnection" and "social corrosion." Along with longer work hours, two-income households, and the strains of the current economic recession and weakening global economy, society has become dependent on cell phones, iPods, BlackBerries, notepad computers, and other technological devices. Rarely is one free from these assistive devices, and distractions are plentiful, causing increasing social disconnects. It has been said that never throughout history have we been so connected and yet socially disconnected as today. Nursing has been impacted by this in that "connecting" with patients has become more difficult, and patient teaching that "sticks" has become a challenge. Goleman (2007) describes the need for practitioners today to develop not only personal "emotional intelligence" but also interpersonal "social intelligence," citing the emerging field of social neuroscience whereby decreased neuronal activity has been found in social situations where certain neurons are activated by the body.

Another societal trend impacting nurses is globalism and the global economy. The NLN's Hallmarks of Excellence in Nursing Education emphasize the need for curriculum to reflect local and global perspectives of societal and health care trends. The NLN defines "global perspective" as follows:

> Knowledge about and critical understanding of global issues that enable an individual to (a) effectively address those issues; (b) acquire values that give priority to ecological sustainability, global interdependence, social justice for all the world's people, peace, human rights, and mutually-beneficial processes of economic, social, and cultural development; (c) develop the will and ability to act as mature, responsible citizens of the world; and (d) develop a commitment to creating acceptable futures for themselves, their communities, and the world. Such a perspective is critical in light of the increasing connectivity and interdependence of the world's social, economic, educational, and other systems. (www.nln.org/Excellence/hallmarks_indicator.htm)

The world has "become smaller" as transcontinental travel has become faster and more common and as telecommunications allows for increased competition and contributes to an expanding global economy. The recent crash in the mortgage industry, with concurrent foreclosures and profit loss in the banking, automotive, and other industries in the United States, caused a global economic crisis. The health care industry is part of this global economy, and the impact on nursing has been great.

Last, the need to develop more energy efficient, clean energy (nonfossil fuel) systems, and sustainable, "green" products are impacting nursing and decisions in the health care field globally. Goleman (2009) describes the need for "ecological intelligence"—to be aware of the hidden impact of foods and products on health and ecological systems.

Nurses who are multilingual, culturally proficient, and sociologically and ecologically intelligent will play an active role in this new economy and make wise decisions for political advocacy. The 1960s phase "Think globally, act locally" has taken on another whole tier of meaning in this new high tech, global economy.

thinking critically

Select three of the societal trends presented. How do you think each will affect your practice as an RN in the future? How will clients be affected? What role can nursing organizations play in the advancement of nursing related to these societal trends?

• NURSING INFORMATICS AND HIPAA

NI is a relatively new area of practice emerging from today's information society. Chaska (2001) cited the need for nurses to assist clients in the new knowledge-based economy, in which individuals are able to have a greater voice in the selection of health care providers and services. NI has been defined by the ANA (2001b) as follows:

> A specialty that integrates nursing science, computer science, and information science to mange and communicate data, information, and knowledge to support patients, nurses, and other providers in their decision-making in all roles and settings. This support is accomplished through the use of information structures, information processes, and information technology. (p. 46)

The ANA updated its publication on NI in 2008 with the text *Nursing Informatics*. As a new field, NI research is examining its impact on patient privacy, ethical decision making, and the nursing profession as a whole. McGonigle and Mastrian (2009) expand on these concepts and those cited by the ANA. They discuss the information and knowledge needs of nurses in the 21st century, ethical applications of informatics, telenursing and the use of e-portfolios, and the use of informatics in health disaster planning and the promotion of community health.

Although younger nursing students are generally more at ease with technology in general, and computer systems in particular, practicing nurses, adult students, and those returning to school later in life may find the challenge greater. As Saba and McCormick (2005) noted, "Nurses are becoming computer literate and the nursing profession is implementing practice standards for its clinical care and data standards for its nursing information technology systems" (p. 3).

The HIPAA was passed in 1996 with compliance required by 2003 to make health care more efficient. It provides portability of medical coverage for preexisting conditions, defines the underwriting process for group medical coverage, and standardizes electronic transmittal of billing and claims information. Because standardization and portability also means that access to patient information has been expanded, a key component of HIPAA is its regulations to maintain confidentiality and security of health data. Tappan, Weiss, and Whitehead (2004) noted the important role of nurse leaders in guarding the privacy of patients and their confidential health information and records. For more information on HIPAA, visit the Web site at www.hippa.com.

Another outcome of advanced technology, informatics, and HIPAA is the tele-health industry. Telehealth is defined as "the use of electronic information and tele-communications technologies to support long distance clinical health care, patient and professional health-related education, public health, and health administration" (Health Resources and Services Administration, n.d.). This has been especially help-ful to patients, nurses, physicians, and other health care professionals in rural areas who are seeking consultative advice from specialists, as well as patient education and professional development opportunities they might not otherwise be able to access.

The Health Care Information and Management Systems Society (HIMSS) was founded in 1961. That HIMSS is "the health care industry's membership organiza-tion exclusively focused on providing global leadership for the optimal use of health care information technology (IT) and management systems for the betterment of health care" (HIMSS, n.d.).

• EXPERIENTIAL WISDOM AND EVIDENCE-BASED PRACTICE

A seminal work by Patricia Benner (1984) was her book titled *From Novice to Expert: Excellence and Power in Clinical Nursing Practice*. Benner argued that although a great deal was known about nursing from a sociological perspective, evidence of that learned through actual clinical practice had not been documented. She described how nurses gain experiential knowledge throughout their clinical practice, from novice beginnings until they become nurse "experts." In the 21st Century, the profession of nursing has broadened its body of knowledge by documenting such evidence-based outcomes of nursing practice since Benner's seminal book.

Documenting the effects of nursing practice, including evidential discovery, can then lead to empirical research on preventive, reparative, and restorative nursing care to improve quality outcomes. This provides rich information for both novice and experienced RNs, and for nursing education reform. As Aveyard and Sharp (2009) note, "The main reason why you need to base your professional practice on the best available evidence (evidence based practice) is that it enables us to deliver the best possible patient/client care rather than out-of-date practice" (p.6). Begun in 1998, the journal *Evidence-Based Nursing* is published quarterly and contains articles of international nursing research for application to the practice of nursing. Numerous articles and books are now published on EBP, ranging from an introduction to EBP for students and nurses who want to know more about EBP and how to collect and use evidence for efficient and effective care (Malloch & Porter-O'Grady, 2006), to full summaries of best practices of nursing procedures organized by clinical special-ties (Lippincott Williams & Wilkins, 2007). Aveyard and Sharp (2009) emphasize, however, that when using EBP, the nurse must also employ clinical/professional judgment, consider patient/client preference, and be mindful of available resources.

• HOLISTIC AND SPIRITUAL CARE

The increasing attention to holistic and spiritual care in nursing is noted by Dossey, Guzzetta, and Keegan (2000), Wilt and Smuker (2001), Norlander (2001),

McSherry (2006), and many others. Providing holistic and spiritual care amidst the increasing complexity of multiethnic client populations, however, poses new challenges for nurses. Although nurses have always cared for their patients' biological, psychological, sociological, spiritual, and other needs, the practice of "holistic nursing" has only become a distinct nursing specialty in recent years.

The American Holistic Nurses Association (AHNA) was formed in 1981 in an effort to bring the concepts of holism to every arena of nursing. Its mission is to "unite nurses in healing." Holistic nursing became officially recognized as a nursing specialty by the ANA in 2006. AHNA then worked with the ANA to define the scope and standards of practice of this specialty, resulting in the foundational document *Holistic Nursing: Scope and Standards of Practice* (2007). As noted on the Web site for AHNA, *Holistic Nursing: Scope and Standards of Practice* is a foundational volume that articulates the essentials of holistic nursing, its activities and accountabilities at all practice levels and settings. The book includes an overview and history of holistic nursing, core values of the profession, educational preparation necessary, standards of practice, and standards of professional performance as well as references and information about complementary and alternative modalities. Holistic nurses honor each patient's subjective experience about health, health beliefs, and values. They integrate self-care, self-responsibility, spirituality, and reflection in their patients' lives. The emphasis is on the nurse facilitating the healing of others, and the AHNA views itself as a bridge between the traditional medical paradigm and universal complementary and alterative healing practices. For more information on holistic nursing, refer to the Web sites for AHNA (www.ahna.org) and ANA (www.ana.org).

Spiritual nursing care is another nursing field that is receiving increased attention. McSherry (2006) noted that the spirituality of the nurse and that of the patient can cause tension. Thus, she provides information on how to provide spiritual care by using a systematic approach, discusses skills nurses need, and describes strategies for overcoming barriers to providing spiritual care. With the increased diversity in culture, ethnicity, and religion among today's nurses, and the inclusion of such concepts in today's nursing curricula whereby nursing students engage in classroom discussions about this topic, the ability to address religious and spiritual preferences and concerns of patients by RNs has been enhanced.

Spiritual nursing is recognized by the ICN as an important element of palliative care in caring for dying patients and their families. Palliative care is the holistic care of patients with advanced progressive illness who are not responsive to curative treatment. Palliative care includes pain management; symptom management; social, psychological, emotional and spiritual support; and support for the patient's caregiver. Hospice nursing is a specialty for nurses particularly interested in palliative care. Established in 1986, the Hospice and Palliative Nurses Association (HPNA) is the nation's largest and oldest professional nursing organization dedicated to promoting excellence in hospice and palliative nursing care. More information can be found on HPNA's Web site at www.hpna.org.

● NURSING ENTREPRENEURISM

Entrepreneurism is somewhat new in the nursing profession. Merriam-Webster (www.m-w.com, retrieved July 6, 2011) defines an entrepreneur as "one who organizes, manages, and assumes the risk of a business or enterprise." Nurse entrepreneurs are risk takers who use their nursing knowledge, expertise, networking, and business skills to assume an independent or collaborative role in a new business or enterprise. Nurses become entrepreneurs for many reasons. Changes in the health care setting, the desire for greater autonomy, and interest in a particular specialty where one wants to devote increased attention are all examples of catalysts that may cause a nurse to become an entrepreneur.

Although nurses are making important contributions to health care reform and quality care, the loss of nurses from clinical practice to entrepreneurism is contributing to the nursing shortage. As Saba and McCormick (2005) noted, "Recent survey data indicate that a growing number of nurses are qualified as information specialists" (p. 3). Others are assuming such roles as legal nurses, lobbyists, diabetic educators, salespersons of a wide array of products, consultants, business owners, and travel and travel agency nurses. As described previously, bioterrorism preparedness and Internet-based entrepreneurial opportunities are also growing.

The Nurse Entrepreneur Network (NeN) was founded by Lea Rae Keyes, RN, to help nurse entrepreneurs start, manage, and grow their businesses. Launched in 2004, NeN is an online network that also helps members form collaborative alliances and promote their businesses. For more information on nurse entrepreneurism, visit the NeN Web site at www.nurse-entrepreneur-network.com.

● HEALTH CARE ADVOCACY AND SERVICE LEARNING

The need for social health care reform (ie, prevention of obesity, diabetes, cancer, AIDS, teenage pregnancy, chemical dependency, etc.) poses new roles and challenges for nursing. Palmer and Savoie (2001) noted the explosion of service learning curricular strands in college educational programs. Service learning experiences provide an opportunity for students to develop civic responsibility by working with individuals and agencies in the community to improve quality of life, assist veterans, serve senior citizens, work with chemical dependency and battered women's shelters, and provide services following disasters (eg, floods, hurricanes) to name a few. The "fit" of this curriculum with nursing's need for more community-based learning experiences is evident. Through such experiences, the nursing student is exposed to health care reform issues and needs and develops an appreciation for the role advocacy plays in such efforts.

● SOCIAL POLICY AND POLITICAL ADVOCACY

Catalano (2005), Ellis and Hartley (2004), Masters (2005), and others have cited the need for nurses to become active in the development of legislation and social policy as they encounter complex ethical dilemmas and confront health care reform issues. Critical and creative thinking is needed to address such issues as biomedical technology, genetic engineering (eg, foods, cloning), robotics, ecologically green and sustainable technologies, and bioethical decision making.

Nurses comprise the nation's largest health care profession. Acting individually and collectively through their organizations, nurses can shape and refine public policy. The ANA Web site (www.ana.org) provides useful information for nurses on how to become involved in important efforts for health care reform and the development of social policy, both as an individual and as members of national nursing organizations.

• CONCLUSION

Nursing has experienced many transitions throughout history. It has evolved based on historical, political, and societal events and has been especially influenced by the changing roles of women, men, and minorities in society. Also important has been nursing's emergence and continuing growth as a profession, with licensure, regulations, standards of practice, ethics, and theories guiding its practice as a science distinct from other health sciences.

The impact of societal trends on nursing cannot be underestimated. There will always be a cause-and-effect on nursing education and practice by what happens in the context of our society. The evolution of nursing is a reflection of society in general. Nurses must have an understanding of their roots and societal trends to better understand the future, prepare for tomorrow's challenges, and provide leadership in advocating for quality health care in all settings.

student exercises

1. Choose an event in the history of nursing that interests you. Research that event more thoroughly and then consider the following points:

   a. What was the general tone in society at that time?

   b. What was the role of both women and men at that time?

   c. What were the functions of nurses, even if not defined in a formal sense?

   d. What drew you to this particular event?

   e. What impact did this event have on the profession of nursing?

2. As you enter the role of professional RN today, reflect on the societal trends presented and how they may impact patients and their families in an area of nursing in which you intend to practice. How will you serve as an advocate for change? What organizations might have an impact, and what actions will you take to become involved in such organizations?

References

American Nurses Association. (1980). *Nursing's social policy statement*. Kansas City, MO: Author.
American Nurses Association. (1985). *Code for nurses with interpretive statements*. Kansas City, MO: Author.
American Nurses Association. (1995). *Nursing's social policy statement*. Kansas City, MO: Author.
American Nurses Association. (2001a). *Code of ethics for nurses with interpretive statements*. Washington, DC: Author. Retrieved June 28, 2007, from http://nursingworld.org/books/ pdescr.cfm?cnum=24; CEN21

American Nurses Association. (2001b). *Scope and standards of nursing informatics practice*. Washington, DC: Author.

American Nurses Association. (2002, April). *Nursing's agenda for the future: A call to the nation*. Washington, DC: Author. Retrieved June 28, 2007, from www.ana.org/naf

American Nurses Association. (2003). *Nursing's social policy statement* (2nd ed.). Washington, DC: Author.

American Nurses Association. (2007). *Holistic nursing: Scope and standards of practice*. Washington, DC: Author. Retrieved August 15, 2010, from www.ahna.org/Resources/Publications/Books/ScopeandStandards/tabid/1938/Default.aspx

American Nurses Association. (2008). *Nursing informatics*. Washington, DC: Author.

American Nurses Association. (2008). *Guide to the code of ethics for nurses: Interpretation and application*. Washington, DC: Author.

American Nurses Association. (2010). *Nursing: Scope and standards of practice*. Washington, DC: Author.

American Nurses Association. (2010). *Nursing's social policy statement: The essence of the profession, 2010 Edition*. Washington, DC: Author.

Anderson, L. W., & Krathwohl, D. R. (Eds.). (2001). *A taxonomy for learning, teaching, and assessing: A revision of Bloom's taxonomy of educational objectives*. New York, NY: Addison-Wesley Longman.

Aveyard, H. & Sharp, P. (2009). *A beginner's guide to evidence-based practice in health and social care*. Berkshire, UK: Open University Press/McGraw-Hill Education.

Barritt, E. R. (1973). Florence Nightingale's values and modern nursing education. *Nursing Forum, 12*(1), 7–47.

Basow, S.A. (2010). Changes in psychology of women and psychology of gender textbooks (1975–2010): Anniversary paper. *Sex Roles, 2010, 62*(3–4), 151–152. Retrieved August 15, 2010, from www.springerlink.com/content/lv763633127m5255

Benner, P. (1984). *From novice to expert: Excellence and power in clinical nursing practice*. Upper Saddle River, NJ: Prentice-Hall.

Benner, P., Sutphen, M., Leonard, V., Day, L., Schulman, L.S. (2010). *Educating nurses: A call for radical transformation*. Stanford, CA: Jossey-Bass.

Burns, J. M. (2003). *Transforming leadership: A new pursuit of happiness*. New York, NY: Atlantic Monthly Press.

Catalano, J. T. (2005). *Nursing now: Today's issues, tomorrow's trends* (4th ed.). Philadelphia, PA: F.A. Davis.

Chaska, N. L. (2001). *The nursing profession: Tomorrow and beyond*. Thousand Oaks, CA: Sage.

Deloughery, G. (1998). *Issues and trends in nursing* (3rd ed.). St. Louis, MO: Mosby.

Dossey, B. M., Guzzetta, C. E., & Keegan, L. (2000). *Holistic nursing: A handbook for practice* (3rd ed.). Gaithersberg, MD: Aspen.

Ellis, J. R., & Hartley, C. L. (2004). *Nursing in today's world: Trends, issues, and management* (8th ed.). Philadelphia, PA: Lippincott Williams & Wilkins.

Ellis, J. R., & Hartley, C. L. (2008). *Nursing in today's world: Trends, issues, and management* (9th ed.). Philadelphia, PA: Wolters Kluwer/Lippincott Williams & Wilkins.

Erickson, J. (2010). Overview and summary: Promoting healthy work environments: A shared responsibility. *OJIN: The Online Journal of Issues in Nursing, 15*(1), manuscript overview. Retrieved August 15, 2010, from www.nursingworld.org/MainMenuCategories/ANAMarketplace/ANAPeriodicals/OJIN/TableofContents/Vol152010/No1Jan2010/Overview-and-Summary-Promoting-Healthy-Work-Environments.aspx

Goleman, D. (1998). *Working with emotional intelligence: Why it can matter more than IQ*. New York, NY: Bantam.

Goleman, D. (2007). *Social intelligence: The new science of human relationships*. New York, NY: Random House.

Goleman, D. (2009). *Ecological intelligence: How knowing the hidden impacts of what we buy can change everything*. New York, NY: Broadway Books.

Grossman, S. C., & Valiga, T. M. (2005). *The new leadership challenge: Creating the future of nursing* (2nd ed.). Philadelphia, PA: F.A. Davis.

Health Resources and Services Administration. (n.d.). *Telehealth*. Retrieved June 28, 2007, from http://www.hrsa.gov/telehealth/

Healthcare Information and Management Systems Society. (n.d.) HIMSS *home page*. Retrieved June 28, 2007, from http://www.himss.org/ASP/index.asp

Hendrix, L. (2004). Paging pointers. *Nursing, 34*(5), 32hn4–32hn6.

Hood, L. (2005). *Leddy & Pepper's conceptual basis of nursing method*. Philadelphia, PA: Lippincott Williams & Wilkins.

Hood, L. (2010). *Leddy & Pepper's conceptual basis of nursing method* (7th ed.). Philadelphia, PA: Lippincott Williams & Wilkins.

International Council of Nurses. (2006). *The ICN code of ethics for nurses.* Geneva, Switzerland: Author.

Joel, L. (2002). Reflections and projections on nursing. *Nursing Administration Quarterly, 26*(5), 11–17.

La Rocco, S. A. (2006). Who will teach the nurses? *Academe, 92*(3). Retrieved July 6, 2011, from www.aaup.org/AAUP/pubsres/academe/2006/MJ/feat/laro.htm

Lindsey, R. B., & Roberts, L. M. (2005). *The culturally proficient school: An implementation guide for school leaders.* Thousand Oaks, CA: Corwin Press, Sage.

Lippincott Williams & Wilkins. (2007). *Best practices: Evidence-based nursing procedures* (2nd ed.). Philadelphia, PA: Author.

Longworth, N. (2003). *Lifelong learning in action: Transforming education in the 21st century.* New York, NY: Routledge/Falmer.

Malloch, K., & Porter-O'Grady, T. (2006). *An introduction to evidence-based practice in nursing and health care.* Boston, MA: Jones and Bartlett.

Masters, K. (Ed.). (2005). *Role development in professional nursing practice.* Sudbury, MA: Jones and Bartlett.

McGonigle, D., & Mastrian, K. (2009). *Nursing informatics and the foundation of knowledge.* Boston, MA: Jones and Bartlett.

McSherry, W. (2006). *Making sense of spirituality in nursing and health care practice: An interactive approach* (2nd ed.). London, UK: Jessica Kingsley.

Moss, M. T. (2005). *The emotionally intelligent nurse leader.* San Francisco, CA: Jossey-Bass.

National League for Nursing. (2006). *Excellence in nursing education model.* New York, NY: Author.

Nightingale, F. (1992). *Notes on nursing: What it is and what it is not.* (A commemorative edition of the first edition published in 1859.) Philadelphia, PA: JB Lippincott.

Norlander, L. (2001). *To comfort always: A nurse's guide to end of life care.* Washington, DC: American Nurses Association.

Palmer, C. E., & Savoie, E. J. (2001). Service learning: A conceptual overview. In G. P. Poirrier (Ed.), *Service learning: Curricular applications in nursing.* Sudbury, MA: Jones and Bartlett.

Parvis, L. (2003). Diversity and effective leadership in multicultural workplaces. *Journal of Environmental Health, 65*(7), 37.

Saba, V. K., & McCormick, K. A. (2005). *Essentials of nursing informatics* (4th ed.). New York, NY: McGraw-Hill.

Tappan, R. M., Weiss, S. A., & Whitehead, D. K. (2004). *Essentials of nursing leadership and management* (3rd ed.). Philadelphia, PA: F.A. Davis.

Wheatley, M. J. (1999). *Leadership and the new science: Discovering order in a chaotic world* (2nd ed.). San Francisco, CA: Berrett-Koehler.

Wilt, D. L., & Smuker, C. J. (2001). *Nursing the spirit: The art and science of applying spiritual care.* Washington, DC: American Nurses Association.

Wright, M., & Vesala-Husemann, M., (2006). Nutrition and disaster preparedness: Focusing on vulnerability, building capacities. *OJIN: The Online Journal of Issues in Nursing,* 11(3), manuscript 5. Retrieved August 15, 2010, from www.nursingworld.org/MainMenuCategories/ANAMarketplace/ANAPeriodicals/OJIN/TableofContents/Volume112006/No3Sept06/tpc31_516086.aspx

Zerwekh, J., & Claborn, J. C. (1997). *Nursing today: Transition and trends* (2nd ed.). Philadelphia, PA: WB Saunders.

Suggested Reading

Chitty, K. K., & Black, B. P. (2011). *Professional nursing: Concepts and challenges* (6th ed.). Maryland Heights, MO: Saunders Elsevier.

Weaver, C. A., Delaney, C. W., Weber, P., & Carr, R. (Eds.). (2006). *Nursing and informatics for the 21st century.* Chicago, IL: Healthcare Information and Management Systems Society.

www.aahn.org: American Association for the History of Nursing. (Last accessed 7.6.2011).

www.nln.org: National League for Nursing. (Last accessed 7.6.2011).

www.ana.org: American Nurses Association. (Last accessed 7.6.2011).

www.aamn.org: American Assembly for Men in Nursing. (Last accessed 7.6.2011).

www.noadn.org: National Organization for Associate Degree Nursing. (Last accessed 7.6.2011).

www.florence-nightingale.co.uk: Florence Nightingale Museum. (Last accessed 7.6.2011).

www.himss.org: Health Care Information and Management Systems Society. (Last accessed 7.6.2011).

www.hrsa.gov/telehealth: U.S. Department of Health and Human Services, Health Resources and Services Administration. (Last accessed 7.6.2011).

www.hipaa.com: Health Insurance Portability and Accountability Act of 1996. (Last accessed 7.6.2011).

www.nln.org/ProfDev/corecompetencies.pdf: National League for Nursing's core competencies of nurse educators with task statements. (Last accessed 7.6.2011).

www.maryseacole.com: Mary Seacole. (Last accessed 7.6.2011).

www.ahna.org: American Holistic Nurses Association. (Last accessed 7.6.2011).

www.nurse-entrepreneur-network.com: Nurse Entrepreneur Network. (Last accessed 7.6.2011).

5

Learning at the ADN Level

● LEARNING OUTCOMES

By the end of the chapter, the student will be able to:

1 Describe learning concepts related to the adult learner.

2 Apply adult learning concepts to oneself.

3 Describe the differences between medical and nursing conceptual models.

4 Give examples of learning activities in each of three learning domains: cognitive, affective, and psychomotor.

5 Discuss the roles of LPN/LVNs and associate degree nurses related to nursing process and nursing diagnosis.

6 Differentiate among the six cognitive learning achievement levels: knowledge, comprehension, application, analysis, synthesis, and evaluation.

7 Differentiate between passive and active learning processes.

8 Identify learning strategies to maximize success in an ADN program.

9 Describe the differences in transition needs of LPN/LVNs entering ADN programs as advanced placement generic, straight-through LPN-to-ADN students, and time-out LPN-to-ADN students.

10 Differentiate between the ADN student and LPN/LVN practice roles.

RN

LPN

v i g n e t t e

George Dobian is fearful of his first nursing course, which he will take in the fall. He has heard from others that nursing school is very different from when he attended LVN school 10 years ago. He was never good at taking tests and that fear has haunted him throughout his adult life. He is afraid of being embarrassed because his employer is paying for his education. He is wondering if he has the wrong study skills or if he has a learning disability. He has talked about his fears to his friend John Scott, a student in his anatomy and physiology class. John has taken a "Success Strategies for the Returning Student" seminar at the community college and speaks openly about his professor's introduction to skills in learning. George is impressed when John says that his test scores and overall memory of materials improved when he began rewriting his notes, discussing course content with others, experiencing problems firsthand during clinical sessions, and participating in teaching projects. George is on his way to sign up for the summer "Success" seminar and has made an appointment to talk with a counselor about determining whether he has a learning disability.

• ADULT LEARNING THEORY

Much has been written about adult learning theory. The knowledge and life experiences you bring with you to the ADN program are valuable assets as you move toward becoming an RN. Perhaps you find yourself in a situation like George's. George has a clear understanding of his goals and motivation mechanisms but really needs help with his transition process. As an adult learner, you need a clear understanding of your goals, learning style, motivational mechanisms, and desired societal roles to aid you in the transition process.

Adult learners draw on a wide variety of life experiences as they pursue additional education. These experiences are a resource and a support to adults in acquiring knowledge. Adults are generally self-motivated and self-directed and have developed a preferred learning style. Unlike the child's learning environment, which is structured and directed by the teacher, the milieu for the adult learner must provide opportunities for self-established goals and learning techniques.

display **5.1**   **Characteristics of Adult Learners**

Adult learners:

- Draw on a variety of life experiences in the educational process.
- Are motivated to learn when they see that such learning solves problems confronting them.
- Are motivated to learn when such learning is needed to fulfill social roles.
- Are self-motivated and self-directed and seek learning to fulfill self-established goals.
- Learn best when the program of learning addresses the individual learning styles they have developed with time.
- Are motivated to learn for purposes of self-actualization and to make a meaningful contribution to society.

Adults are motivated to learn when they see the meaning and relevance of learning in fulfilling societal roles or solving daily problems faced at home or on the job. In addition, many variations exist among adult learners based on their learning styles, gender, ethnicity, socioeconomic, and cultural backgrounds. Wlodkowski (1999) emphasized the role that intrinsic motivation plays in learning. He described how one's intrinsic motivation is based on emotions, which are socialized through culture, and therefore, influences the degree to which one engages in and is motivated by various learning activities. The same learning activity that frustrates you may be enjoyed by another student, and vice versa, based on your social and cultural backgrounds and life experiences. Recognizing your emotional response, accepting it, and moving forward will minimize stress in the learning process. The key characteristics of adult learners are provided in Display 5.1.

Experiential Knowledge and the Adult Learner

As an LPN/LVN and an adult with a wide variety of life experiences, you bring to the ADN program a great deal of knowledge, including expertise in specific content areas of the curriculum. This extensive experiential knowledge enhances the educational process in several ways.

First, having both theoretical and practical knowledge, skills, and abilities provides you with the self-confidence to tackle new areas of learning and venture into new clinical experiences.

Second, your areas of expertise will be a rich resource to peers, as theirs will be to you, as you participate in learning activities and work in groups to fulfill course objectives and meet clinical competencies at the RN level.

Third, your rich experiential background provides a wealth of information for making connections between prior learning experiences and new ones, problem solving, and analyzing and synthesizing new theoretical content and practical applications.

Meaning and Relevance of New Knowledge

Adult learners are motivated to learn when what they are learning is relevant and useful in their work and home lives. The LPN/LVN who returns to school to pursue an ADN often does so for monetary reasons or for increased autonomy or career mobility. However, once in the transition process, this same nurse discovers the increased ability she or he has to plan and implement individualized care to clients. Wlodkowski (1999) stated:

> Competence is the most powerful of all motivational conditions for adults. Competence is our reality check: it tells us what is possible by our own will. As adults we have a deep desire to be competent and often seek learning as a means to this end. Across cultures, this human need for competence is not one to be acquired but one that already exists and can be strengthened or weakened through learning experiences. (p. 240)

The ability to make nursing diagnoses, solve problems, and work collaboratively with physicians and other health care workers to provide comprehensive client care results in additional motivation and the incentive to continue pursuit of this increased scope of practice. The increased independence and ability to solve problems and accept new challenges in their everyday world creates even greater motivation for LPN/LVNs to further their learning.

thinking critically

Reflect on an experience when some new knowledge had particular meaning and relevance to you in your personal or work life. How did this motivate you to learn even more?

Personal and Professional Achievement and Self-Actualization

A parallel but different motivational force in adults pursuing further education is self-fulfillment or self-actualization. To self-actualize is to realize fully one's potential (*Merriam-Webster OnLine*, n.d.). Whether for personal or professional achievement, one motivation for LPN/LVNs to seek ADN education is to realize their potential as nurses, to acquire the knowledge, skills, and abilities to practice at the RN level. Covey (2004) noted that when one finds his own voice, effectiveness is enhanced and one is able to go from good to great. Perhaps your pursuit of a professional degree and professional practice is this desire to find your own voice for self-actualization.

thinking critically

Reflect on the factors that have motivated you to pursue an ADN. When things get tough from time to time throughout the program, how can you draw on these resources to maintain that motivation?

Self-Directed, Individualized Learning

In addition to a wealth of experiential learning, the adult learner has gained insight into the means by which she or he learns best. Individualizing your approach to new content can offer many possibilities for maximizing the learning process.

The adult learner is self-directed and seeks learning to fulfill self-established goals. The LPN/LVN who sets personal goals related to the accomplishment of competencies and objectives of the ADN program is more likely to experience success than are those who are not self-directed.

• PRACTICAL/VOCATIONAL AND ASSOCIATE DEGREE NURSING EDUCATION: A COMPARISON

Although the educational programs for the LPN/LVN and the ADN student may appear to be similar, close examination reveals major differences between the two. Masters (2005) described that role development in professional nursing practice includes theory, philosophy, ethics, critical thinking, clinical judgment, informatics, resource management, quality management, and economics, to name a few, as the nursing student develops as an individual nurse, cares for individual and family clients, and works collaboratively with other health care team professionals.

You may at first think the only difference between the two programs is some additional science background and technical skill development with more complex procedures. However, you will find that developing professional competence involves learning and thinking in a whole new way. McAuliffe (2006) noted that qualities of professional competence include initiative, sensitivity to one's own sensitivity, evidence-based decision making, and self-evaluation. He stated, "Professional competence is not achieved by simply applying clear, technical, and universally applicable solutions to practical problems, but by being able to make evidence-based decisions that emerge from the consideration of multiple perspectives. Professional competence is a product of this reflective capacity. It is not consistent with unquestioned allegiance to routine and tradition" (p. 477).

Philosophies and Conceptual Models

Each nursing program is built on a philosophy developed and shared by that program's nursing faculty. Although both levels of nursing programs (LPN/LVN and ADN) set forth beliefs about the practice of nursing in their philosophy statements, the ADN program's philosophy generally provides greater depth in its view of nursing, defining such central concepts as man (client or person), health, environment, nursing, caring, teaching, and learning.

The conceptual model is the template of theoretical concepts and principles that is a basis for developing the curricular content for the nursing program. The conceptual model is derived from the program's philosophy and guides the development of course objectives and competencies. Many LPN/LVN programs are built on a medical model, in which the LPN/LVN operates as a member of the nursing profession, providing care to clients with medical disorders or dysfunctions. As a directed care provider, the LPN/LVN carries out physicians' orders and contributes to the planning, implementation, and evaluation of care to individual clients based on nursing diagnoses established by the RN. The LPN/LVN programs that use a nursing model (ie, based on nursing theory and nursing diagnoses rather than medical diagnoses) often choose a human needs approach because this model fits well with the directed scope of practice of the LPN/LVN. ADN programs often use an integrated nursing model for their conceptual framework, drawing on the research of nurse theorists and incorporating nursing diagnoses to guide the developing autonomous practice of the RN student. These models allow for the nurse with an associate degree to practice both independently and collaboratively with other health care providers, within their scope of practice.

---

display **5.2**	**Core Components of Nursing Practice for Graduates of ADN Programs**

1. Professional behaviors
2. Communication
3. Assessment
4. Clinical decision making
5. Caring interventions
6. Teaching and learning
7. Collaboration
8. Managing care

Curricular Frameworks

The curricular frameworks for each of these levels of nursing programs are consistent with their nurse practice acts, National Council of State Boards of Nursing (NCSBN) test plans (NCSBN, 2009, 2010), and competencies identified by such professional organizations as the National League for Nursing (NLN). Each state's Nurse Practice Act outlines the educational preparation needed for the LPN/LVN and RN practice levels. Each nursing school's curricula must be approved by the state board of nursing to be accredited so that program graduates will be eligible for licensure through the NCLEX after completion. In addition, most ADN programs have adopted student learning outcomes for each course, for the program, and for conferring of a degree consistent with the college's institution-level student learning outcomes (SLOs) as required by the regional accrediting body.

The NLN (2004) identified eight core components of nursing practice for graduates of ADN programs (Display 5.2). These components are essential to the work of the entry-level RN and inherent in the three roles of professional nursing practice (provider of care, manager of care, and member within the discipline of nursing). They provide the framework for organizing educational outcomes of graduates of ADN programs.

Curricular Content and Learning Domains

In the mid-1900s, Benjamin S. Bloom (1956) identified three learning domains into which curricular content falls and from which educational objectives are written. The cognitive domain is the area of learning in which you acquire knowledge. The affective domain is the area of learning involving values and attitudes. The psychomotor domain is the area of learning in which you develop manipulative skills in the discipline.

thinking critically

To gain a better understanding of the three learning domains, think about the last time you attended a nursing in-service at work. What cognitive learning took place? What words, procedures, and rules did you need to learn and apply to participate in the in-service? What affective learning took place? What attitudes did you need to change or develop? How did your beliefs or views about nursing and the type of people involved change? What psychomotor learning took place? What hands-on skills did you need to learn?

Both LPN/LVN and ADN education programs contain curricular content in all three learning domains. For example, both programs require knowledge of body structure and function (cognitive domain), an appreciation for the self-image changes confronting the aging individual (affective domain), and the ability to take accurate vital signs (psychomotor domain). However, more in-depth content in each domain is included in the ADN program curriculum. A review of the curriculum content in each of the two program levels reveals that additional content or course work is required for the ADN program in such areas as the biological and behavioral sciences; computational, communication, and language skills; advanced medical–surgical nursing; psychiatric nursing; and management and leadership skills.

Learning Achievement Levels

Within the cognitive domain, Bloom (1956) identified six learning achievement levels: knowledge, comprehension, application, analysis, synthesis, and evaluation. Bloom developed the Taxonomy of Educational Objectives to differentiate the various types of thinking. Objectives were developed for the cognitive, affective, and psychomotor domains, and educators have used these for curriculum planning over the decades. During the 1990s, Lorin Anderson (a former student of Bloom) led a team of cognitive psychologists to review and revise the Taxonomy for the 21st Century, including the terminology, structure, and emphasis within the cognitive domain. Display 5.3 shows a comparison of Bloom's original and Anderson's revised Taxonomy of Educational Objectives (Anderson & Krathwohl, 2001; Bloom, 1956). Competencies at the LPN/LVN level include the knowledge, comprehension, and application of content within the scope of practice of the LPN/LVN. Competencies at the ADN level include all six cognitive learning achievement levels. Whether your ADN program uses the original or the revised taxonomy, the ability to analyze, synthesize, evaluate, and create is essential to the RN in thinking critically to establish nursing diagnoses, design nursing care plans, and manage client care. Curriculum content and learning activities in the ADN program support learning achievement at these higher levels of thinking.

---

display 5.3   **Comparison of Bloom's Original (1956) and Anderson's Revised (2001) Taxonomy of Educational Objectives in the Cognitive Domain**

BLOOM'S ORIGINAL TAXONOMY	ANDERSON'S REVISED TAXONOMY
Knowledge	Remembering
Comprehension	Understanding
Application	Applying
Analysis	Analyzing
Synthesis	Evaluating
Evaluation	Creating

Adapted from Bloom, B. S. (Ed.). (1974). The taxonomy of educational objectives: Affective and cognitive domains. New York, NY: David McKay; Anderson, L. W., & Krathwohl, D. R. (Eds.). (2001). A taxonomy for learning, teaching, and assessing: A revision of Bloom's taxonomy of educational objects. New York, NY: Longman.

Nursing Process and Nursing Diagnosis

Taylor, Lillis, LeMone, and Dynn (2008) described the nursing process as a systematic method that helps the nurse and client develop a plan to meet the client's needs. Nursing process progresses through its scientific steps in five phases: assessment, diagnosis/analysis, planning, implementation, and evaluation. Both the LPN/LVN and the RN participate in the nursing process within their respective scopes of practice. However, the roles played by each differ. Table 5.1 provides a comparison of the roles of LPN/LVNs and RNs with regard to nursing process and nursing diagnosis. The LPN/LVN collects data, assists with patient assessment, contributes to the planning phase, implements basic therapeutic and preventive measures outlined in the plan, and evaluates the effectiveness of such measures. The RN collects data and performs patient assessment, analyzes and groups data, draws conclusions and uses judgment in establishing diagnoses, designs a plan of care collaborating with other health care providers, develops an implementation plan with short- and long-term goals, and provides outcomes of the plan, redesigning as needed.

table
5-1   COMPARISON OF THE ROLE PLAYED BY LPN/LVNS AND RNS IN NURSING
PROCESS AND NURSING DIAGNOSIS

Nursing Process Phase	Role of LPN/LVN	Role of RN Beyond LPN/LVN Scope of Practice
Assessment	Gathers data Performs patient assessment Identifies patient strengths	Gathers more extensive biopsychosocial data Groups and analyzes data Researches additional data needed Identifies client resources
Nursing Diagnosis	Not applicable	Draws conclusions Uses judgment Makes diagnoses
Planning	Contributes to development of care plans	Sets short- and long-term client goals Establishes priorities Collaborates and refers
Implementation	Provides basic therapeutic and preventive nursing measures Provides client teaching Record client information	Manages client care (performs and delegates) Provides client and family teaching Provides referrals Records and exchanges client information with health team
Evaluation	Evaluates effects of care given	Evaluates effectiveness of overall plan; analyzes new data Modifies, redesigns plan Collaborates with other health team members

The test plan for the NCLEX-PN (NCSBN, 2010) outlines the role of this practitioner in relation to the nursing process:

> The practical/vocational nurse uses a clinical problem-solving process (the nursing process) to collect and organize relevant health care data, assist in the identification of the health needs/problems throughout the client's life span, and contribute to the interdisciplinary team in a variety of settings. The entry-level practical/vocational nurse demonstrates the essential competencies needed to care for clients with commonly occurring health problems that have predictable outcomes. "Professional behaviors, within the scope of nursing practice for a practical/vocational nurse, are characterized by adherence to standards of care, accountability of one's own actions and behaviors, and use of legal and ethical principles in nursing practice." (NAPNES, 2007)

The entry-level practical nurse acts in a more dependent role when participating in the planning and evaluation phases of the nursing process and acts in a more independent role when participating in the data collecting and implementing phases of the nursing process.

In contrast, the test plan for the National Council Licensure Examination for Registered Nurses (NCSBN, 2009) recognizes the role of the RN in all five phases of the nursing process, including the analysis (nursing diagnosis) phase. Nursing process as well as the caring, communication and documentation, and teaching/learning processes are integrated throughout the client needs areas (safe and effective care environment, health promotion and maintenance, psychosocial integrity, and physiological integrity). Test questions are based on the job analysis study of practicing RNs (NCSBN, 2008). More in-depth information on Nursing Process is covered in Chapter 10.

Differences in the Learning Process

As you enter the ADN program, you may discover differences in the learning process from that encountered in the LPN/LVN program you attended. These differences may be attributed partly to the length of time between the programs, especially if it has been many years since your participation in the LPN/LVN program. However, even if you just recently completed the LPN/LVN program, you will encounter differences attributable to the areas discussed in this chapter: program philosophies; conceptual models; curricular frameworks; curricular content within learning domains; addition of the analysis, synthesis, and evaluation learning achievement levels; and role in nursing process and nursing diagnosis. Curry (2008) cites that as a returning student, you may not be familiar with nursing theory and the "abstract nature of theory may elicit anxiety in students who previously learned in concrete and structured educational modes and functioned professionally with technical expertise" (p. 16).

Because the goal of the ADN program is to enable you to function in the independent and interdependent (collaborative) modes, use higher-level thinking skills, and make nursing diagnoses using analysis and judgment, you will experience two key differences in the educational process: (a) an active learning process will mostly likely be the mode of operation and (b) learning activities will include a focus on developing your ability to analyze and synthesize curricular content and to achieve learning outcomes.

Active learning is the act or process of acquiring knowledge or skills by being engaged in action or activity. As Kearney-Nunnery (2008) notes, "Active participation can be a distinct advantage in learning. It can clarify thoughts and observations, prompt interactions, and lead to insights" (p. 19). The active learning environment of the ADN program, when compared perhaps to your LPN/LVN training, will require you to be resourceful, disciplined, self-directed, and proactive in seeking those learning opportunities that will build both your confidence and your competence to function as a professional nurse. Wlodkowski (1999) stated,

> Today's world of work increasingly requires people who can capably self-direct in their jobs. However, sometimes instructors encounter adults who seem dependent, lacking in self-confidence, or reluctant to take responsibility for their learning. There are a number of possible reasons for this. Three of the most common are that (1) these adults have not been socialized to see themselves as in control of their own learning, (2) their experience in school or in the particular domain of learning has been generally negative or unsuccessful, and (3) they do not believe they have a free choice as to whether or not they engage in the learning or training experience. This last reason, very common among adults, is a *personal security* issue. In many instances, adult learners need courses and training not so much because they want them but because they need the jobs, the promotions, and the money for which these learning experience are basic requirements. This is the reality for many adults, and it may be one about which they feel they have little choice. "Just tell me what to do," is their common refrain. (p. 241; italics added)

At times, you may feel this way within the active learning environment of the ADN program.

In addition to traditional lecture, laboratory, and clinical experiences, learning activities in the ADN program include classroom activities and out-of-class assignments that require active participation. Sather (2009) describes the value of professional learning teams where students learn from one another and improve their professional practice. She acknowledges that working in teams may be a new process and may be a challenge for some members who may find themselves questioning their own values, beliefs, and practices. Such exercises are designed to build self-confidence, develop communication skills, develop analytical skills, and foster critical thinking to prepare you for the autonomous professional role you will be expected to assume after graduation. No longer will the correct response be to report findings to the RN or physician. You will now need to analyze information, think critically, use judgment, establish nursing diagnoses, confront ethical issues, take action, manage client care, and delegate interventions while maintaining responsibility for clients under your care. The active learning process in the ADN program and learning activities that focus on developing your ability to analyze and synthesize curricular content will prepare you for these new challenges. Your nursing instructors and other faculty on campus teaching at the associate degree level are preparing you for today's world of work where problem solving, critical thinking, and lifelong learning are vital to your success as an RN. Contemporary teachers focus less on teaching and more on facilitating learning so that both you and the teacher are focused on your learning. As Weimer (2002) wrote, "Learner-centered teachers connect students and resources. They design activities and assignments that engage learners. They facilitate learning in individual and collective contexts" (p. 76). Weimer (2002) outlined what teachers do when instruction is learner centered, identifying seven principles of the faculty role in learner-centered

display **5.4**	**Seven Principles of the Faculty Role in Learner-Centered Teaching**

1. Teachers do less learning tasks.
2. Teachers do less telling; students do more discovery.
3. Teachers do more design work.
4. Teachers do more modeling.
5. Teachers do more to get students to learn from and with each other.
6. Teachers work to create climates for learning.
7. Teachers do more with feedback.

Adapted from Weimer, M. (2002). *Learner-centered teaching: Five key changes to practice*. San Francisco, CA: Jossey-Bass.

teaching (Display 5.4). Longworth (2003) added that the old method of imposing large quantities of information onto students and hoping they remember it is obsolete. The world is changing at a more rapid pace and the need for lifelong learning means that "what to think" is superseded by "how to think."

● LEARNING STRATEGIES FOR SUCCESS

As an adult learner, you can adopt learning strategies that will maximize your success in the ADN program by increasing your self-awareness, establishing self-directed goals, becoming an active learner, and adopting techniques to stimulate your thinking.

Self-Awareness

ADDRESSING YOUR LEARNING STYLE

In Chapter 1, you learned about learning styles and how individuals have different ways in which they best learn in an educational setting. You reflected on this material to determine your own learning style(s) or ways you learn best. Are you an auditory, visual, or kinesthetic learner? Do you need to role play or in other ways "experience" the content you are trying to learn? Exploring new forms of study habits or redesigning group study sessions to address your learning style(s) will enhance your success. Learners must know how they learn best and be aware of their strengths and weaknesses in the learning process. This self-awareness then leads to being a more confident and self-directed learner (Weimer, 2002). In addition, make sure your instructor knows how you learn best. When teachers are aware of your particular learning style they can focus on teaching methods and strategies that will be particularly helpful to you. Santrock and Halonen (2010), however, note that it is good for you to diversify your learning style and try new methods as a strategy to achieve success in both current and future learning activities.

ACCOMMODATING FOR DISABILITIES

Many individuals with physical, mental, or learning disabilities have experienced success in pursuing a career at the ADN level. The law requires all educational institutions to provide reasonable accommodation to individuals with disabilities, but it is up to the individual to request such accommodation.

Some students may have experienced difficulty in school without knowing they had a learning disability. Several indicators of possible learning disabilities are shown in Display 5.5.

The key to overcoming a learning disability and achieving success in the ADN program is to identify and understand the learning disability, and then, seek

---

display 5.5   **Indicators of Possible Learning Problems or Learning Disabilities**

VISUAL PERCEPTUAL PROBLEMS

- Reverses letters and order of letters
- Omits endings of words
- Cannot edit own work
- Mismarks computerized scoring sheets
- Loses place while reading (marks place with finger or piece of paper)
- Has difficulty lining up numbers correctly (uses graph paper to do math)
- Is confused by complex visual fields (when doing a work sheet, blocks out all but essential item)

AUDITORY PERCEPTUAL PROBLEMS

- Cannot differentiate sounds (e and i, m and n)
- Has difficulty sounding out unknown words
- Is poor at spelling
- Is highly distracted by background noise
- Cannot locate stress in words or sentences

SPATIAL PERCEPTUAL PROBLEMS

- Has trouble differentiating left from right
- Has trouble following directions (gets lost easily)
- Is slow to learn dance routines

VISUAL–MOTOR PROBLEMS

- Miscopies information
- Has poor handwriting

INTEGRATION PROBLEMS

- Understands concepts but forgets facts, dates, and names
- Frequently has difficulty recalling commonly known words
- Is poor at spelling (cannot remember order of letters)
- Understands mathematical concepts but cannot remember the order of steps to solve math problems
- Has poor organizational skills

ATTENTION DEFICIT

- Has trouble sitting still for an extended time
- Is highly distractible
- Is unable to concentrate for an extended time
- Jumps from task to task

accommodation for the disability. Each college provides testing to identify learning disabilities as well as support services and referrals for students with disabilities. Norwich (2008) describes dilemmas associated with differences, inclusion, and disabilities. The college learning disability specialist can work with you and your instructor to identify effective accommodation strategies for you.

ADDRESSING AGE, GENDER, SEXUAL ORIENTATION, AND CULTURAL DIFFERENCES

As described in Chapter 1, LPN/LVNs enrolling in ADN programs may experience barriers to achievement of course objectives and competencies because of age, gender, sexual orientation, or cultural differences in relation to other students or social roles. The re-entry nurse may feel uncomfortable if classmates or peers in study or clinical groups are much younger. The male student who acquired his LPN/LVN through military service may be participating for the first time in an educational setting where peers and instructors are predominantly female. He or his peers may be uncomfortable in group learning activities, or he may be called on in the clinical area to help move patients or do other physical activities, thus impeding his ability to work on clinical objectives and competencies in his student role.

Cultural mores may also hamper success in the program. The dependent role of women in some cultures may prevent such female students from teaching male clients, developing autonomy, collaborating with physicians, and developing leadership and management skills. Cultural views of time, acceptable verbal and nonverbal communication skills, and proxemics (comfort in spatial relations) may prevent the student from meeting clinical competencies involving these areas of interpersonal skills and responsibilities.

Strategies for success for students experiencing difficulties because of age, gender, sexual orientation, or cultural differences (Display 5.6) include

1. identifying situations that generate discomfort
2. discussing these areas with the instructor(s)
3. sharing and confronting such issues openly in class discussions and clinical conferences
4. exploring successful coping and accommodation strategies that have been used by other students and nurses

Many resources are now available to assist minority students on how to succeed on a majority campus. Books, periodicals, and online resources discuss success strategies for minority students, including those who are gay, lesbian, or bisexual; how to

---

display 5.6   Strategies for Success for Students Experiencing Difficulties Because of Age, Gender, Sexual Orientation, or Cultural Differences

1. Identify situations that generate discomfort.
2. Discuss these areas with the instructor.
3. Share and confront such issues openly in class discussions and clinical conferences.
4. Explore successful coping and accommodation strategies that have been used by other students and nurses.

deal with racism; and moral and ethical decisions students may face based on their ethnic, cultural or religious values.

Self-Directed Goals

A second strategy for maximizing success is to establish self-directed goals. Chapter 1 describes breaking up reading and other learning activities into smaller time blocks and scheduling time in advance for study as important in the goal-setting process. Doing research online or preparing questions for discussion before a study group session will enhance your learning at the session. Proactively seeking clinical skills during each clinical session will ensure completion of clinical skill checklists by the end of the term.

Active Learning

The ADN program will include learning activities for students to work with peers and other health care professionals in a variety of ways. There are many benefits of active participation by adult learners who are often distracted by personal problems, yet have a wealth of first hand experience to contribute. Active participation in class enables you to put other worries and issues in your personal life aside while you engage in course content. This focus will strengthen what you learn and improve retention of content for later use on exams and in the clinical area. Through the active learning process, students develop the ability to apply curricular content, analyze and problem solve, think critically, and perform independently, as they advance from the LPN/LVN to the RN level of practice.

A variety of active learning activities may be included in the design of the ADN educational program. Commonly found are such activities as brainstorming, small group discussion, role playing, and formal debates. The student who takes a proactive approach in creating her or his own active learning strategies will enhance success. Forming study groups, posing problems to solve, writing study questions to exchange with peers, and designing care plans in a collaborative process are examples of ways you can strengthen the learning process for both you and your peers.

thinking critically

If you have started courses in the registered nursing program, examine the learning activities and assignments in the course syllabus. Are these different than those you experienced in your LVN/LPN training? Do some of these involve active learning? How is the instructor guiding you into an active learning model?

Techniques to Stimulate Thinking

A similar learning strategy for success is to develop techniques to stimulate thinking about curricular content in each of the three learning domains. One of the best strategies for stimulating thinking is to continually ask yourself questions about the learning being acquired (the what, where, why, who, how, and what if questions). Other strategies for developing your critical thinking skills are addressed later in this text in Chapter 9. Example questions follow for each of the three learning domains.

COGNITIVE DOMAIN

What is the meaning of this content? How does it relate to last week's learning? How does it relate to prior content or courses? How would I explain this to someone else? How would I apply this in practice? How would this apply to clients of different ages, the opposite gender, different cultures, or those who are disabled? What are opposing viewpoints to this content?

AFFECTIVE DOMAIN

How would I feel if I or a family member was experiencing this disorder, dysfunction, or difficulty? How would I react if this were happening to someone close to me? How do I value this type of response or behavior? How might someone experience this whose age, gender, cultural background, or sexual orientation was different than mine? What values or beliefs underlie this patient's or nurse's comments? What ethical dilemmas might arise in this situation, and how would I confront them?

PSYCHOMOTOR DOMAIN

What are the principles underlying this procedure (aseptic techniques, ethical considerations, protection of privacy, body mechanics, energy conservation, resource conservation, and therapeutic effect)? How else could this be performed while maintaining these principles? How would I teach this to a client? How could this be done in a home environment? What verbal and nonverbal communication is occurring? What shortcuts can I take to save time or supplies while still maintaining the principles involved?

In addition to these learning strategies for success, you will want to take into account your individual uniqueness. Later in this text, you will have an opportunity to draw on these strategies and others in designing your own individualized learning plan.

NCLEX–RN *Might Ask*

5.1

The nursing student is teaching a client with a colostomy about irrigation of the stoma. The type of learning domain the student would use to teach the client is

    A. Cognitive.
    B. Psychomotor.
    C. Affective.
    D. Communicative.

• See Appendix A for correct answer and rationale.

● TRANSITION NEEDS UNIQUE TO THE LPN/LVN-TO-ADN STUDENT

In this chapter, you have been learning about the process of transitioning from the LPN/LVN role to the ADN student role. As an LPN/LVN, you are entering the ADN program in one of three entry patterns. Transition needs of LPN/LVNs vary among the three patterns.

LPN/LVNs Entering a Generic ADN Population

The generic ADN student starts at the beginning of the ADN program and progresses through the curriculum to completion of the program. Generic ADN students are provided with an orientation at the start of the program and learn about the history and development of ADN and registered nursing in general. An overview of the program philosophy, conceptual model, and curriculum framework is usually presented, and the student is socialized into the role and expectations of the RN scope of practice.

The LPN/LVN who enters a generic ADN class is usually advance placed 25% to 50% of the way through the program. She or he may be a lone enrollee or may be accompanied by others advance placed at this point of entry. The orientation and socialization (transition) process varies according to nursing program policies and practices, but most programs provide only a minimal orientation/socialization process. Material and student exercises presented in this text are designed to enhance the success of both students who have and have not been provided with a formal transition course or process.

The unique needs of LPN/LVNs entering a generic ADN population center on socialization not only into the program culture but also into the class culture. These cultures include the unwritten and written rules and acceptable behaviors of student participants. The LPN/LVN who takes a proactive approach in seeking assistance from faculty and classmates in getting to know the ropes and trying to fit in with study groups increases her or his chance of success.

Straight-Through LPN/LVN-to-ADN Students

The straight-through LPN/LVN-to-ADN student is one who has participated in the school's LPN/LVN program and has continued directly into the ADN program (usually at the second year level). When large groups of students are involved in this entry pattern, or if the college offers only a career ladder (LPN/LVN-to-RN) "bridge" program and no generic program, the transition may be smoother. The culture of the school will be familiar, including instructional support areas (eg, library, computer lab, and skills center), and the student may know faculty in the program. The ADN program generally provides a formalized orientation or transition course for these students. This text's design allows for its use in this entry pattern as well.

The unique needs of LPN/LVN-to-ADN students in this entry pattern center on the role transition required to move to the registered nursing scope of practice. The learning environment may shift from a more passive learning process to a more active learning process. Performance that was considered acceptable and competent in the LPN/LVN program is suddenly inadequate, as faculty foster independent thinking, problem solving, and self-directed learning in these students.

Time-out LPN/LVN-to-ADN Students

The time-out LPN/LVN-to-ADN student completes an LPN/LVN program and then works (or not) before embarking on the ADN program. The time out may be as short as 1 year or as long as a decade or more. Thus, the needs of these students are individualized according to the length of time out, whether the individual worked as an LPN/LVN and in what job role, and whether the individual is attending the same or a different school. This text is organized to enable the time-out LPN/LVN-to-ADN student to meet her or his individual needs.

• DIFFERENTIATING ADN STUDENT AND LPN/LVN PRACTICE ROLES

A difficulty encountered by most LPN/LVNs returning to school to pursue the ADN is the role confusion that emerges in the clinical setting. Emerson (2007) provides an overview of rights and responsibilities of students in the clinical setting. She notes that the student must abide by laws in that state, policies of the clinical agency, and of the nursing school. Often this means that procedures you are used to performing in your LPN/LVN practice are "off limits" in your new role. Issues of liability, legal parameters, and the level of autonomy can be confusing and problematic for the ADN student who is an LPN/LVN.

Issues of Liability

As a student in the ADN program, the LPN/LVN is bound by contract language in the agreement between the school and the clinical agency, policies of the clinical agency, policies of the ADN program, and course-by-course objectives and competencies in the curriculum. For example, the LPN/LVN may work at an agency other than that of the clinical assignment as an ADN student. Differences in policies, standardized procedures, and protocol between the two agencies may cause frustration for the student, particularly if she or he is still employed as an LPN/LVN on days alternating with the student experience and thus is operating out of two different agencies. As a second example, procedures the LPN/LVN performs regularly in her or his licensed practice because she or he has had additional training (eg, intravenous therapy) may be beyond the curriculum level or contract language for the course in which she or he is enrolled in the ADN program and not allowed. Keeping in close contact with the instructor at the clinical site and verifying interventions planned are essential when dealing with liability issues; it also helps minimize frustration.

Legal Aspects

In addition to these liability issues, several legal aspects must be considered by the LPN/LVN in the ADN student role. While in the student role, the LPN/LVN is not functioning as a licensed person but rather as a student in the ADN program. As such, she or he practices as all other program students within the legal parameters of that role. Handling controlled substances and signing for insulin, blood, and narcotics should be performed by the LPN/LVN in the student role under the same guidelines as such procedures would be performed by other nonlicensed ADN students.

Autonomy and Parameters for Instructor Supervision

LPN/LVNs in the ADN student role may also experience a feeling of loss of autonomy at the very time faculty are advocating increased autonomy in the RN role. In particular, the time-out LPN/LVN-to-ADN student who has gained clinical expertise and has been given increasing responsibilities in the practice setting may experience this loss the greatest. Patient assessment and nursing interventions that the LPN/LVN has been performing independently may now have to be done under the supervision of the instructor, such as procedures and medication administration. The instructor may also notice poor practices that need to be corrected, which can cause even further frustration. The LPN/LVN-to-ADN student must have a clear understanding of the level of independence allowed in relation to nursing care activities according to program policies and each course's clinical guidelines and must discuss areas of role conflict with the instructor.

NCLEX–RN *Might Ask*   5.2

The LPN/LVN-to-RN student nurse is assigned to a client in an ambulatory surgical setting. The LPN in this setting is held to the legal accountability of a(n)

   A. Layman.
   B. Student.
   C. LPN.
   D. RN.

· *See Appendix A for correct answer and rationale.*

● CONCLUSION

This chapter is built on information presented in previous chapters about ADN education programs. This chapter also examines adult learning theory and how you as an adult learner can enhance your success in the ADN program. The LPN/LVN and ADN education programs are compared in the areas of philosophies and conceptual models, curricular frameworks, curricular content and learning domains, learning achievement levels, nursing process and nursing diagnosis, and differences in the learning process.

Learning strategies for success are covered, including addressing your learning style; accommodating for disabilities; addressing differences in age, gender, sexual orientation, and cultural background; establishing self-directed goals; engaging in active learning activities; and adopting techniques to stimulate thinking. Transition needs unique to a variety of LPN/LVNs pursuing ADN education are also addressed, including a discussion of the difference in the licensed versus student roles played by these LPN/LVNs entering an ADN program.

student exercises

Obtain a school catalog or access an online catalog with course descriptions of the curricula for the ADN program you are planning to enter (or have entered). Review nursing and non-nursing course titles, course descriptions, and breakdown of lecture and laboratory time spent in each course. In the following space, write key concepts or phrases from the course descriptions that indicate learning you will gain in each of the three learning domains as you complete course work for the program.

LEARNING DOMAIN	COURSE NUMBER	KEY CONCEPTS/PHRASES
1. Cognitive domain (knowledge)		
2. Affective domain (values, attitudes)		
3. Psychomotor domain (skills)		

References

Anderson, L. W., & Krathwohl, D. R. (Eds.). (2001). *A taxonomy for learning, teaching, and assessing: A revision of Bloom's taxonomy of educational objects*. New York, NY: Longman.

Bloom, B. S. (Ed.). (1956). *Taxonomy of educational objectives: The classification of educational goals*. New York, NY: David McKay.

Covey, S. R. (2004). *The 8th habit: From effectiveness to greatness*. New York, NY: Free Press.

Curry, B. D. (2008). Coping with returning to school. In R. Kearney-Nunnery (Ed.), *Advancing your career: Concepts of professional nursing* (Chapter 2). Philadelphia, PA: F.A. Davis.

Emerson, R. J. (2007). *Nursing education in the clinical setting*. St. Louis, MO: Mosby.

Kearney-Nunnery, R. (2008). *Advancing your career: Concepts of professional nursing*. Philadelphia, PA: F.A. Davis.

Longworth, N. (2003). *Lifelong learning in action: Transforming education in the 21st century*. New York, NY: Routledge/Falmer.

Merriam-Webster OnLine (n.d.)

Masters, K. (2005). *Role development in professional nursing practice*. Boston, MA: Jones & Bartlett.

McAuliffe, G. (2006). The evolution of professional competence. In C. Hare (Ed.), *Adult development and learning* (Chapter 21). Oxford, UK: Oxford University Press.

National Association for Practical Nurse Educators and Service (NAPNES). (2007). *Standards of practice and educational competencies of graduates of practical/vocational nursing programs*. Silver Spring, MD: Author.

National Council of State Boards of Nursing. (2009). *Report of findings from the 2008 RN practice analysis: Linking the NCLEX-RN examination to practice*. Chicago, IL: Author.

National Council of State Boards of Nursing. (2009). *2010 NCLEX-RN Test Plan National Council Licensure Examination for Registered Nurses (NCLEX-RN Examination)*. Chicago, IL: Author.

National Council of State Boards of Nursing (2010). *2011 NCLEX-PN test plan: Test plan for the National Council Licensure Examination for Practical/Vocational nurses (NCLEX-Plan Examination)*. Chicago, IL: Author.

National League for Nursing. (2004). *Educational competencies for graduates of associate degree nursing programs*. New York, NY: Author.

Norwich, B. (2008). *Dilemmas of difference, inclusion, and disability: International perspectives and future directions*. London, UK: Routledge Taylor and Francis Group.

Santrock, J. W., & Halonen, J. S. (2010). *Your guide to college success: Strategies for achieving your goals*. Boston, MA: Wadsworth Cengage Learning.

Sather, S. E. (2009). *Leading professional learning teams*. Thousand Oaks, CA: Corwin.

Taylor, C., Lillis, C., LeMone, P., & Dynn, P. (2008). *Fundamentals of nursing: The art and science of nursing care* (5th ed.). Philadelphia, PA: Lippincott Williams & Wilkins.

Weimer, M. (2002). *Learner-centered teaching: Five key changes to practice*. San Francisco, CA: Jossey-Bass.

Wlodkowski, R. (1999). *Enhancing adult motivation to learn: A comprehensive guide for teaching all adults* (Rev. ed.). San Francisco, CA: Jossey-Bass.

Suggested Reading

Bloom, B. S. (Ed.). (1974). *The taxonomy of educational objectives: Affective and cognitive domains*. New York, NY: David McKay.

Browne, M. N., & Keeley, S. (2000). *Striving for excellence in college: Tips for active learning*. Upper Saddle River, NJ: Prentice-Hall.

Carter, C. (2002). *Keys to college studying: Becoming a lifelong learner*. Upper Saddle River, NJ: Prentice-Hall.

Carter, C., Bishop, J., Bixby, M., & Kravitz, S. L. (2001). *Keys to study skills: Opening doors to learning*. Upper Saddle River, NJ: Prentice-Hall.

Covey, S. R. (2004). *The 8th habit: From effectiveness to greatness*. New York, NY: Free Press.

National League for Nursing, Council of Associate Degree Programs. (1990). *Educational outcomes of associate degree nursing programs: Roles and competencies*. New York, NY: Author.

National League for Nursing, Council of Practical Nursing Programs. (1999). *Entry-level competencies of graduates of educational programs in practical nursing*. New York, NY: Author.

Tileston, D. W. (2000). *10 best teaching practices: How brain research, learning styles, and standards define teaching competencies*. Thousand Oaks, CA: Corwin Press.

On the (WEB)   *www.m-w.com:* Merriam-Webster OnLine. (Last accessed 7.6.2011).

www.ncsbn.org: National Council of State Boards of Nursing. (Last accessed 7.6.2011).

www.nlnac.org: National League for Nursing Accreditation Commission. (Last accessed 7.6.2011).

www.nsna.org: National Student Nurses Association. (Last accessed 7.6.2011).

6

Individualizing a Plan for Role Transition

● **LEARNING OUTCOMES**

By the end of this chapter, the student will be able to:

1 Assess preparedness for the student role based on information learned in previous chapters.

2 Describe learning style(s) based on information learned in previous chapters.

3 Assess your own uniqueness as an adult learner based on information learned in previous chapters.

4 Identify prior cognitive, affective, and psychomotor learning achieved through formal education and experience.

5 Design a personal education plan (PEP) to enhance success in the ADN program.

6 Apply concepts learned to establish an effective instructor–student partnership.

● KEY TERMS

experiential learning	mutual goal setting	standardized test
feedback mechanism	nonstandardized test	strategic learner
instructor–student	personal education	student success
partnership	plan (PEP)	strategy
mentor	proactive learner	time management

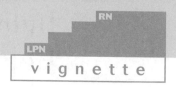

vignette

Sherry Williams is an LPN in her first semester of ADN school and is meeting with her nursing advisor. Sherry has opted to take an advanced placement course via the Internet and is not sure where to start with a needs assessment that she has been assigned to perform.

ADVISOR: Hi, Sherry. Thank you for scheduling an appointment with me. I enjoy seeing my students, but sometimes they don't come in until after the first exam. How can I help you?

SHERRY: I see you have sent me a needs assessment. I'm not sure why we are doing this, and I'm a little intimidated with the length of the form. Can you help me understand why I'm doing this and how to do it?

ADVISOR: Because you have opted to take the advanced placement course for LVNs via the web, the faculty wants to tailor your course so that it concentrates on your needs. For example, if you're a whiz at math, we want to spend less time on that and more on, say, nursing planning—especially if your exposure to that has been minimal in your current position.

SHERRY: So, this is similar to how we deal with teaching a patient with diabetes. If the client and family know about insulins and can return demonstrate an injection, we might concentrate more on their diet, especially if blood sugars aren't under control.

ADVISOR: Exactly. We realize that our students in this course come from a wide variety of backgrounds. Some haven't been in school for years, some have been away for only a few years, and some are fresh out of LPN school.

SHERRY: I didn't realize that. I guess it is sort of like a new employee working at our nursing home. Everyone comes with different experiences, and being new, you have to get adjusted. We have learned a lot from people just out of school as well as from other workplaces.

ADVISOR: The same will be true with this course. I will send everyone a list of course participants' e-mail addresses so that even though you won't meet each other face to face, you can "talk" to each other online. I hope this will help you share experiences.

SHERRY: Okay, now on to the assessment...

ADVISOR: The reason this is so in-depth is that it makes you think about what you are good at. Perhaps you are an expert at administering tube feedings or inserting urinary catheters but need more help with fluid and electrolytes or medication theory. If so, we can concentrate more on these topics, and you may want to attend the parallel course that meets here on campus for more hands-on work in the lab or more classroom work as needed.

SHERRY: I see now. It's all falling into place... I think I can take it from here.

ADVISOR: Great. Let's do the first page together. You can either finish outside my office and hand it in now or you can mail or e-mail it to me in a day or two.

SHERRY: I have to pick my kids up now, so I will e-mail it to you by tomorrow. Thanks for your help.

Throughout Unit I, we explore the concepts of transition and change. Chapter 1 discusses lifelong learning and your return to school. Chapter 2 examines role development and transition, including the phases of role transition and how they apply to you as you move from the role of an LPN/LVN to that of an RN. Chapter 3 discusses the process of change, the effects of change, and ways to adjust to change. In applying these concepts to your LPN/LVN-to-RN role transition, you have looked at the positive outcomes you will experience in the change process.

Chapter 4 provides you with a historical account of the transitions that have been experienced in the discipline of nursing, including the evolution of ADN. Chapter 5 focuses on learning at the ADN level and how it differs from LPN/LVN training.

In Chapter 6, you are given the opportunity to apply knowledge gained from these preceding chapters to yourself, assess prior knowledge and experience, and design a personal education plan (PEP) specific to your individual needs. You will assess your preparedness for the student role, examine your learning style, and reflect on the unique characteristics and needs you bring to the ADN program. As described in Chapter 1, and noted by Campbell, Cignetti, Melenyzer, Nettles, and Wyman (2011), the PEP you develop in this chapter can become part of your portfolio as you meet with your nursing adviser to plan for your return to school and success in pursuit of your RN.

Several methods for assessing your theoretical and experiential knowledge and abilities are discussed in this chapter, and you will also use these in developing your PEP at the end of this chapter (Display 6.1) to enhance success in the ADN program and on the NCLEX-RN, which you will take after you complete the ADN program.

Also presented in Chapter 6 is a discussion of the instructor–student partnership. Strategies for fostering a successful partnership are explored, as are techniques for individualizing your learning activities and strengthening your clinical practicum in the ADN program. Such concepts as mutual goal setting and feedback mechanisms are presented, and as part of your PEP development, you will outline areas for discussion with your faculty advisor at your individual conference.

• ASSESSING PREPAREDNESS FOR THE STUDENT ROLE

The first step in individualizing a plan for role transition is to examine your preparedness for the student role, as discussed in Chapter 1. If you just recently completed the LPN/LVN nursing program or have been recently completing course work and receiving academic advising in preparing for the ADN program, you may

| display **6.1** | **Personal Education Plan for Successful LPN/LVN-to-RN Role Transition** |

Name _____   Date _____

School I will be attending

Review the Thinking Critically sections of the chapter, and use your written responses to complete the following plan.

I. Action Plan: Preparedness for the Student Role

A. Overcoming re-entry barriers

Examine the demographics of the ADN program you will enter (eg, ages, gender mix, culture diversity, and generic vs. advance placed members).

1. Identify strengths you will bring to the class based on your personal uniqueness and how these can be used.

_____
_____
_____
_____
_____
_____
_____
_____
_____

2. Identify potential barriers you anticipate, based on your personal uniqueness (eg, cultural background, fears, and self-confidence) and your plan to overcome these potential barriers.

_____
_____
_____
_____
_____
_____
_____
_____

B. Preparing for the school setting
   1. List the areas with which you need to locate and familiarize yourself on campus. Obtain a campus map, and plot a self-guided tour.

_____

_____

_____

_____

_____

_____

_____

_____

_____

   2. List the campus processes or systems with which you need to familiarize yourself and who you need to see or where you need to go to obtain information.

_____

_____

_____

_____

_____

_____

_____

_____

Process/System	Who or Where

3. List the library and research skills you need to acquire to become oriented to the library and to use it effectively. Be sure to include online services.

_____

_____

_____

_____

_____

_____

_____

_____

_____

_____

C. Developing student success strategies

1. List the texts and other resources you will need to buy or borrow to prepare for the nursing program.

_____

_____

_____

_____

_____

_____

_____

_____

2. List the traits (characteristics) and roles of mentors and study groups that will enhance your success at the ADN level.

_____

_____

_____

_____

_____

_____

_____

_____

Mentor Traits   **Mentor Roles**

_____

_____

_____

_____

_____

_____

_____

_____

_____

_____

Study Group Traits   **Study Group Roles**

_____

_____

_____

_____

_____

_____

_____

_____

D. Time management

Write down your action plan for effective time management as you transition to the student role. Include elements of the win/win agreements you established with significant others.

_____

_____

_____

_____

_____

_____

_____

_____

_____

_____

II. Action Plan for Needed Course Work

List all course work needed to complete ADN requirements and college graduation requirements. Note course work completed or in progress. If course work was completed at another school or if you received equivalency or advance standing credit, indicate course(s) or experience for which you were granted that status. For course work needed, indicate the term and year you plan to take each course.

Nursing and Graduation Requirements	Course Completed Name of School	Course Planned
At This School (Term/Year) (IP = In Progress)	Another School Equivalency (Course, School)	Term/Year (IP = In Progress)

already feel comfortable with or settled into the student role. In assessing your preparedness for the student role, four areas of preparedness should be examined:

- The re-entry process
- The school setting
- Student success strategies
- Time management

Re-entry Process

For those who have been away from the educational setting for some time or who have acquired their LPN/LVN license in a pathway other than formal education (eg, military or other service experience), moving into the college student role may feel awkward and uncomfortable. It is important to find out the demographics of the ADN program you plan to enter to know how your characteristics and biases will fit with the class you will enter. What have the age, gender, and ethnic distributions of classes been during the last few years at this nursing school? How many other LPN/LVNs will be entering this class, and what percentage of the class as a whole will be represented by the LPN/LVN constituency? Are the LPN/LVNs in this group advanced placement, straight-through, or time-out students (as described in Chapter 5)?

thinking critically

Write down how you are similar to and different from the typical student in the ADN program you will enter. Consider age, gender, ethnicity, and nursing experience. In areas in which you are different, cite strengths you will bring to the class to enhance others' learning, and identify actions you can take to develop comfort with the re-entry process. (Save this information for use in designing your PEP.)

The School Setting

Feeling prepared to enter (or re-enter) the school setting develops self-confidence and comfort in the student role. "Knowing the ropes" or knowing where to find things on campus and how to function within the processes and systems of the school can assist you in this process. Chapter 1 describes strategies for success in the student role. Ask yourself these questions: Do you have a campus map? Do you know the location of such areas as counseling, registration, student services, health center, child care services (if needed), nursing office, library, computer lab, and bookstore? Do you know how to register for classes, apply for financial aid or scholarships, and seek assistance for disabilities or for tutoring? Do you know how to use the library, research a topic, and use online systems and the Cumulative Index for Nursing and Allied Health Literature (CINAHL) to locate periodical (journal) articles? If you do not have a computer, do you know where on campus you can access one to complete an assignment? Do you know where and how to access copying services? Are there any orientation sessions, printed materials, or student success courses you can take to prepare yourself better for the school setting? How much of the above can you access online to develop familiarity with such resources prior to arriving on campus?

Student Success Strategies

As described in previous chapters, many strategies can be used to support your success in the ADN program. Preparing for the student role involves identifying student success strategies that meet your individual needs and with which you feel comfortable. A variety of student success strategies follow.

Take a moment to reflect on the previous questions. Write down several actions you can take to prepare yourself better for the student setting. (Save this information for use in designing your PEP.)

LEARNING TECHNIQUES

Have you developed effective learning techniques and study skills to be successful in this more complex ADN course work? Meeting objectives and achieving learning outcomes and competencies identified for this program will necessitate that you not only gain knowledge, comprehension, and the ability to apply content learned but that you also analyze data, draw conclusions, use judgment, synthesize information, and make decisions by thinking critically about course content during learning activities. Critical thinking and clinical decision making are discussed later in this text. What learning techniques do you possess, and what resources have you developed to support you in this process?

BECOMING A PROACTIVE LEARNER

Have you learned how to be a proactive learner? The proactive learner seeks experiences to add knowledge, skills, and abilities to her or his expertise. Carter, Bishop, and Kravitz (2002) identified techniques for becoming a lifelong learner, describing the "strategic learner" as one who puts her/himself into new learning situations to help achieve one's identified goals. They noted that knowledge in every field is doubling every 2 to 3 years. This is certainly true in nursing! Thus, lifelong learning is essential. One must become self-directed, resourceful, and a critical and creative thinker. Carter et al. (2011) provide tools to assist the student in developing 21st Century workplace skills, including the use of social media and strategies for applying that learned to workplace situations, using analytical, creative, and practical skills. Are you taking advantage of college resources, Web resources, college orientation and success courses, and textbooks to access these learning opportunities in alignment with your goals? Are you assessing those clinical skills you will want to seek once you are in the clinical setting to brush up on your techniques? These are all aspects of becoming a proactive learner.

Assess your study skills and resources. Identify those you possess and those you need to develop to support yourself in the ADN program. Are you a strategic learner? What can you do to develop yourself in this area? (Save this information for use in designing your PEP.)

DEVELOPING MENTORS

In addition to study skills and resource materials, developing mentors and participating in study groups are strategies that increase your chances of success. Sinetar

(1998) described mentoring as "the act of encouragement." Vance and Olson (1998) discussed the "mentor connection" in nursing:

> We believe that mentoring is essential to our full development as human beings and as professionals. It is possible, of course, to have a productive career without a significant mentor, but mentoring promotes career success faster and easier. Mentor relationships have a profound impact on self and career development. Mentor relationships shape and nourish us. They have the capacity to transform the path of our human journey. (p. 3)

A mentor is someone with whom you can consult, who will give you advice, and who will counsel, guide, and help you in the learning process. More advanced students, program graduates, instructional aides, and learning resource specialists are examples of people who may be appropriate mentors for you. A good mentor will be honest with you, assist you in times when you are "stuck," and offer you moral support when you are discouraged, frustrated, or have lost confidence. Huston (2006) describes the importance of a mentor to remove barriers and "fight for you," as well as pointing out your strengths at important times to build confidence.

Much has been written in recent years about the value of mentoring, especially in today's world where information changes rapidly and job turnover often occurs every 2 to 3 years. Fletcher (2000) defined mentoring as

> the potential of a one-to-one professional relationship that can simultaneously empower and enhance practice. Mentoring means guiding and supporting trainees to ease them through difficult transitions; it is about soothing the way, enabling, reassuring as well as directing, managing, and instructing. It should unlock the ways to change by building self-confidence, self-esteem and a readiness to act as well as to engage in ongoing constructive interpersonal relationships. (p. 1)

When choosing a mentor, you must decide on qualities in prospective mentors that will enhance your success based on your individual learning style and personality. An individual who is a good mentor for one student may be a poor one for another. For example, do you want a mentor who will challenge you with prodding questions about program content or one who will act as a sounding board for your ideas? Do you want a mentor who will be nurturing and offer words of encouragement or one who will challenge you and assist you in disciplining yourself to study? What role(s) do you want your mentor to play?

Choosing a mentor is another area in which you need to be proactive. Duff (1999) emphasized the importance of

- Women mentoring women as career professionals with job and personal lives
- Not "waiting" for a mentor to appear, but rather taking the initiative to seek a mentor
- Overcoming the fear of appearing demanding, needy, or weak or the fear of being rejected
- Choosing a mentor you admire, respect, can confide in, and whose values are those with which you feel comfortable

You should not be hesitant to ask a new program graduate or experienced RN to be your mentor. In fact, the nurse you ask will most likely be honored and will gain as much from the mentor–mentee relationship as you will.

STUDY GROUPS

Forming or joining a study group can greatly enhance thinking, problem-solving, and decision-making skills. However, selecting or forming a study group must take into account your preference(s) for learning. The ground rules for the study group must be clear. For example, does each member read all material and then discuss it with the group, or does each member take a portion of the assignment and then present or teach it to the others? Will the purpose of the study group be to meet frequently and discuss the content or infrequently bringing only answered questions or problems to the group? What will be the format of the sessions? How small or large will it be? These questions must be addressed early in the process to avoid conflict and ensure the time spent enhances your learning.

thinking critically

Think about the type of learning required in an ADN program and the strengths and growth needed to achieve this learning level. On a piece of paper, make a large box with four quadrants. Label each of the four quadrants as follows: mentor characteristics, mentor role, study group characteristics, and study group role. Fill in each box, and examine your results. Do you know anyone who will meet your needs to be your mentor? Do you know classmates with whom you might work well in a study group? (Save this information for use in designing your PEP.)

Time Management

A last important area to examine in assessing your preparedness for the student role is the area of time management. Often, the LPN/LVN entering an ADN program must balance a number of roles, such as spouse, parent, student, worker, and community citizen. The nursing program can be demanding at times. As discussed in Chapter 1, preparing for the student role involves such time management success strategies as balancing personal, career, and student roles; reassessing commitments to committees, boards, and service groups; and enlisting the support of significant others through the use of win/win agreements.

Covey, Merrill, and Merrill (1994) advocated completing a weekly time map that includes your goals and highest priorities for each of your roles (worker, spouse, parent, community service person, student, etc.) so that the most important tasks are accomplished rather than just the urgent ones. This will minimize feeling like you are operating in a crisis mode and the likelihood of your neglecting one or more important roles. For further reading on time management, see Chapter 14.

thinking critically

On a sheet of paper, identify your roles, group commitments, and significant others. Write an action plan for time management that takes into account these three items and the win/win agreements you developed in Chapter 1. (Save this action plan for use in designing your PEP.)

● ASSESSING LEARNING STYLE

The second step in individualizing a plan for transition from the LPN/LVN to the ADN level is to assess your learning style. In previous chapters, you learned about the characteristics of adult learners and that we each learn best in different ways. Some people are visual learners, whereas others are auditory learners. Some learn best through teaching strategies in which the learner uses manipulative skills or body kinetic (motion) or kinesthetic (sensory) approaches to learn course content. Take a moment and review the four styles of learners presented in Chapter 1 and the characteristics of adult learners discussed throughout Unit 1.

thinking critically

Based on material learned and exercises completed in Chapter 1 and reflecting on learning activities that have been the most helpful to you in the past, assess and write in your own words a description of your learning style. Give examples of learning activities that fit your learning style. (Save this information for use in designing your PEP.)

● THE REFLECTIVE PROCESS: ASSESSING ADULT LEARNER UNIQUENESS

The third step in individualizing a plan for role transition is to identify your unique characteristics as an adult learner. In Chapter 5, you learned about the characteristics of adult learners and driving forces that motivate such learners in the educational setting. Adult learners bring with them to the educational setting a variety of personal and professional life experiences. Bastable (2008) emphasizes the importance of assessing learning needs, including knowledge gaps, and being aware of learning styles. She notes that it is also important for the learner to be exposed to different methods of learning methods so that it will be less stressful in future situations. Friend and Bursuck (2009) stress the need to also include any special needs you have as you develop your PEP.

Each adult learner has developed values, biases, and fears; each is motivated by her or his own unique driving forces. Each has identified personal and career goals that guide her or him in the learning process. As you transition to the RN role you will assume more of a leadership role where others will be taking directions from you and following your lead. In order to assume a lead role, it is important to see yourself in that role. As you begin your transition from the LPN/LVN to the RN role, how do you view yourself? Can you see yourself in the lead role?

thinking critically

Reflect on yourself as an adult learner. Write down specific areas of nursing expertise you believe that you have developed in the practice of nursing, things that motivate you to learn in classroom and clinical settings, and personal goals you hope to achieve by participating in the ADN program. (Save this information for use in designing your PEP.)

• ASSESSING PRIOR LEARNING: STANDARDIZED AND NONSTANDARDIZED TESTS

The fourth step in individualizing a plan for role transition from the LPN/LVN to the ADN level is to assess your prior learning. You acquire knowledge, skills, and abilities in the cognitive, affective, and psychomotor domains through formal education and experiential learning processes. (For a discussion of the three learning domains, refer to Chapter 5.)

In addition to a review of transcripts for course work completed, assessment tests are available to assist you in assessing your knowledge base and to guide you as you pursue a career as an RN. Many standardized tests are available for individual use, and many nursing schools use standardized or nonstandardized tests for assessment and selection purposes. A standardized test has undergone numerous validity and reliability research studies to ensure that content is valid and unbiased and that test takers would provide the same answers if the same test was administered again or by a different test administrator. It has also been administered to several populations, resulting in available normative data (information on the norms from various populations of test takers). Standardized tests are often published by formal organizations and are usually copyrighted. In contrast, nonstandardized tests are locally prepared (often by a teacher or school) and may contain regional questions.

Assessment Tests for General Education

Many standardized tests are available to assess reading, writing, and mathematical computation skills. Most 2-year colleges require some form of general education assessment in their college admissions process. You will need to find out if any tests are required by the college or your nursing program. Some commonly used tests are as follows:

ACT	American College Test
SAT	Scholastic Achievement Test
TABE	Test of Adult Basic Education
NET	Nurse Entrance Test
DET	Diagnostic Entrance Test
RNEE	Registered Nurse Entrance Exam
COMPASS	Computer Adaptive Placement Assessment and Support System
TOEFL	Test of English as a Foreign Language

Some of these tests can be taken more than once, and many have workbooks, textbooks, and workshops for preparing for the exam that are available on the Internet and may be available at the college bookstore. Conley (2005) noted that students must be academically prepared to be successful in college and that re-entry students may not do as well in general education classes as those straight out of high school. General education test preparation workbooks, textbooks, and workshops can strengthen your knowledge base as you return to school.

Subject Area Assessment Tests for Nursing and Support Curricula

Assessment tests are available to assist LPN/LVNs in assessing knowledge in specific nursing curricular areas. Test areas include nursing fundamentals, medical–surgical nursing, obstetric nursing, pediatric nursing, nutrition, pharmacology, anatomy and physiology, microbiology, and the behavioral sciences. Your nursing school may require some of these, but you also may want to take some of these on your own. Professional organizations (eg, NLN and ANA) and the private sector (eg, American College Testing and College-Level Examination Program) have assessment tests for specific subject areas in the discipline of nursing.

Integrated Nursing Assessment Tests

Many books have been written on test-taking strategies. Nugent and Vitale (2008) have provided excellent suggestions for nursing students on how to take multiple-choice tests. Because many tests you will take during your ADN education (and ultimately the NCLEX-RN) are in this format, it may help you to examine your skill in this area. The author's suggestions include how to read questions well, understand the intent of the question, and eliminate answer choices as a result, in order to select the correct answer. Other strategies for test-taking can be found in your college library or learning resource center as well as online. More specific examples of types of test questions are covered in Chapter 7.

Nursing Review Tests

An additional self-evaluation technique LPN/LVNs have found useful in assessing their prior learning in preparation for role transition to the ADN level is published review texts. Subject-specific and integrated nursing review texts are available, providing you with the opportunity not only to assess strong and weak areas in your knowledge base but also to practice answering multiple-choice test questions in preparation for the nursing program and the NCLEX-RN, which you will take after you complete the ADN program.

---

thinking critically

Examine the course work in the ADN program for which you will receive challenge or equivalency credit (or beyond which you will be advance placed). Reflecting on your own learning needs identify in writing the methods or tests you would like to use and those required by your nursing program to assess your prior learning in nursing. Contact your school's nursing department, counseling office, bookstore, or testing center to determine the process for accessing the assessment tests you have identified. (Save this information for use in designing your PEP.)

● INSTRUCTOR–STUDENT PARTNERSHIP

Throughout this chapter, you have worked through several Thinking Critically exercises for self-assessment. In preparing to develop your PEP, you have assessed your preparedness for the student role, learning style, adult learner uniqueness, and prior learning. As you use this information to design your plan, another area to consider will be the instructor–student partnership. Wlodkowski (1999) stated, "For most adults, the first sense of the quality of the teacher–student relationship will be a feeling, sometimes quite vague, of inclusion or exclusion. Upon awareness of exclusion, adult learners will begin to lose their enthusiasm and motivation" (p. 90). The culturally responsive teacher will utilize what Wlodkowski and Ginsberg (2003) describe as a motivational framework, which includes four intersecting motivational goals: establishing inclusion, developing attitude, enhancing meaning, and engendering competence. For this reason, it is important to establish a positive rapport with your faculty advisor early in the program. Your relationship with your faculty advisor will be critical for all of these four motivational goals and will serve as a positive resource to you if you are struggling during the program.

The goal of the instructor–student partnership is the growth and success of the student. The more the instructor understands your learning style, strengths, areas for growth, and individual uniqueness, the more the partnership will be able to meet your learning needs. Lofmark and Wikblad (2001) studied nursing students to determine from their view which factors facilitated and which obstructed learning in clinical practice and reported the following results:

> The students emphasized responsibility and independence, opportunities to practice different tasks, and receiving feedback as facilitating factors. Others perceived promoting factors included perceptions of control of the situation and understanding of the "total picture." Examples of obstructing factors were the nurses as supervisors not relying on the students, supervision that lacked continuity, and lack of opportunities to practice. Perception of their own insufficiency and low self-reliance were drawbacks for some students. (p. 43)

Do you share some of these same perceptions?

Scheele (2005) noted that returning students often make one of two errors: either overplaying their role by reminding instructors that they too have experience or underplaying it (acting dumb). Scheele stated,

> While returning students might feel they should be more equal in status to the faculty, they are still dependent on advice and guidance. So in many ways they are equivalent to the traditional student and should not lead with a sense of their greater maturity. On the other hand, if you are a returning student, you should not make the mistake, out of fear of failing, of falling back into a completely subservient student role. It is easy to regress from your actual age of thirty or forty to become, in effect, an anxious adolescent, reverting to the emotional age you were when you were last in school. These errors are easy to fall into, but they are still a costly mistake. Accept your student status, but preserve your mature adult self. (p. 27)

Meeting with your instructor/advisor early and sharing your PEP, including information about how you learn best, your fears, your goals, barriers to overcome, accommodations needed, clinical experiences needed, and methods of feedback that are most helpful to you, will maximize the ability of your partnership with the instructor to reach its goal: your success. This is also an opportunity to share with the instructor your strengths, your clinical and life experiences and the contributions you can make to the class and learning experience. Last, you can each determine how to contact each other (phone, e-mail, etc.) in case the need arises.

● CONCLUSION

In this chapter, you have been presented with the opportunity to apply knowledge gained from the preceding chapters to yourself. You've been asked to assess prior knowledge and experience and design a PEP specific to your individual needs. Assessing your preparedness for the student role, examining your learning style, and reflecting on the unique characteristics and needs you bring to the ADN program are critical for your success. The PEP you develop in this chapter can become part of your portfolio as you meet with your nursing adviser to plan for the successful pursuit of your RN.

Several methods for assessing your theoretical and experiential knowledge and abilities were discussed in this chapter, and you were asked to use these in developing your PEP (Display 6.1). These should enhance your success in the ADN program and on the NCLEX-RN, which you will take after you complete the ADN program.

Finally, the discussion of the instructor–student partnership and strategies for fostering a successful partnership were explored, as were techniques for individualizing your learning activities and strengthening your clinical practicum in the ADN program. Your success will depend on you focusing on the concepts of mutual goal setting and feedback mechanisms as they were presented, and as part of your PEP development. With these tools in hand you should have everything you need for building a successful and mutually satisfying instructor–student partnership.

student exercises

1. Now that you have completed the Thinking Critically sections of this chapter, you are ready to develop your PEP (Display 6.1). Gather all exercises you have completed throughout the text for entry into your PEP and complete all sections.

2. Schedule an appointment with your instructor/advisor to review the PEP, and you have already made some great first steps toward success in your new role as you embark on the transition to professional registered nursing practice!

References

Bastable, S. B. (2008). *Nurse as educator: Principles of teaching and learning for nursing practice* (3rd. ed). Sudbury, MA: Jones and Bartlett.

Campbell, D. M., Cignetti, P. B., Melenyzer, B. J., Nettles, D. H., & Wyman, R. M., Jr. (2011). *How to develop a professional portfolio: A manual for teachers* (5th ed.). Boston, MA: Pearson.

Carter, C., Bishop, J., & Kravitz, S. L. (2002). *Keys to college studying: Becoming a lifelong learner.* Upper Saddle River, NJ: Prentice-Hall.

Carter, C., Bishop, J., & Kravitz, S. L. (2011). *Keys to success: Building analytical, creative, and practical skills.* (7th ed.). Upper Saddle River, NJ: Prentice-Hall.

Conley, D. T. (2005). *College knowledge: What it really takes for students to succeed and what we can do to get them ready.* San Francisco, CA: Jossey-Bass.

Covey, S. R., Merrill, A. R., & Merrill, R. R. (1994). *First things first: To live, to love, to leave a legacy.* New York, NY: Simon & Schuster.

Duff, C. S. (1999). *Learning from other women: How to benefit from the knowledge, wisdom, and experience of female mentors.* New York, NY: AMACOM, American Management Association.

Fletcher, S. (2000). *Mentoring in schools: A handbook of good practice.* London, UK: Kogan Page.

Friend, M., & Bursuck, W. D. (2009). *Including students with special needs: A practical guide for classroom teachers* (5th ed.). Upper Saddle River, NJ: Pearson.

Huston, C. J. (2006). *Professional issues in nursing: Challenges and opportunities.* Philadelphia, PA: Lippincott Williams & Wilkins.

Lofmark, N. J., & Wikblad, K. (2001). Facilitating and obstructing factors for development of learning in clinical practice: A student perspective. *Journal of Advanced Nursing, 34*(1), 43–50.

Nugent, P. M., & Vitale, B. A. (2008). *Test success: Test-taking techniques for beginning nursing students* (5th ed.). Philadelphia, PA: F.A. Davis.

Scheele, A. M. (2005). *Launch your career in college: Strategies for students, educators, and parents.* Westport, CT: Praeger.

Sinetar, M. (1998). *The mentor's spirit: Life lessons on leadership and the art of encouragement.* New York, NY: St. Martin's Press.

Vance, C., & Olson, R. K. (Eds.). (1998). *The mentor connection in nursing.* New York, NY: Springer.

Wlodkowski, R. (1999). *Enhancing adult motivation to learn: A comprehensive guide for teaching all adults* (Rev. ed.). San Francisco, CA: Jossey-Bass.

Wlodkowski, R. J., & Ginsberg, M. B. (2003). *Diversity and motivation: Culturally responsive teaching.* San Francisco, CA: Jossey-Bass.

Suggested Reading

Brown, H., & Edelmann, R. (2000). Project 2000: A study of expected and experienced stressors and support reported by students and qualified nurses. *Journal of Advanced Nursing, 31*(4), 857–864.

Kolb, A. Y., & Kolb, D. A. (2005). Learning styles and learning spaces: Enhancing experiential learning in higher education. *Academy of Management Learning and Education, 42*(3), 193–212.

Palmer, P. J. (1998). *The courage to teach: Exploring the inner landscape of a teacher's life.* San Francisco, CA: Jossey-Bass.

On the (**WEB**)   *www.daytracker.com:* A good site for organizational calendars. (Last accessed 7.6.2011).

www.aamn.org: American Association for Men in Nursing. (Last accessed 7.6.2011).

www.back2college.com: A Web site with answers to frequently asked questions for individuals returning to school. (Last accessed 7.6.2011).

7

Test Success for the LPN: Challenge of NCLEX-RN Questions

● LEARNING OUTCOMES

By the end of this chapter, the student will be able to:

1 Describe the benefits of CAT.

2 List the four main categories of client needs according to the NCLEX-RN test blueprint.

3 Describe the components of a test question.

4 Identify the differences between the NCLEX-PN and the NCLEX-RN.

5 Identify the complexity of questions used from knowledge through analysis.

6 Understand why alternate questions are used.

7 Develop a plan for success on exams using before-, during-, and after-test strategies.

● KEY TERMS

acronym	computerized adaptive	NCLEX-RN blueprint
acrostic	testing (CAT)	reciprocal teaching
alternate item formats	correct option	test distracter
analysis questions	knowledge questions	test item
application questions	metacognition	test option
comprehension	mnemonics	test stem
questions	NCLEX-RN	

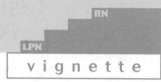

vignette

Randy Caruthers has been an LVN for 15 years and is a serious, hardworking student. He has sacrificed financially by going part time to complete his schooling. It worries him that he has given up time with his 5-year-old son to complete his course requirements. He has just received the results of his first nursing test and is dismayed to see that he is barely passing. He is confused about what to do and where to start first. He approaches his course professor with a bewildered and frustrated look.

RANDY: What is it with these nursing tests? I have an A average in all my other courses, and with the time I put into this, I believe that I should have had a better grade!

PROFESSOR: You seem angry and upset! And I know you need to work through these feelings, but I'm not the enemy. I am here to help.

RANDY: You bet I'm angry. I've been working at this for over 3 years! And now, I don't know whether I can do this!

PROFESSOR: What we need to do, Randy, is to sit down and look at your test together. I know that you attended the test review after the test, and I know that you take your studies seriously. But we need to channel that anger and frustration into action. Together we can assess your strengths and needs, look at your current study habits, and develop a plan that might help you be more successful. As with the nursing process though, the first step is to assess your needs.

RANDY: I was relying on this first test to help increase my average in the course. Come to think of it…I didn't do very well on my PN tests either. I sure would appreciate the extra help.

The situation Randy and his professor are engaged in is an event that plays out many times in nursing schools throughout the United States. Test taking is an anxiety-producing situation for both the test taker and the test designer. In a fast-paced world where students carry such heavy personal and professional loads, failure to live up to expectations on an exam can take a heavy toll on the student's psychosocial state and future. No one wants a student to fail. Entry into nursing school is competitive. The nursing school has a vested interest in not only the recruitment but also the retention of students. Students often need help to be successful, and there are many tools available to aid them. To help increase the odds of success, we have developed this chapter to review the development of the NCLEX-RN and its test blueprint. We will describe the wording used in a test item, identify components of Bloom's Taxonomy of Educational Objectives, and describe helpful hints to take those difficult nursing tests with more accuracy and confidence. To do this, we walk you through what to do before, during, and after a test.

● DEVELOPMENT OF THE NCLEX-RN

It is important to review the history of the NCLEX-RN development to aid the student in understanding why nursing tests are different from other college examinations. As an LVN/LPN, you are familiar with the testing processes used in nursing. However, if you have not graduated recently, you may not be aware of changes that have been made to the NCLEX. In this section, we review a brief historical development of the NCLEX-RN and computerized adaptive testing (CAT), as well as how the NCLEX adapts to an ever-changing health care environment.

Historical Development of the NCLEX

Nursing has always used testing in one way or another to verify minimal safe standards at the bedside. Testing is designed for one main point: It ensures the public a safe practitioner. The NCLEX-RN is only one part of the critical information needed by the state board of nursing to issue a license to practice. "NCLEX-RN is administered to graduates of nursing school to test the knowledge, abilities, and skills necessary for entry-level safe and effective nursing practice" (Billings, 2011, p.2). Although the NCLEX is designed with safety in mind, it only tests minimal competency level (Display 7.1).

If you graduated in the 1960s to early 1990s, you are familiar with the paper-and-pencil style of the NCLEX-PN. As a PN, you have already established a minimum competency level by successfully passing the NCLEX-PN. To be a candidate for the NCLEX-PN, you had to take proficiency tests in school and graduate. After graduation, the date and time of the NCLEX-PN was given to you. To take the test, you had to physically sit with other graduates in a proctored setting in a large institution. Sometimes you had to wait weeks to months to take the exam. This was very stressful. It was also detrimental because it has been proven that the time from graduation to test taking has a negative impact on your success (Norton, Relf, Cox, Farlly, & Tucker, 2006). After the test, you had to wait weeks to months for your results. If you failed, you had to wait for the next sitting of the exam.

Obviously, this way of testing had many disadvantages. It took longer to test and longer to get results. The stress on the new graduate nurse was intense; you were in limbo for weeks waiting for results. The test took longer to grade because

---

display 7.1   **Important Points About the NCLEX-RN**

- The NCLEX-RN is designed to provide public assurance of a safe practitioner.
- The NCLEX-RN determines minimal competency level of an applicant.

each graduate PN answered the same amount of questions. The end result was that it took longer to produce functioning nurses in the field. At a time when more safe practitioners in the nursing field are critical, this system is not efficient enough.

COMPUTERIZED ADAPTIVE TESTING

In 1994, CAT was implemented for testing on the NCLEX-RN. This was the first time that the state boards of nursing used computers for testing. CAT allowed nursing graduates to be tested at multiple sites more frequently, therefore decreasing the "downtime" between graduation and taking or retaking the examination. CAT was different in that it was individualized and tailor made for the test taker. Each test question in CAT was, and still is, based on successfully answering the question before it. With CAT, if a candidate answers a question successfully, the next question is more difficult. If a candidate answers a question incorrectly, he or she gets an easier question next. The difficulty of test questions is predicated on answers given until the computer determines it has enough data to either pass or fail the student. Before CAT, a student could go back on a paper-and-pencil test and change an answer. With CAT, there is no "going back" to change an answer. The advantage of this is that the new graduate can get through the test faster. The minimum number of questions a test taker can receive is 75. Once the computer determines the minimum safe competency level, the test is ended (Display 7.2).

HOW QUESTIONS ARE FORMED AND CHANGED

The NCLEX-RN is revised every 3 years by a job analysis done by working RNs, educators, and managers. Skills, interventions, and critical incidents of the nursing practice are reviewed by the NCSBN through the National Council Examination Committee. This process supports the clinical relatedness and validity of the examination. The focus of the job analysis and committees is on the knowledge of graduate nurses who have an entry level of practice. Questions are written by pragmatic educators and put through a rigorous examination by the committee. Questions are then carefully added to the test pool for the NCLEX after trial use in the NCLEX exams. It is through this that the NCLEX-RN blueprint is reviewed and revised if needed. The NLN has just revised its test blue print

display **7.2** **Advantages of CAT Testing**

- Quick
- Individualized
- Multiple sites of administration
- Multiple times of administration
- Retake time is faster
- Time between graduation and first taking is faster

in 2010. You can see the blue print by visiting the NCSBN Web site at https://www.ncsbn.org/1287.htm

● MAIN CATEGORIES OF THE NCLEX-RN BLUEPRINT

The NCLEX-RN blueprint is similar to a blueprint for a house or building. Much like an architectural blueprint provides the direction or the step-by-step plan for the building, the NCLEX-RN blueprint is a roadmap the faculty and student can follow to determine priorities for content on a nursing exam. The NCLEX-RN test blueprint follows the nursing process but has four main categories of client needs. It is important for the student to know about the blueprint in order to anticipate the content, scope, and areas covered by test plans. Occasionally students will feel as if questions and nursing professors are "out to get 'em." If students are encouraged to visit the NCSBN and if faculty are willing to share their test plans, it goes a long way to settle nerves. Nursing instructors need to share the test blueprint with students before the test to enlist their understanding that the test examines important nursing concepts (McDonald, 2007). As an LPN/LVN, the same blueprint provided a path for faculty to follow in developing your exams.

Four Main Categories of Client Needs

The NCLEX-RN blueprint shows us four main "beams or trusses" that support the building of the NCLEX-RN test. These are described as main categories of client needs (Table 7.1). Students taking a nursing school exam and the NCLEX-RN can anticipate demonstrating their competence on nursing examinations in these areas. In addition, nursing tests are also based on subcategories of the fundamentals of nursing practice that are listed in Display 7.3. So, you can see that there is a process or logic, if you will, on how those tests are designed. It is not just an arbitrary process that is instructor driven.

table
7-1 FOUR MAIN CATEGORIES OF CLIENT NEEDS

Client Needs	Subcategories
1. Safe, effective care environment	Management of care Safety and infection control
2. Health promotion and maintenance	
3. Psychosocial integrity	
4. Physiological integrity	Basic care and comfort Pharmacologic and parental therapies Reduction of risk potential Physiological adaptation

Available at the NCSBN Web site at www.ncsbn.org.

NCLEX-RN *Might Ask (Alternate Item Format)*   7.1

Place a check mark in front of the four main categories of the NCLEX-RN test blueprint.

Caring
Nursing Process
Teaching/Learning
Safe, Effective Care Environment
Health Promotion and Maintenance
Psychosocial Integrity
Physiological Integrity

---

display 7.3   **Fundamental Process of Nursing Practice**

Caring
Communication and documentation
Cultural awareness
Nursing process
Self-care
Teaching/learning

Available at the NCSBN Web site at https://www.ncsbn.org/1287.htm

● TEST LINGO: KEY COMPONENTS TO A TEST

Now that we have covered the NCLEX-RN test blueprint, you need to know more about the design of the questions themselves. Randy's professor would certainly be reviewing this with him to increase his understanding of the questions and what they are testing. Understanding the "lingo" or construction of the test is like understanding the structure of a sentence. To correctly format a sentence, the writer and reader must know about its construction. So if the test blueprint is the plan, the test questions themselves are the nails and boards that build the house. If the nails and boards (test questions) are not of good quality, the house will fall down (tests will not test what they are designed to do). To understand questions, the student needs to know the structure of a test question.

---

display 7.4   **Structure of a Multiple-Choice Question**

The nurse is performing a physical assessment on a client with a pneumothorax. The nurse palpates a crackling, popping sound   THE TEST ITEM
under her hands near a chest tube site. This finding indicates

A. tactile fremitus	DISTRACTOR
B. subcutaneous emphysema	**CORRECT OPTION**
C. egophony	DISTRACTOR
D. whispered pectoriloquy	DISTRACTOR

---

display 7.5   **Differences in Test Questions**

Non-NCLEX Style Question	NCLEX Style Question
A risk factor for coronary artery disease includes A. height B. cancer C. weight **D. high cholesterol**	The nurse is assessing a patient for risk factors for coronary artery disease. Which of the following would indicate a higher risk for this potential health problem? A. Height B. Cancer C. Weight **D. High cholesterol**

Bold indicates the correct option.

The test question is called an item. The part of the test item that states the problem is called the test stem. In a multiple-choice question, all potential choices to the question are called test options. The options that the student must eliminate, or the incorrect answers, are called the distracters. In a multiple-choice exam, there are three incorrect distracters and one correct option (Display 7.4).

Students need to carefully read each question on the exam, eliminate the distracters, and choose the correct option. In addition to this, nursing questions need to be written so that they involve a simulated nurse/patient situation. Because of this scenario style, nursing questions can become quite long and involved. Paraphrasing what the test item is actually asking becomes key to answering the question and can be challenging for the student. Nursing tests may look familiar to other types of tests students have taken, but they are truly different (Display 7.5).

To make matters more complex, nursing instructors need to change the level of difficulty from simple to complex so that questions are designed to simulate the critical thinking and problem solving needed by the nurse in the "real world." To do this, students need to know a bit more about how the level of difficulty is determined.

thinking critically

Look at the question in Display 7.5. In the NCLEX style question, identify the test stem, test options, and distracters.

● BLOOM'S TAXONOMY AND LEVEL OF DIFFICULTY

There have been many different theories that educators have used to help categorize the level of difficulty for test items. The one that is most widely used, and also used by the NCSBN, is Bloom's Taxonomy of Educational Objectives (Bloom, Englehart, Furst, Hill & Krathwohl, 1956). The structure that Bloom created goes from simpler questions that are knowledge based to ones that are quite complex, involving evaluation of information. The NCSBN designs nursing questions so that they include the knowledge through evaluation levels (Table 7.2). Let us now take a trip through question design using these various levels. The levels should look familiar to you from Chapter 5.

table
7-2

COMPARISON OF BLOOM'S TAXONOMY AND NCLEX-RN STYLE QUESTIONS

Benjamin Bloom's Taxonomy	NCLEX-RN Taxonomy
Knowledge	Knowledge
Comprehension	Comprehension
Application	Application
Analysis	Analysis
Synthesis	
Evaluation	

Knowledge Questions

Information that a student has filed or stored in the brain and that is easily recallable is called knowledge. Knowledge is concrete and easily identified in the form that it was learned. It also requires the fewest steps by the student to determine the answer. A student either knows the answer or does not know it. Types of knowledge questions that may be used are

- Definitions
- Steps in a procedure
- Common terms or facts
- Identifying a medication, a normal dose, or its side effects

Students usually believe that these are the easiest questions to answer, but the success of answering these correctly depends on memorizing material. Knowledge questions can be made more difficult if the concept being tested is one that is difficult to understand. For example, many pathophysiology questions are difficult if they involve the endocrine system. An example of a knowledge level question would be

The nurse knows a patient's hemoglobin value normally is
A. 10–20%
B. 25–35%
C. 35–45%
D. 55–65%

To demonstrate how a similar question in content areas can be changed to reflect a higher level of difficulty, we use the example of a hemoglobin test in the following sections.

Comprehension Questions

The second type of question a student will need to answer is called a comprehension question. These are a step more difficult than knowledge questions. They require a student to know the material and to understand the importance of the information by paraphrasing it in her or his own words. Types of comprehension questions that may be used are

- Understanding a definition or term
- Telling why a lab result is important
- Recognizing what and why a step in a procedure is important
- Identifying why or how a medication will work

Students usually believe that these questions are a bit more difficult to answer. However, answering them correctly depends not only on memorizing material but also on truly understanding the material and its importance to nursing practice. An example of a comprehension-level question would be

The nurse is assessing a patient's complete blood cell count. The hematocrit value is a reflection of
A. the number of red cells circulating in the body
B. the type of anemia a patient has
C. the percentage of red cells to serum
D. the infection fighting ability of the body

In this question, the student needs to translate the meaning this value has with the functioning of the patient.

Application Questions

A third type of question a student will need to answer on a nursing test is called an application question. These questions are a step higher and more difficult than both knowledge and comprehension questions. They require a student not only to know the material but also to understand and apply it to a given and often new situation. An application question may ask the student to solve a problem, change a nursing action, or manipulate variables in a given situation. Types of application questions that may be used are

- Apply a definition or term to a new situation
- Assess the importance of a lab result in relationship to a disease
- Prioritize what steps in a procedure are important or when they occur
- Evaluate a response to a medication

Students usually believe that these questions are among the most difficult to answer. Successful elimination of distracters and identification of the correct answer depends on memorizing and understanding the material, and applying it to a new nursing situation. An example of an application question would be

The nurse is evaluating a patient's complete blood cell count after administration of a unit of packed red blood cells. The hematocrit value is 75%. This value indicates
A. too much circulating volume
B. a decrease in circulating serum levels
C. a higher level of circulating oxygen
D. not enough red blood cells

In this question, the student needs to know the normal value of the hematocrit and what its role is in the vascular component of the blood. She or he also has to apply this material to the definitions given in the distracters. This is a three-step process requiring the student to think critically and integrate previous taxonomy levels.

Analysis Questions

The last type of question and the most difficult to answer is the analysis question. This type of question has much information a student needs to break down into components for understanding. It will require the student to understand the complex relationships of constituent parts. It requires knowledge, understanding, and the ability to apply, dissect, and scrutinize elements. It also requires the student to arrive at an answer by eliminating among all possibly correct answers and arriving at the best or highest priority. Types of analysis questions that may be used are

- Choosing the *best* definition or term to a new situation
- Anticipating lab test results with a client's history/diagnosis
- Prioritizing the first step of action to perform when a given set of symptoms occurs
- Identifying the best medication to give a client according to his or her symptoms and variables given in the stem

To students, these questions require a high degree of critical thinking. The correct answer is predicated on the previous types of cognitive-level questions. A successful elimination of distracters depends on identifying the data delivered in the stem and eliminating many variables. There is also a tendency to read into the questions and not focus on important aspects given. An example of an analysis question would be

The nurse is evaluating the complete blood cell counts of four patients. One of the patients has a hematocrit value of 75%. This value is MOST REFLECTIVE of which of the following patients?

A. A 45-year-old male with sickle cell disease in crisis

B. A 55-year-old man with a history of chronic lung disease admitted with shortness of breath

C. A 65-year-old female with ovarian cancer

D. A 75-year-old female with chronic right-sided heart failure

If the student is to answer the previous question successfully, she or he must know what a hematocrit value is and *predict* which client would be most likely to have it. It requires a student to know about the diseases listed and the *anticipated* value of each client. It is quite discriminating in its scope and therefore very complex. This question also simulates a judgment call a nurse would make in screening lab data in which he or she would consider which one is consistent with the patient's problem. See Table 7.3 for a review of the taxonomy levels.

table
7-3 .... LEVELS OF COMPLEXITY AND TYPES OF NCLEX-RN QUESTIONS

Taxonomy	Definition	Types of Questions
Knowledge	Recallable Learned by memorization/repetition	Definitions Steps in a procedure Common terms/facts Medication doses, side effects
Comprehension	Understanding Paraphrasing Meaning/intent Translate Interpret	The hows and whys of information use
Application	Using information that is understood	Using information in a new setting by demonstrating, solving, changing, and modifying it. Making judgments
Analysis	Looking at information and examining the essential features in relationship to each other Priority setting Recognizing effects	Comparing and contrasting information Best or better answer Highest priority or initial response

● HOW THE NCLEX-RN DIFFERS FROM THE NCLEX-PN

Because you have had the benefit of taking the NCLEX-PN already, you have probably seen many questions that have included knowledge, comprehension, and application. Most of the questions on the NLCEX-PN were of the latter two: comprehension and application. The ones that you have not seen are the analysis questions. Also, the number of questions in the NCLEX-RN test will predominately be in the application and analysis range (Table 7.4). The change in the type of question delivered by the NCLEX-RN is more reflective of the more complex nature of the level of judgment needed by the RN.

table
7-4 .... DIFFERENCE BETWEEN NCLEX-RN AND NCLEX-PN COGNITIVE LEVELS

NCLEX-PN	NCLEX-RN
Knowledge	Knowledge
Comprehension*	Comprehension
Application*	Application*
	Analysis*

*Indicates majority of the questions.

table
.... ALTERNATE ITEM FORMATS
7-5

Types of Questions	Examples
Fill in the blanks: Student must provide an answer rather than select it from options	Calculating medication Prioritizing nursing actions
Multiple response: Students must identify multiple correct answers	Performing steps in a procedure Selecting correct nursing interventions for a particular diagnosis
Mathematical calculations	Calculating intake and output Performing a medication calculation Determining a score on a Glasgow Coma Scale or Braden Scale
Use of graphic images, pictures, charts, or tables (sometimes called "hot spot" questions)	Determining the location of bronchial breath sounds Calculating the amount of potassium in a renal diet

• ALTERNATE ITEM FORMATS

We have now completed the history of the NCLEX-RN and the types of cognitive domain that may be reflected in the questions that you can anticipate in your nursing exams. In 2003, technology evolved so that CAT could include questions other than multiple-choice ones. These new, innovative questions are called alternative item formats (AIFs). There are no established norms for the number of questions using this format to be included on the NCLEX-RN and the NCLEX-PN, but initially there should only be about 2% (NCSBN, 2010). AIF questions include

- Fill in the blanks
- Identifying multiple correct answers
- Mathematical calculations
- Use of graphic images, pictures, charts, or tables

Examples of these are included in Table 7.5.

• PREPARATION FOR A NCLEX-RN STYLE EXAM

Needless to say, preparation for class and exams is an important function for the students and professors in your program. Nursing school is very competitive and you have been accepted because the faculty believe in your ability to succeed. However, it is up to you to do the work involved in clearing the pathway to successful achievement in your nursing courses. To achieve success, you need to know effective ways of preparing before, during, and after a nursing examination.

Before the Exam

A wise man once said, "Planning is everything, but the plan itself is nothing." In other words, you do not have to be a slave to the plan, but planning is something you have to do for some kind of control over your life.

PLANNING

Once you get the syllabus and course outline, you should immediately use a planning tool to write down due dates for exams and projects. At a minimum, for every hour you spend in class, 2 hours should be devoted to study and preparation. Thus, if you have a 3-hour nursing lab, a minimum of 6 hours a week should be devoted to studying for that lab alone. So, in your planning tool, block out times during the week to devote to this all-important prep time. Planning is a part of good study habits and provides the backbone to the discipline required in such a robust, rigorous program.

The ideal study time is in 1.0- to 2-hour blocks of uninterrupted time. With a busy lifestyle, you also want to use any downtime to your advantage. When Randy and his professor looked at his class schedule, they blocked out weekly time so that Randy could be consistent in his study habits. (This is similar to the Critical Thinking activity done in Chapter 1.) Randy and his professor also found some extra study time for Randy. Randy had a long commute to school, so his professor suggested that he tape important concepts missed in his first exam and play them in the car. Randy also found that he could download and listen to some of his instructor's lectures (Podcast) on his iPod while working out at the gym each week. Together they also found extra study time while he waited for his son to complete his karate lessons. Although Randy had to answer questions from curious onlookers, they became a much needed support group as his program progressed.

USING CLASS/PROFESSOR TIME WISELY

During your study time, you should be reading for comprehension. You should be asking yourself, "Do I understand this material?" Keep a tablet and pencil nearby when you read. Write down what you do not understand. Most professors will start a lecture, class, or lab by asking if there are any questions; use this time as an opportunity to ask questions. Do not feel alone. Chances are that if you do not understand the material, there are at least five other students who do not understand it either. Do be assertive in your learning needs. If there are a lot of questions and you do not want to "soak up class time," set up a regular appointment to meet with the professor outside class. This serves many purposes. It gets your questions answered and your needs met. It decreases problems with other classmates, and it allows the instructor to get to know you as an individual, therefore becoming familiar with your needs as well as the classes'.

MEMORIZATION

After reading the levels of Bloom's Taxonomy, it should be clear that memorization of material is necessary to pass nursing examinations. There are many memory aids that you can use to help with what seems to be an overwhelming amount of information. Mnemonics such as acrostics and acronyms are helpful in both visualizing and jogging your memory. A mnemonic is any device that provides an easy way to increase memory. It helps you retain your lower-level knowledge. An acrostic is an arrangement of words into a phrase that helps you to recall information. Here are two types of acrostics that are helpful for students:

We evolve **Ape To M**an

Aortic
Pulmonic
Erb's point
Tricuspid
Mitral

The letters APE T and M in "ape to man" can help a student remember what the heart values are for auscultation of heart sounds.

Another type of acrostic is

Conk, **R**apidly **P**lease **O**ld **M**an

C = **Consciousness**
R = **Respiratory pattern**
P = **Pupillary size and responses**
O = **Oculocephalogyric reflexes**
M = **Motor response to pain**

The letters CRPOM correspond to the evaluation of coma. Students do not need to rely on previously produced acrostics and may develop their own.

Another type of memory enhancer is an acronym that is a word that is made up to remind you of other words. Some common ones are

PEARRL: **P**upils **E**qual **A**nd **R**ound and **R**eactive to **L**ight
UNLOADME (the acronym for treating heart failure): **U**pright positioning, **N**itrates, **L**asix, **O**xygen, **A**lbuterol, **D**obutamine, **M**orphine, and **E**xtremities
White on the right (arm), **snow** (white electrode) over **grass** (green electrode), **smoke** (black electrode) over **fire** (red electrode) = the lead placements on the chest for telemetry.

If these words are coupled with a picture or diagram, they enhance learning for both auditory and visual nursing students.

New mnemonics do not work for every student; in fact, learning the mnemonic can sometimes be more difficult for students than learning the material. Try to stick with what works for you, but if you have not tried this, give it a chance because it works as a powerful memory tool for many. For example, Randy's professor noted that he was creative and could develop mnemonics that worked well for him. Randy started writing mnemonics on index cards and took them with him while his son went to dental and medical appointments. He also used them for breaks between his classes. He got his wife involved with quizzing him while they both prepared supper and fed their son. It made his wife happy that she was involved, and she took over typing up his cards and drawing pictures that crystallized the facts. Randy, with instructor encouragement, decided to share his learning techniques with the class. The reception was both humorous and positive for all involved. It also started other more artistic students down this same pathway for developing their learning materials.

MAKING READING COME ALIVE

Reading a textbook is a very passive process. There is no manipulation or action on the part of the reader. One of the keys to successful learning is to interact with the textbook. Ways this can be accomplished are by using a highlighter, talking to the textbook, forming study groups, and using any interactive tools that come with it. If you have time and it works for you, you might try to write notes about the more difficult parts. Writing information down helps you interact and think about the materials.

USING A HIGHLIGHTER

Most students know that using a highlighter to mark key concepts helps you remember and understand them. The use of a highlighter makes you think critically about the material and determine which information is most important. It also makes the review process much easier. However, it can become a problem when you look back and the entire page is highlighted. This is jokingly called "highlighteritis" or "highlighter hyperplasia." Students become so overwhelmed with the volume of information presented that they are infected with the use of the highlighter. There are some guidelines that you can follow to prevent highlighteritis.

First, pretend that there is a shortage of ink and that you are using your only highlighter. This will force you to identify and mark only the critical information. Second, read with the understanding that only five lines on a page can be highlighted. What are the critical points? How would a nurse put this information to use?

TALKING TO THE TEXTBOOK

Another way to make reading more interactive is to have a conversation with the author while reading. If the author was in the same room while you were reading, what would you want to ask him or her? What is as clear as mud? What doesn't make sense to you? Keep a tablet near your text and write these questions out. Use this list as a starting point at the beginning of your professor's lecture. Most instructors are more than happy to answer questions and clarify important nursing concepts. If you are in a study group with other students, use these questions as study topics to get another person's viewpoint. If the textbook has concepts listed in either the front or the back of the chapters, make sure you understand their meaning. They are a path for students to follow to make the journey easier to understand. Look at the end-of-chapter questions or the study guide that goes with the text. Do you understand why an answer is correct or incorrect? If not, again, write these questions down to discuss with the instructor either in class or during office hours. Do not be afraid to be assertive in seeking meaning. Chances are that if you do not understand the concept, there are others in your class in the same situation; you are not alone.

FORMING STUDY GROUPS

Study groups will also help you become a more active learner. Study groups allow you to teach information to each other. This is called reciprocal teaching or "each one teach one." Whether you know it or not, if your instructor has a post conference, this is a type of study group that applies learning to the clinical situation.

Independent student study groups should structure their meetings so that each participant takes a chunk of the material, summarizes it in his or her own words, teaches it to other students, and then makes up multiple-choice questions that stress the importance of the information. You can also try to design mnemonics, draw pictures, or use information from clinical days to help the learning process. This approach forces each participant to talk out loud, hear oneself think, and manipulate information. This also forces the participant to defend his or her answer. The rationale for this is that "more brains are better than one."

USING INTERACTIVE TOOLS

Most textbooks come with some type of learning tool. Many times these are workbooks, online sources, and interactive discs. These tools add to the student workload, but they are also designed to aid the learner in a more active process. Workbooks force the learner to answer questions by filling in crosswords or filling in blanks and using case studies to manipulate information. They reinforce those "need to know" versus "nice to know" brain synapses. Online resources point the learner to material that may also require interaction.

These learning tools encourage the student to interact with nursing material. They take the learner from a passive state to one of active participation. This is important because what you hear, you forget; what you see, you sometimes remember; but what you do, you learn for a lifetime. These learning tools are also helpful in studying for the course and preparing for clinical. They will structure your time and help prevent cramming before the examination. Cramming does not increase learning. It may help you with knowledge questions but rarely helps at the application and analysis levels. An organized plan of study will be of critical benefit for that all-important exam day. Thus, we next cover what to do before, during, and after a nursing examination.

● IMMEDIATELY BEFORE THE EXAM

There are some key things to do before you take an exam. Prepping your body to take the test should be similar to an athlete preparing for a contest. Most important, get a good night's sleep. You have organized your study time and have participated in active study techniques. Stop studying in the early evening and do something enjoyable. You will not give top performance if you are tired from an all-night cram session. Get everything that you need for the exam ready to go and put it in a convenient place before you leave. These items may include #2 sharpened pencils, calculator, extra paper, watch, earplugs, and/or examination book if needed (Nugent & Vitale, 2008).

Next, eat a well-balanced breakfast. A good breakfast is something with carbohydrates and proteins that will last you through the morning. A glass of milk and a bagel or cereal with fruit are foods that will help make your blood sugar rise slowly and keep it elevated without peaks and valleys.

display 7.6	Tips for Success Before an Examination

1. Prepare items needed for the exam the night before. If need be, pack your car that night!
2. Get a good night's sleep.
3. Eat a well-balanced breakfast.
4. Arrive early.
5. Consider a brisk walk before the exam if your peers upset you and make you nervous.
6. Ask whether you can use earplugs during the exam.
7. Synchronize your watch to the classroom.

Leave from home early and arrive early. Nothing will stress you out more than an unexpected bus delay or traffic jam. If other students are talking negatively and worrying you before the examination, try to avoid them. If you are anxious and nervous, try to walk it off before the exam. A brisk 10-minute walk will stimulate your sympathetic nervous system, making you more alert and expending some of that nervous energy that may block your understanding and critical thinking ability. Also, synchronize your watch to the exam room clock. If students turning the test in early tend to distract you, ask the proctor if you can wear earplugs. A little bit of preplanning can go a long way toward helping you feel relaxed and ready to concentrate on the exam (Display 7.6).

During the Exam

There are some important things that you can do during the exam to increase your likelihood of succeeding. Skim through the exam. If there are short answers or alternative-type questions at the end of the exam, do those first. The professor will often write on the exam how the questions are weighted or how the points are spread. Because multiple-choice questions are usually quicker to answer and may be weighted less, try to leave the multiple-choice section for last.

Once you have skimmed the exam, back track and read each question carefully. You should first respond to the easier knowledge-based questions. If a question takes you longer than 2 minutes to do, leave it and proceed to the next question. If you spend too much time on one question, it can leave you worried and thus affect the answer to the next question. You can also waste valuable minutes on a timed test. Also, something in the next question may jog your memory to help you with the correct response. So, do not ruminate; proceed through the exam.

For the harder questions, ask if you can use a highlighter to write on the exam. If you can, highlight the important words. This will help you focus on key items in the exam, making you less inclined to read things into the exam that are not present. Paraphrase the question. What is it asking? What important nursing concepts apply? Cross out the distracters one by one. If you can, physically strike off the answer on the test itself to give you a visual cue of your choices. Think of why you are eliminating it. If time permits, write short memory jogs on why you chose that particular answer. In a test review after the exam, this will help you identify any display **7.7**   **Tips for Success During the Examination**

1. Skim through the test answering what you know is absolutely correct.
2. Read each question carefully.
3. Skip questions that are confusing.
4. Ask the proctor if you do not understand a question.
5. For harder questions, use a highlighter if allowed.
6. Paraphrase the question: What is it asking?
7. Cross out the distracters.
8. If two distracters seem equally correct, what nursing concepts make one better than the other?
9. Watch out for absolutes.
10. Do not change the answers.
11. Look for the best answer.

faulty thinking on your part. Once you have made your choice, stick with it. This is called "going with your glimmer." Meaning that the first choice, or your "gut reaction," is usually the best.

What should you do if you "don't have a clue" what the question is asking? Most important, do not panic. Definitely leave the question for the end of the test. Remember, in multiple-choice questions, you have a 25% chance of getting the correct answer. If a distracter is partially incorrect, the entire choice is incorrect. Eliminate any "all or every" answers. There are rarely any absolutes as answers. If all choices seem correct, then look for similarities in the options; if two are similar, then cross them off. If the question refers to the best choice, choose the one that is all encompassing or the broader focused choice (Display 7.7).

Before You Turn in the Exam

There are some things that you should do before you turn in the exam. First, remember to write your name on it. Second, look at the bubbles on a multiple-choice exam, making sure you have filled them in and have not left any blank. Third, review any alternate questions, making sure you have answered them to your best ability. Do not forget the backside of the pages. Because tests are often double sided, instructors will remind you to check the backsides when you turn in the exam. If your instructor has included alternative questions, answer those first as they require recall not recognition. If you need to later, go back to these; something might have jogged your memory during the multiple-choice part of the test.

● AFTER THE EXAM

Once you have turned in the exam, take the time to do something good for yourself. You cannot change the outcome now, but you can reward yourself for doing the best job that you could do. Talk a long-delayed hike, read a passage in your favorite book, enjoy an ice cream cone, take a jog in the park, or buy something special.

Treat yourself for a job well done, at least the best you could do. Forget about the test until it becomes time to get it back. Then you can spring right back into action!

Once you have gotten your grade, examine your study patterns for the test. Did you do all reading assignments and any homework associated with them? Did you use chapter vocabulary and concepts, lecture outlines and notes, and any adjunctive study aides? If you have done these things and get a good score, you are headed in the right direction. Pat yourself on the back and continue with your plan. If you have not done as well as you had hoped, perhaps the problem is more complicated and will require the help of an expert to get you back on track. Perhaps you have a full plate of things that have been keeping you occupied—family, friends, or crises at work. If life does get in the way, perhaps you will have to settle for the C when you've been a B student. Or you will have to develop support systems to help with life.

Getting Help

The first person to contact is the course instructor. Schedule an appointment right after the first exam. The instructor's office hours are designed so that they are available to students who need that person-to-person help. If you schedule the appointment ahead of midsemester, your instructor will be available and will get to know you. The instructor will also be better able to evaluate your progress over several weeks and before the time constraints placed on everyone at semester's end. Remember that the course instructor designs the test and is the content expert. Although the entrance to nursing programs is competitive, faculty has a vested interest in retaining you as a student. They do not want to fail you; they want you to succeed! However, they are also required to maintain nursing standards.

Ask to review the exam with the instructor so that he or she can determine the types of questions you are missing as well as your subject matter strengths and needs. Ask if you can meet on a regular basis. If an NCLEX-RN review text is not required, ask if there is one that the faculty person recommends.

Use any and all ancillaries that come with your textbooks. Many texts now provide online resources, free nursing journal articles, help with medication math calculation, and animations and case studies that are interactive. These can be invaluable in helping you master pathophysiological concepts and complex procedures and getting more nursing NCLEX-RN questions under your belt. There is a lot out there; you need to find time to use it.

Also, ask if there are other services available at the college to help you in mastery of NCLEX-RN questions. Many schools have a variety of support systems designed for the nursing student. Support for students may include student tutors (especially for math and English), learning specialists (for time management, anxiety-reducing techniques, learning style, and general tips for test taking), outside testing agencies (e.g., Kaplan or ATI Testing), and nursing question resources that are often computer based and do not require the assistance of a specialist. Use these services as many are free to you and are covered in your tuition. These tutors are nonthreatening and available at many liberal time intervals. They won't have to give you a grade so they don't hold a perceived power position like a nursing instructor so students need to use these services to help them conquer the more difficult aspects of nursing courses like writing the dreaded term paper or special help with medication math calculations.

thinking critically

For additional study tips for the NCLEX exam, visit the NCSBN Learning Extension at http://learningext.com/groups/880ce6ef50/summary. Explore this Web site. What does it say about general study tips, test-taking hints, and relaxation techniques? Which of these have you incorporated into your study routine? Which of these could you use to help you study? Does it have questions you could incorporate into your study routines?

● CONCLUSION

Test-taking skills are ones that are not easily acquired for all nursing students. Because the style of CAT and NCLEX-RN test questions may not be familiar, you may need help in achieving your desired success with them. To maximize your success, it is important to review how the NCLEX-RN was developed, what it entails, and the overall test blueprint developed by the NCSBN. Test question complexity is based on Bloom's Taxonomy, and although it is not important to memorize each step, students need to know that they have to study in different ways to decrease their test anxiety. Furthermore, a bit of knowledge regarding test construction will help students understand the need to paraphrase what the question is really asking. Last, applying important tips for before, during, and after the examination will benefit the student in decreasing test phobia.

student exercises

1. If possible, arrange to meet with one of your instructors. Have him or her review your first test, and try to take five questions identifying the key components of the test items. Make a list of the questions you missed. According to Bloom, what level of the taxonomy were they? What subject matter were they? Are there any trends you can identify that will be helpful for the next exam?

2. Keep a diary of how you feel before the test. What did you do? How did you prepare? What made you nervous? What calmed you down? Keep track of these over the semester. What did you find about your test-taking preparation that's good? What needs to be changed? Discuss these in a group setting.

3. Meet with a group of students in the class. Discuss the following: What was your "nightmare test?" What made it that way? What was your best testing experience, and what made it that way? What are the strategies you are using that help you master material before an exam? Have someone make a typed copy of your findings. Share this information with your course instructor, and see if he or she has other words of wisdom to help with nursing tests.

4. Visit the NCSB e-learning site at http://ncsbn.hivelive.com/pages/95062efc57 (last accessed 7.6.2011). It looks at the 10 best practices for e-learning. Do you use any of these? Does your group use any of these? What has been helpful/harmful? If you could add to this list, what would you add?

References

Billings, D. (2011). *Lippincott's review for NCLEX-RN* (10th ed.). Philadelphia, PA: Lippincott Williams & Wilkins.

Bloom, B. S., Englehart, M. B., Furst, E. J., Hill, W. H., & Krathwohl, D. R. (1956). *Taxonomy of educational objectives. The classification of educational goals. Handbook I: Cognitive domain.* New York, NY: Longmans Green.

McDonald, M. (2007). *The nurse educator's guide to assessing learning outcomes* (2nd ed.). Boston, MA: Jones and Bartlett.

National Council State Board of Nursing (NCSBN). (2010). *NCLEX-RN® examination: Test plan for the National Council Licensure Examination for Registered Nurses.* Chicago, IL: Author. Retrieved January 31, 2010, from https://www.ncsbn.org/1287.htm

Norton, C., Relf, M., Cox, C., Farlly, J., & Tucker, M. (2006). Ensuring NCLEX-RN success for first-time test-takers. *Journal of Professional Nursing, 22*(5), 322–326.

Nugent, P., & Vitale, B. (2008). *Fundamentals success: A course review applying critical thinking to test taking* (2nd ed.). Philadelphia, PA: F.A. Davis.

Suggested Reading

Bruck, L., Labus, D., & Mayer, B. H. (Eds.) (2005). *Springhouse review for NCLEX-RN* (6th ed.). Philadelphia, PA: Author.

Dunham, K. (2004). *How to survive and maybe even love nursing school: A guide for students by students* (2nd ed.). Philadelphia, PA: F.A. Davis.

James, E. (2006). NCLEX success. *Advance for Nurses, 8,* 25, 31.

Lippincott Williams & Wilkins. (2006). *NCLEX-RN 250 new-format questions* (2nd ed.). Philadelphia, PA: Lippincott Williams & Wilkins.

Lippincott Williams & Wilkins. (2010). *NCLEX-RN review made incredibly easy!* (5th ed.). Philadelphia, PA: Lippincott Williams & Wilkins.

Nugent, P. & Vitale, B. (2008). *Test success: Test-taking techniques for beginning nursing students* (5th ed.). Philadelphia, PA: F.A. Davis.

Ohman, K. (2010). *Davis's NCLEX-RN success.* Philadelphia, PA: F.A. Davis.

Silvestri, L. (2010). *Saunders comprehensive review for the NCLEX-RN® examination* (5th ed.). Philadelphia, PA: Elsevier Saunders.

Wilfong, D., Szolis, C. & Haus, C. (2007). *Nursing school success: Tools for constructing your future.* Sudbury, MA: Jones and Bartlett Publishers.

On the WEB *http://learningext.com/pages/e1405788a0:* NCSBN learning extension for students. (Last accessed 7.6.2011).

https://www.ncsbn.org/1287.htm: Provides students and educators with a blueprint for exams. (Last accessed 7.6.2011).

www.howtostudy.org: Provides practical resources for students on the best ways to study. (Last accessed 7.6.2011).

Core Competencies for Professional Nursing Practice

8

Practicing Within Regulatory Frameworks

● **LEARNING OUTCOMES**

By the end of this chapter, the student will be able to:

1 Relate the differences between regulations, policies, and standards of practice in nursing.

2 Identify boundaries and restrictions of practice of the LPN/LVN.

3 Describe the differences between LPN/LVN and RN scopes of practice.

4 Discuss the meaning of and need for regulation language in nurse practice acts.

5 Write a statement that reflects the scope of practice of the RN in the United States, after examining the nurse practice acts.

6 Differentiate among directed, autonomous, and collaborative nursing practices.

7 Analyze sample situations to determine directed, autonomous, and collaborative nursing practices in action.

8 Describe mechanisms for identifying differences in the knowledge and roles of LPN/LVNs and RNs.

9 Differentiate between the NCSBN test plans for PNs and RNs.

10 Differentiate between the roles of the LPN/LVNs and RNs in the nursing process.

11 Contrast the differences between core competencies for the LPN/LVN and those for the RN.

● KEY TERMS

affective learning
American Nurses Association
autonomous nursing practice
cognitive learning
collaborative nursing practice
competency
directed nursing

practice
evidence-based practice
learning domains
National League for Nursing
NCLEX-PN
NCLEX-RN
nurse practice act
nursing diagnosis

nursing process
permissive language
policy
psychomotor learning
regulation
restrictive language
scope of practice
standards of practice
state board of nursing

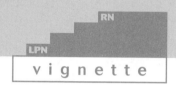

vignette

Lori Ann Dietz, LPN, is talking with another LPN-to-RN student about entering an ADN program. The discussion has centered on validation for clinical practice.

LORI ANN: I have been a licensed practical nurse for 20 years. In that time, I have done multiple catheterizations, charted on hundreds of clients, monitored rhythm disturbances by telemetry, and passed medications effectively and safely. Why do I have to do this all over again? Why do I have to demonstrate performance in skills I have already mastered as an LPN?

As you enter the RN program, you are embarking on a whole new scope of practice level. Perhaps you have felt like the LPN in the vignette. As an LPN/LVN, you have practiced under the direction of the RN or the physician to whom you have reported. Your role has been a directed role, for the most part restricted by state law to performing certain nursing procedures, administering medications (depending on the state), and perhaps even (with additional certification) performing some intravenous therapy procedures.

To answer the question of this nursing student, your scope of practice as an RN will not only be broader in the types and complexity of procedures you perform but will also require additional knowledge, independent thinking, and problem-solving skills. Increasingly, you will be expected to use research to maintain and upgrade your nursing practice. This is called evidence-based practice. You will acquire the ability to collaborate with other health care team members to design plans for comprehensive care to patients and clients, and to foster prevention and self-care among these health care consumers.

● REGULATIONS, POLICIES, AND STANDARDS

Regulations, policies, and standards all play a role in defining the practice of the RN. A thorough understanding of each is essential as you embark on an RN educational program.

Regulations

Regulations are those guidelines for nursing practice established through the state boards of nursing in the United States and colleges of nursing in Canada. State legislatures grant power through statutory laws by regulations. According to the National Council of State Boards of Nursing (NCSBN, 2002, 2006), nursing regulation is "enacted through state legislative action and state legislatures delegate many enforcement activities to state administrative agencies" (p. 1). Regulation of nursing practice matters because nursing is one of the health professions that poses risk of harm to the public if practiced by someone who is unprepared and incompetent. The public may not have sufficient information and experience to identify an unqualified health care provider, and is vulnerable to unsafe and incompetent practitioners (NCSBN, 2002, 2006). State and federal regulations exist to govern various aspects of the health care industry and health care professionals.

Regulations at the state level define the scope of practice, requirements for licensure and relicensing, certification and continuing education requirements, and disciplinary consequences for health care practitioners. Regulations that define the practice of individuals licensed in a particular area are called practice acts. Nursing practice acts are laws established in a state or province to regulate the practice of nursing. Although practice acts may differ from state to state or province to province, much similarity and support of reciprocity are increasingly evident as states attempt to meet the needs of consumers, health care workers, and the health care industry. Extensive use of the NCLEX-RN throughout the states is an example of this effort. In many states, a single nurse practice act defines the practice of RNs and LPN/LVNs. Some states have two separate practice acts for these two levels of practitioners.

Regulations, especially those with the purpose of defining the scope of practice of various health care professionals, can be written with either restrictive or permissive language. Restrictive language restricts the practitioner to performing only the functions and procedures outlined in the regulation. LPN/LVN practice acts are often written in this manner.

Permissive language in regulations allows practitioners to use judgment and make decisions to serve their purpose in performing their roles. Display 8.1 contrasts restrictive and permissive language in LPN/LVN and RN practice acts in the state of Kansas. Permissive language is used for the more autonomous practice of the RN. Similar restrictive and permissive language for LPN/LVN and RN practice acts, respectively, exists in many other states.

thinking critically

Differentiate between restrictive and permissive language in other rules you have encountered in your life, and describe the difference in your ability to think and act independently in each.

---

display **8.1**   **Restrictive and Permissive Language in Practical/ Vocational and Registered Nurse Practice Acts in the State of Kansas**

RESTRICTIVE LANGUAGE FOR THE PRACTICAL NURSE

60-16-102 Scope of Practice for Liscensed Practical Nurse Performing Intravenous Fluid Therapy

(a) A licensed practical nurse under the supervision of a registered professional nurse may engage in a limited scope of intravenous fluid treatment, including the following:
   (1) Monitoring;
   (2) maintaining;
   (3) discontinuing intravenous flow and an intravenous access device not exceeding three inches in length in peripheral sites only; and
   (4) changing dressings for intravenous access devices not exceeding three inches in length in peripheral sites only. (p. 41)

PERMISSIVE LANGUAGE FOR THE REGISTERED NURSE

The practice of professional nursing as performed by a registered professional nurse for compensation or gratuitously... means the process in which substantial specialized knowledge derived from the biological, physical, and behavioral sciences is applied to: the care, diagnosis, treatment, counsel and health teaching of persons who are experiencing changes in the normal health processes or who require assistance in the maintenance of health or the prevention or management of illness, injury or infirmity; administration, supervision or teaching of the process as defined in this section; and the execution of the medical regimen as prescribed by a person licensed to practice medicine and surgery or a person licensed to practice dentistry. (p. 5)

Kansas State Board of Nursing. (2009, July). *Nurse Practice Act statutes & administrative regulations.* Topeka: Author. Retrieved January 23, 2010, from http://www.ksbn.org/npa/npa.htm

---

Policies

To implement and enforce regulations, governing bodies (often in the form of appointed boards) are established to develop policies. A policy is "a high-level over-all plan embracing the general goals and acceptable procedures especially of a governing body" (*Merriam-Weber Dictionary*, 2011). In nursing, each state establishes a state board of nursing to develop guidelines for interpreting regulations. The state boards of nursing also ensure implementation of regulations with continuity. They include members of the public on their boards of directors to ensure consumer protection as regulations are implemented. With few exceptions, most states have a single state board of nursing for governing the practice of the LPN/LVN and the RN.

An example of a regulation by the Pennsylvania State Board of Nursing is shown in Display 8.2. The policy is a guide for nursing schools to ensure that the regulation is implemented with continuity throughout the state.

---

thinking critically

Describe the difference between a rule (regulation) and an interpretation (policy) related to one or more rules that you have seen in an organization, service club, charity group, or social organization. What confusion or differing interpretations of the rule led to the need for the policy to be developed?

---

display **8.2**   **Administrator, Faculty and Staff Requirements for the Pennsylvania State Board of Nursing**

(a) A nursing education program shall employ a sufficient number of qualified faculty, faculty assistants, allied faculty and staff to accomplish the objectives of the curriculum and the systematic evaluation plan. The minimum faculty and staff requirements are as follows:
   (1) Full-time nurse administrator.
   (2) Full-time faculty members in the areas of practice encompassed within the curriculum.
   (3) Additional faculty members as needed.
   (4) Allied faculty members as needed.
   (5) Adequate personnel to provide program support services, including administrative, clerical, library, admissions, financial aid, and student services.
(b) The nurse administrator's credentials shall be submitted to the Board for approval. The nurse administrator's qualifications are as follows:
   (1) The nurse administrator of a baccalaureate degree nursing education program shall hold at least one graduate degree in nursing. The nurse administrator shall hold an earned doctoral degree or have a specific plan for completing doctoral preparation within 5 years of appointment. The nurse administrator shall have experience in nursing practice, nursing education, and administration. A professional nurse who does not hold at least one graduate degree in nursing, but who has experience in nursing practice, nursing education, and administration, may be considered on an individual basis.
   (2) The nurse administrator of an associate degree or diploma program shall hold at least one graduate degree in nursing. The nurse administrator shall have experience in nursing practice, nursing education, and administration. A professional nurse who does not hold at least one graduate degree in nursing, but who has experience in nursing practice, nursing education, and administration, may be considered on an individual basis.
   (3) The length of appointment of an interim or acting nurse administrator of a nursing education program may not exceed 1 year.
   (4) The nurse administrator shall hold either a temporary practice permit to practice professional nursing or be currently licensed as a professional nurse in this Commonwealth.
(c) Faculty qualifications are as follows:
   (1) Faculty members teaching required nursing education courses shall hold at least one graduate degree in nursing, shall be currently licensed as professional nurses in this Commonwealth, and shall have expertise in their areas of instruction.

(continued)

(2) Faculty members without a graduate degree in nursing shall be designated faculty assistants. Faculty assistants shall be currently licensed as professional nurses in this Commonwealth. Faculty assistants may teach required nursing education courses only when fully qualified faculty are not available and shall teach under the direct guidance of a faculty member qualified as set forth in paragraph (1). Faculty assistants shall have a baccalaureate degree in nursing and shall give evidence of a plan for obtaining a graduate degree in nursing. A person may teach as a faculty assistant in a nursing education program in this Commonwealth for a maximum cumulative period of 5 years.

(3) Faculty members without a degree in nursing, but who hold at least one graduate degree in a subject area pertinent to their area of teaching, shall be designated as allied faculty members. Allied faculty members may teach basic sciences or specialized areas of health care practice.

(4) Faculty employed to teach dietetics-nutrition shall be currently licensed to practice dietetics-nutrition in this Commonwealth.

(5) An individual who enhances faculty-directed clinical learning experiences by guiding selected clinical activities shall be designated as a clinical preceptor. A clinical preceptor shall hold a current license to practice professional nursing in the state of the clinical experience.

　(i) Faculty shall have input into the selection of preceptors.

　(ii) Faculty shall retain responsibility for planning and evaluating student learning experiences when students are engaged in clinical activities with a preceptor.

　(iii) If a faculty member is not physically present in the area in which students are practicing, a faculty member shall be immediately available by telephone or other means of telecommunication when students are engaged in clinical activities with a preceptor.

(d) Program support personnel shall be qualified by education and experience to serve in the capacity in which they are employed.

Standards

When nurses became more independent and accountable for their actions, they began to develop standards of practice. The practice of nursing is controlled through the standards of practice, licensure, and nurse practice acts. "Standards of practice are essential because they serve as guidelines for providing and evaluating nursing care" (Craven & Hirnle, 2009, p. 42). They further defined the actions that constitute safe, prudent care for which the nurse is accountable. Regulations and policies denote only minimal requirements for licensed nurses. Professional organizations play a key role in further defining the discipline of nursing, identifying entry-level competencies, and establishing standards of practice for the discipline. A standard is a measurement that denotes the degree or worth of an action.

The American Nurses Association (ANA) and the National League for Nursing (NLN) are two professional organizations that establish standards of practice for the discipline of nursing. Other specialty organizations, such as the American Association of Critical-Care Nurses, have standards that are based on the general standards but are more specific for nurses who work in a specialty area, for example, in the critical care units. Many states have a state chapter of each organization (eg, Pennsylvania Nursing Association [PNA], Pennsylvania League for Nursing). One of the most notable publications by the ANA (2010) is its *Nursing's Social Policy Statement*. An excerpt from this document is shown in Display 8.3. The first social policy statement was ground breaking and provided clarity on the definition of nursing as a discipline, identifying it as an entity discrete from medicine, with its own unique purpose and autonomous practice. This social policy statement was updated and expanded in 1995 and 2003.

Both the ANA and the NLN, each of which is composed of nurses who pay dues as members of the discipline, continue to set standards and publish documents that identify nursing's role in the health care industry, entry-level competencies of practitioners in the discipline of nursing, and professional accrediting standards for nursing education programs.

thinking critically

Visit the ANA Web site at http://nursingworld.org
Choose the ANA site on safe patient handling. What is safe patient handling? What does it say about safe patient handling? What are the educational resources available regarding safe patient handling? What is the ANA doing about this problem? The federal government.

display 8.3   Nursing's Social Policy Statement

The ANA has drafted its *Nursing's Social Policy Statement*, which defines nursing as its own discipline, separate from medicine. Following are the standards of practice and professional performance for nurses listed in the statement.

SIX STANDARDS OF PRACTICE

(1) Assessment
(2) Diagnosis
(3) Outcomes Identification
(4) Planning
(5) Implementation
(6) Evaluation

NINE STANDARDS OF PROFESSIONAL PERFORMANCE

(1) Quality of Practice
(2) Education
(3) Professional Practice Evaluation
(4) Collegiality
(5) Collaboration
(6) Ethics
(7) Research
(8) Resource Utilization
(9) Leadership

From American Nurses Association. (2010). *Nursing's social policy statement* (3rd ed.). Washington, DC: Author.

NCLEX–RN *Might Ask*   (8.1)

> An RN is explaining to a family about how the scope of his or her practice is governed by the state nursing practice acts. These acts are considered
>
> A. Regulations.
> B. Policies.
> C. Permissive language.
> D. Standards of care.
>
> * See Appendix A for correct answer and rationale.

• NURSE PRACTICE ACTS

Nurse practice acts exist in each state as part of the state's regulations (laws) (Taylor, Lillis, LeMone, & Lynn, 2011). Nurse practice acts vary in length, from a simple document only several pages in length to complex documents many pages in length for each practice level (eg, the LPN and RN practice acts in Pennsylvania). States provide additional clarity and interpretation of the practice of nursing through policies established by the state boards of nursing. Most state nurse practice acts are available online. If you do not know how to access yours, just use a search engine such as Google or Mozilla Firefox to find it.

Changing regulations (laws) requires a lengthy political process. The choice of the extent to which specifics of nursing practice are incorporated into law is at the discretion of the state and may or may not be desirable, depending on the state's desire for flexibility and ease of change of such language. However, policies can be changed by the state board of nursing as needed. Because the role of nurse practice acts and subsequent policies by the state board of nursing for implementing and enforcing such laws is to protect the consumer, public hearings are often held when major regulation or policy changes are proposed.

The ANA has played a key role in shaping nurse practice acts and providing guidance to states in restructuring nurse practice act language. Nurses need to keep in contact with their state boards of nursing and the ANA to continue to make an impact on the continually evolving nurse practice acts.

• DIRECTED, AUTONOMOUS, AND COLLABORATIVE NURSING PRACTICE

A key factor differentiating the scopes of practice of LPN/LVNs and RNs is the extent of independence legislated by nurse practice act language.

Directed Nursing Practice

The restrictive language used in outlining the scope of practice of the LPN/LVN delimits this nurse's practice to a directed role. Directed, as defined by the *Oxford English Dictionary* (2010), means "aimed, addressed or guided." Although many

LPN/LVNs have achieved a great deal of independence in their practice, particularly as it relates to caring for patients with common disorders or dysfunctions, their practice remains by law a directed nursing practice. Practical/vocational nursing has been defined by the ANA (1980) as follows:

> The practice of practical nursing means the performance for compensation of technical services requiring basic knowledge of the biological, physical, behavioral, psychological, and sociological sciences and of nursing procedures. These services are performed under the supervision of a registered nurse and utilize standardized procedures leading to predictable outcomes in the observation and care of the ill, injured and infirm; in the maintenance of health, in action to safeguard life and health; and in the administration of medications and treatment prescribed by any person authorized by state law to prescribe. (p. 6)

Inherent in this definition is the standard that the educational preparation of the LPN/LVN provides this practitioner with the basic knowledge for practice in a directed role. It also allows the LPN/LVN to use standardized procedures within that directed role.

Consistent with ANA's definition of nursing is NLN's (1989) *Entry-Level Competencies of Graduates of Educational Programs in Practical Nursing*, which defines the role of the practical/vocational nursing program graduate:

> The graduate of the practical/vocational nursing programs is eligible to apply for licensure. Licensed practical/vocational nurse's practice under the guidance of a registered nurse or licensed physician/dentist. The primary role of the licensed practical/vocational nurse is to provide nursing care for clients experiencing common, well-defined health problems in structured health care settings. In their roles as members of the discipline of nursing, practical/vocational nurses actively participate in and subscribe to legal and ethical tenets of the discipline. (p. 1)

Autonomous Nursing Practice

Merriam-Webster's Dictionary (2010) defines autonomous as "having the right or power of self-government." Autonomous nursing practice is engaging in the practice of nursing independently, without external supervision. The ANA (1980) contrasted the practice of nursing (ie, registered nursing) with the practice of practical nursing:

> The practice of nursing (ie, registered nursing) means the performance for compensation of professional services requiring substantial specialized knowledge of the biological, physical, behavioral, psychological, and sociological sciences and of nursing theory as the basis for assessment, diagnosis, planning, intervention, and evaluation in the promotion and maintenance of health; the case finding and management of illness, injury, or infirmity; the restoration of optimum function; or the achievement of a dignified death. Nursing practice (ie, registered nursing) includes, but is not limited to, administration, teaching, counseling, supervision, delegation, and evaluation of practice and execution of the medical regimen, including the administration of medications and treatments prescribed by any person authorized by state law to prescribe. Each RN is directly accountable and responsible to the consumer for the quality of nursing care rendered. (p. 6)

The substantial specialized knowledge enables the RN to exercise judgment, design and implement plans of care, and engage in various independent functions.

NCLEX–RN *Might Ask*   8.2

In working with clients, the nurse uses the resources of many other health care workers to achieve acceptable outcomes in client care. In this role, the nurse is working
A.   Independently.
B.   As an advocate.
C.   Autonomously.
D.   Collaboratively.

· *See Appendix A for correct answer and rationale.*

thinking critically

Compare and contrast the areas in your personal life in which you perform in a directed role versus an autonomous role. What additional specialized knowledge enables you to exercise judgment and perform independently when in the autonomous role?

Collaborative Nursing Practice

Collaboration among health care providers is essential for meeting an array of client needs and fostering health in a holistic manner. As defined by *Merriam-Webster* (2010), to collaborate is to "to work jointly with others or together especially in an intellectual endeavor." Collaborative nursing practice, also called interdependent nursing practice, is working jointly with others (often physicians) in performing nursing roles within the legislated scope of practice.

The nurse and the physician practice autonomously in making nursing diagnoses and medical diagnoses, respectively. However, collaboration improves comprehensiveness, efficiency, and consistency in fostering health in clients. Many states have created practice act language to allow for the development of standardized procedures, developed jointly by physicians and nurses. Standardized procedures enhance the nurse's ability to function independently. Standardized procedures are developed for use in organized health care systems (eg, hospitals, clinics, home health agencies, community health services, physicians' offices). Display 8.4 depicts a sample of standardized procedure guidelines from the California Nursing Practice Act (California Board of Registered Nursing, 2010).

● MECHANISMS FOR IDENTIFYING DIFFERENCES IN KNOWLEDGE AND ROLES

Although there is a common core of knowledge and competencies in the practice of LPN/LVNs and RNs, the knowledge base and practice roles differ between these two licensed health care providers. How does an individual, organization, council, or licensing board determine the knowledge and roles of a specific practitioner? How do the knowledge and roles of the LPN/LVN differ from those of the RN?

What expectations should an employer have of these two levels of practitioners? What additional knowledge and role abilities should the LPN/LVN expect to gain by participating in and completing an ADN educational program? What knowledge, skills, and abilities should be tested under the governance of the state boards of nursing to assure the public that individuals are competent to be licensed to practice within the scope of practice outlined in state law? These questions are

---

display 8.4 — **California Nurse Practice Act (2010) Standardized Procedure Guidelines**

1470: PURPOSE

The Board of Registered Nursing in conjunction with the Medical Board of California (see regulations of the Medical Board of California, Article 9.5, Chapter 13, Title 16 of the California Code of Regulations) intends, by adopting the regulations contained in the article, to jointly promulgate guidelines for the development of standardized procedures to be used in organized health care systems which are subject to this rule. The purpose of these guidelines is as follows:
(a) To protect consumers by providing evidence that the nurse meets all requirements to practice safely.
(b) To provide uniformity in development of standardized procedures.

1474: STANDARDIZED PROCEDURE GUIDELINES

Following are the standardized procedure guidelines jointly promulgated by the Medical Board of California and by the Board of Registered Nursing:

(a) Standardized procedures shall include a written description of the method used in developing and approving them and any revision thereof.
(b) Each standardized procedure shall
  (1) Be in writing, dated, and signed by the organized health care system personnel authorized to approve it.
  (2) Specify which standardized procedure functions registered nurses may perform and under what circumstances.
  (3) State any specific requirements that are to be followed by registered nurses in performing particular standardized procedure functions.
  (4) Specify any experience, training, or education requirements for performance of standardized procedure functions.
  (5) Establish a method for initial and continuing evaluation of the competence of registered nurses authorized to perform standardized procedure functions.
  (6) Provide for a method of maintaining a written record of people authorized to perform standardized procedure functions.
  (7) Specify the scope of supervision required for performance of standardized procedure functions, for example, immediate supervision by a physician.
  (8) Set forth any specialized circumstances under which the registered nurse is to immediately communicate with a patient's physician concerning the patient's condition.
  (9) State the limitations on settings, if any, in which standardized procedure functions may be performed.
  (10) Specify patient record keeping requirements.
  (11) Provide for a method of periodic review of the standardized procedures (p. 65).

California Office of Administrative Law. (2009). *Title 16: California Code of Regulations. Division 14: Board of Registered Nursing. California Nurse Practice Act.* Sacramento, CA: Author. Available online at http://www.rn.ca. gov/regulations/title/16.shtm #1470 and 1474 (last accessed 7.7.2011).

addressed in this chapter as the knowledge and roles of the LPN/LVN and the RN are explored, explained, compared, and contrasted. Several mechanisms are used to identify such differences in knowledge and roles. These include periodic job analysis studies, licensure examination test plans, licensure requirements and nurse practice acts, and professional organization standards.

Job Analysis Studies

An important mechanism for determining the knowledge needed and the roles played by a particular licensed health care provider is to survey those already in the work setting who are licensed to practice at that level. Such job analysis studies have been conducted for LPN/LVNs and RNs.

Kane and Colton (1988) conducted the initial job analysis of newly licensed LPN/LVNs to examine the entry-level practices of such nurses. Activities these respondents cited were analyzed in relation to the frequency of their performance, their impact on maintaining client safety, the various settings in which they were performed, and the age ranges of clients. A framework for entry-level performance was established, incorporating the nursing process, specific client age and needs, and the practice setting. This job analysis was updated in 1997 by Yocom (1997). The framework continues to be used by the NCSBN in designing the NCLEX-PN.

Chornick, Yocom, and Jacobson (1993) conducted a similar job analysis study of entry-level performance of RNs. This work continues to be updated every 3 years. The survey results in these studies were similarly analyzed, resulting in a framework for entry-level performance that incorporated the nursing process and specific client needs. The latest job analysis was done in 2009 and is available online at https://www.ncsbn.org/2008_RN_Practice Analysis.pdf (last accessed 7.11.2011). The NCSBN is using the framework from this recent study to design the NCLEX-RN.

---

thinking critically

Visit the above NCSBN Web site. Scan through the document especially toward the end. The NCSBN lists may procedures that newly graduated RNs need to know and do. Write down five of them and discuss them in a group. Did any of them surprise you?

Licensure Examination Test Plans

As described previously, job analysis studies play a key role in the design of licensure examination test plans. It is critical that such test plans identify the knowledge and roles of practitioners at the designated licensure level. Thus, in addition to job analysis studies, the NCSBN examines the scope of practice for that licensure level by its member jurisdictions and uses item writers (nurses and nurse educators) to operationalize the test plan for actual test construction. The NCLEX-PN differs from the NCLEX-RN in relation to the results of the respective job analyses, the scopes of practice as defined by member jurisdictions, and the levels of knowledge, skills, and abilities tested (see Chapter 7).

Licensure Requirements and Nurse Practice Acts

Nurse practice acts in each state outline eligibility and requirements for licensure within that state. Although not required, most states use the NCLEX-PN and NCLEX-RN to determine eligibility for licensure. Minimum examination scores needed for licensure eligibility are determined according to the nurse practice act language in each state.

Nurse practice acts in each state also delineate the nursing education program content and clinical experience needed for the program to be accredited by the state board of nursing and for the program graduate to be eligible for licensure. Any additional knowledge or course work required for licensure beyond that in the LPN/LVN or RN program is also outlined in the nurse practice act (Beauchamp, Walters, Kahn, & Mastroianni, 2008; Guido, 2006). In addition to behavioral and biological sciences and core nursing content, some states specify a certain number of hours of education in such areas as communication skills, communicable diseases, pharmacology, child and elder abuse, and substance abuse. Nurse practice acts may also designate specific roles for LPN/LVNs and RNs related to such areas as medication administration, intravenous therapy, blood administration or withdrawal, and chemotherapy.

Professional Organization Standards

Although job analysis studies identify activities being performed by newly licensed LPN/LVNs and RNs and state boards of nursing establish licensure eligibility, these represent only minimal competencies for licensed practice. An additional mechanism for identifying differences in the knowledge and roles of LPN/LVNs and RNs is the standards set by professional organizations.

---

d i s p l a y 8.5 **Roles and Competencies of the RN**

ROLES

Provider of care
Manager of care
Member of the discipline

CORE COMPETENCIES OF THE GRADUATE ENTRY-LEVEL RN

(1) Professional behaviors
(2) Communication
(3) Assessment
(4) Clinical decision making
(5) Caring interventions
(6) Teaching and learning
(7) Collaboration
(8) Managing care

National League for Nursing, Council of Associate Degree Nursing. (2000a). *Educational competencies for graduates of associate degree nursing programs.* Sudbury, MA: Jones and Bartlett.

NLN's (1989) *Entry-Level Competencies of Graduates of Educational Programs in Practical Nursing* describes the role and competencies that should be expected from the graduate LPN/LVN. Likewise, NLN's (2000b) *Educational Outcomes of Associate Degree Nursing Programs: Roles and Competencies* defines three interrelated roles and eight core competencies of the associate degree nurse. Knowledge critical to each role and the expected competencies of graduates are outlined in the document. Display 8.5 provides an overview of the roles and competencies.

• NATIONAL COUNCIL LICENSURE EXAMINATIONS
Practical/Vocational Nursing Test Plan

The *Test Plan for the NCLEX Examination for Practical Nurses* (NCSBN, 2008) provides a concise summary of the content and scope of the NCLEX-PN examination and serves as a guide for candidates preparing to write the examination and for those individuals involved in developing it. The test plan provides the foundation for the development of each licensure examination, so that each NCLEX-PN examination reflects the knowledge, skills, and abilities essential for the application of the phases of the nursing process to meet the needs of clients with commonly occurring health problems having predictable outcomes.

As indicated, the test plan designed by the NCSBN (2008) is based on the job analysis study originally conducted by Yocom (1997). The NCLEX-PN examination includes test items at the cognitive levels of knowledge, comprehension, and application, with most items at the comprehension and application levels.

The test plan notes that the LPN functions in a directed role, contributing to care planning and participating in the nursing process. The NCSBN/NLN (1989) stated:

> The entry-level practical/vocational nurse, under appropriate supervision, provides competent care for the clients with commonly occurring health problems having predictable outcomes. The practical/vocational nurse uses the nursing process to collect and organize relevant health care data to assist in the identification of health care needs/problems of clients throughout the clients' life span and a variety of settings. (p. 3)

The NCSBN (2011) test plan details client needs that can be addressed by the LPN/LVN and emphasizes that this level practitioner requires "basic" knowledge of nursing in four major categories: safe, effective care; health promotion and maintenance; psychosocial integrity; and physiological integrity. The following elements are integrated throughout the NCLEX-PN: caring, communication, cultural awareness, documentation, nursing process, self-care, and teaching/learning. You can visit this Web site to look at the entire plan at the NCSBN by typing the following URL into your browser: https://www.ncsbn.org/2011_PN_TestPlan.pdf

Registered Nursing Test Plan

The *Test Plan for the NCLEX Examination for Registered Nurses* (2010), similar to that for practical nursing, serves as a guide for those preparing to take the NCLEX-RN examination and for item writers in their development of the exam. The test plan

NCLEX–RN *Might Ask*   **8.3**

An LVN is asking an RN about the NCLEX-RN test. The LVN is correct when he or she states to the RN that passing NCLEX-RN demonstrates
- A.   Specialty competency.
- B.   Excellence in practice.
- C.   Average competency.
- D.   Minimal competency.

· *See Appendix A for correct answer and rationale.*

was developed on the basis of the job analysis study by Hertz, Yocom, and Gawel (2000). In contrast with the test plan for the NCLEX-PN, test items for the NCLEX-RN are at the cognitive levels of knowledge, comprehension, application, and analysis, with most items at the application and analysis levels.

The test plan for registered nursing delineates this practitioner's role in nursing process, noting (in contrast with that of practical nursing) autonomous functions, such as assessment, nursing diagnosis, plan development, and evaluation; and collaborative functions, such as planning with other health team members, delegating, and providing referrals. Similar to the test plan for practical nursing, the test plan for registered nursing outlines the knowledge, skills, and abilities needed to address client needs. However, unlike the practical nursing test plan, the test plan for registered nursing calls for a more in-depth knowledge base and skills in teaching, communication, and management. For more information on the differences in the two examinations, refer to Chapter 7. You can also visit the NCSBN RN Test Plan Web site by inserting the following URL into your browser: https://www.ncsbn.org/2010_NCLEX_RN_TestPlan.pdf

• PRACTICAL/VOCATIONAL NURSING ROLES AND COMPETENCIES

Practical/Vocational Nursing Roles

The NLN (1989) defines the roles of the LPN/LVN as follows:

> The primary role of the licensed practical/vocational nurse is to provide nursing care for clients who are experiencing common, well-defined health problems in structured health care settings. In their roles as members of the discipline of nursing, practical/vocational nurses actively participate in and subscribe to the legal and ethical tenets of the discipline. (p. 1)

This definition clearly designates two roles for the LPN/LVN: care provider and member of the discipline of nursing.

Competencies in the Care Provider Role

Within the care provider role, the NLN (1989) outlined competencies of the LPN/LVN in each of the four phases of the nursing process: assessment, planning, implementation, and evaluation.

ASSESSMENT

In the assessment phase, the LPN/LVN assesses basic needs of clients by collecting data and identifying deviations from normal. She or he documents these data and communicates findings.

PLANNING

In the planning phase, the LPN/LVN contributes to the development of nursing care plans, determines client care need priorities, and assists in revising such care plans. She or he uses established nursing diagnoses in this planning process for clients with common, well-defined health problems.

IMPLEMENTATION

In the implementation phase, the LPN/LVN provides care using effective communication, collaborating with other health team members, and instructing clients regarding health maintenance. She or he uses accepted standards of practice and records and reports implementation activities. The LPN/LVN also maintains the privacy and dignity of clients.

EVALUATION

In the evaluation phase, the LPN/LVN seeks guidance and continues collaboration with others in modifying nursing approaches and revising nursing care plans.

Competencies in the Member of the Discipline Role

As a member of the discipline of nursing, the LPN/LVN, as delineated by the NLN (1989), describes her or his role in the health care delivery system and complies with the state's nurse practice act. She or he identifies personal strengths, weaknesses, and potential, using educational opportunities; she or he not only adheres to nursing's code of ethics but also functions as a health care consumer advocate.

● ASSOCIATE DEGREE NURSING ROLES AND COMPETENCIES

Associate Degree Nursing Roles

In 1990, the NLN identified three interrelated roles of the associate degree nurse: provider of care, manager of care, and member within the discipline of nursing. With the 2000 document, the NLN Council of Associate Degree Competencies Task Force believed that the role expectancies would be simpler and duplication would be avoided by organizing expected competencies into eight core components that crossed the traditional boundaries of the three roles of provider of care, manager of care, and member within the discipline of nursing. The three roles and eight core components depicted in Display 8.5 provide an organizing framework for expected RN entry-level competencies, and therefore, the educational outcomes for graduates of ADN programs.

Competencies in the Care Provider Role

The associate degree nurse uses the nursing process when engaging in the care provider role.

ASSESSMENT

In addition to competencies specified at the practical nursing level, the associate degree nurse conducts a more extensive data collection process, using various resources. She or he contributes this information to a database and is able to identify changes in the client's health status.

DIAGNOSIS

Unlike the practical nurse, the associate degree nurse has the educational preparation to analyze and interpret data, identifying actual or potential health care needs and selecting nursing diagnoses.

PLANNING

In addition to competencies at the practical nursing level, the associate degree nurse establishes client-centered goals, develops client-specific care plans, and develops individualized teaching plans in collaboration with other health care workers.

IMPLEMENTATION

In addition to competencies at the practical nursing level, the associate degree nurse initiates nursing interventions, implementing care plans according to priorities of goals and making adjustments as client situations change. The associate degree nurse also fosters a health-supportive environment, promoting rehabilitation potential, providing for physical and psychological safety, and using communication techniques that assist clients with coping and problem solving. Individualized, client-centered care management and teaching plans are implemented, providing continuity of care, and referrals are provided as needed.

EVALUATION

The associate degree nurse evaluates the client's progress toward goals and the effects of interventions, revising care plans as needed.

Other Core Competencies

The NLN task force identified 68 expected competencies of the entry-level RN, including the nursing process steps described previously, inherent in the care provider, manager, and member of the discipline roles. The task force organized these competencies under eight core component headings: professional behaviors, communication, assessment, clinical decision making, caring interventions, teaching and learning, collaboration, and managing care (Display 8.5). Specific competencies in each of these eight components can be found in NLN (2000a).

• LICENSED PRACTICAL/VOCATIONAL VERSUS REGISTERED NURSE KNOWLEDGE, SKILLS, AND ABILITIES

The knowledge, skills, and abilities of those in the nursing profession progress along a continuum, with increasing complexity at each practice level. The educational curricula for the LPN/LVN, the RN, and the baccalaureate and higher degree nurse prepare these health care providers to perform within the scope of the practice prescribed by law and in the roles identified by professional organizations, such as the NLN.

As discussed in Chapter 5, in the mid-1900s Benjamin Bloom and others identified three learning domains that provided a basis for the development of educational curricula for decades to follow. These learning domains were cognitive (knowledge), affective (values), and psychomotor (manipulative skills) learning abilities. Within the cognitive learning domain, six increasingly complex learning achievement levels are identified: knowledge, comprehension, application, analysis, synthesis, and evaluation.

Nursing process, nursing diagnosis, and nursing care plan design require abilities in all six of the cognitive learning levels and in the affective and psychomotor domains. Related to these abilities in the three learning domains, LPN/LVNs and RNs demonstrate different competencies within their roles. As cited, the *Test Plan for the NCLEX Examination for Practical Nurses* (NCSBN, 2011) includes test items at the knowledge, comprehension, and application levels; subsequent editions include some analysis questions. The *Test Plan for the NCLEX Examination for Registered Nurses* (NCSBN, 2010) includes some test items at the knowledge level, but mostly at the comprehension, application, and analysis levels. More emphasis is now being placed on the higher analysis level. This reflects the increased complexity inherent in the scope of practice and job analysis study for registered nursing. Chapter 5 describes ADN curricular content and learning activities in each of the three learning domains and in the six achievement levels of the cognitive domain.

• CONCLUSION

This chapter examines the scopes of practice of the LPN/LVN and the RN. A differentiation among regulations, polices, and standards of practice in nursing is provided, along with discussion of restrictive and permissive language. Directed practice, autonomous practice, and collaborative practice are described, and sample language from states' nurse practice acts illustrates the difference in scopes of practice of the LPN/LVN and the RN.

This chapter also compares and contrasts the knowledge and roles of LPN/ LVNs and RNs. Four mechanisms for identifying the knowledge and roles of these two practitioners are described: job analysis studies, licensure examination test plans, licensure requirements and nurse practice acts, and professional organization standards. NCSBN's test plans for PNs and RNs are compared and contrasted. ADN and LPN/LVN roles are discussed, including competencies and each practitioner's role in the nursing process.

student exercises

1. Search the Web to review the LPN/LVN and RN nurse practice acts from your state. What are the differences in permissive and restrictive languages? The many state boards of nursing throughout the United States are easily accessed through the ANA Web site.

2. Outline several RN activities that fall within each of the three practice functions: directed, autonomous, and collaborative practice.

3. Write in your own words a broad definition of the scope of practice of the RN in the United States.

4. Develop a chart comparing and contrasting the care provider role competencies in each phase of the nursing process for the LPN/LVN and the associate degree nurse.

5. Research a nursing organization of your choice. Does it have standards of care? How are they different from the standards of nursing practice in scope?

References

American Nurses Association. (1980). *The Nursing Practice Act: Suggested state legislation.* Kansas City, MO: Author.

American Nurses Association. (2010). *Nursing's social policy statement* (3rd ed.). Washington, DC: Author.

Beauchamp, T., Walters, L., Kahn, J., & Mastroianni, A. (Eds). (2008). *Contemporary issues in bioethics.* Belmont, CA: Thomson Wadsworth.

California Board of Registered Nursing. (2010). *Title 16: California Code of Regulations. Division 14: Board of Registered Nursing. California Nurse Practice Act.* Sacramento, CA: Author. Retrieved July 2, 2007, from http://www.rn.ca.gov/npa/title16.htmOUT

Chornick, N., Yocom, C., & Jacobson, J. (1993). *1993–94 Job analysis study of newly licensed entry-level registered nurses.* Chicago, IL: National Council of State Boards of Nursing.

Craven, R., & Hirnle, C. (2009). *Fundamentals of nursing: Human health and function* (6th ed.). Philadelphia, PA: Wolters Kluwer/Lippincott Williams & Wilkins.

Guido, G. (2006). *Legal & ethical issues in nursing* (4th ed.). Upper Saddle River, NJ: Pearson, Prentice-Hall.

Hertz, J., Yocom, C., & Gawel, S. (2000). *Linking the NCLEX-RN examination to practice: 1999 practice analysis of newly licensed registered nurses in the U.S.* Chicago, IL: National Council of State Boards of Nursing.

Kane, M., & Colton, D. (1988). *Job analysis of newly licensed practical/vocational nurses: 1986–87.* Chicago, IL: National Council of State Boards of Nursing.

Kansas State Board of Nursing. (2009, July). *Nurse Practice Act statutes & administrative regulations.* Topeka, KS: Author. Retrieved January 23, 2010, from http://www.ksbn.org/npa/npa.htm

Merriam-Webster Dictionary. (2011). Merriam-Webster OnLine. Retrieved January 31, 2010, from http://www.m-w.com/dictionary Oxford English Dictionary On-Line

National Council of State Boards of Nursing. (2002). *Model nursing practice act and nursing administrative rules.* Chicago, IL: Author.

National Council of State Boards of Nursing. (2006). *Nursing regulation and the interpretation of nursing scopes of practice*. Retrieved from July 1, 2007, from https://www.ncsbn.org/ NursingRegand InterpretationofSoP.pdf

National Council of State Boards of Nursing. (2008). *Test plan for the NCLEX examination for practical nurses*. Chicago, IL: Author.

National Council of State Boards of Nursing. (2009). *2008 RN Practice Analysis: Linking the NCLEX-RN Exam to Practice*. Chicago, IL: National Council State Board of Nursing.

National Council of State Boards of Nursing. (2010). *Test plan for the NCLEX examination for registered nurses*. Chicago, IL: Author.

National League for Nursing, Council of Practical Nursing Programs. (1989). *Entry-level competencies of graduates of educational programs in practical nursing*. New York, NY: Author.

National League for Nursing, Council of Associate Degree Nursing. (2000a). *Educational competencies for graduates of associate degree nursing programs*. Sudbury, MA: Jones and Bartlett.

National League for Nursing, Council of Associate Degree Programs. (2000b). *Educational outcomes of associate degree nursing programs: Roles and competencies*. New York, NY: Author.

Taylor, C., Lillis, C., LeMone, P., & Lynn, P. (2011). *Fundamentals of nursing: The art and science of nursing care* (7th ed.). Philadelphia, PA: Lippincott Williams & Wilkins.

Yocom, C. (1997). *1997 job analysis study of newly licensed entry-level practical/vocational nurses*. Chicago, IL: National Council of State Boards of Nursing.

Suggested Reading

Bloom, B. S. (Ed.). (1956). *Taxonomy of educational objectives: The classification of educational goals*. New York, IL: David McKay.

Bloom, B. S. (Ed.). (1974). *The taxonomy of educational objectives: Affective and cognitive domains*. New York, NY: David McKay.

On the WEB

www.m-w.com/dictionary: Merriam-Webster On-Line. (Last accessed 7.6.2011).

www.nln.org: National League for Nursing. (Last accessed 7.6.2011).

www.ncsbn.org: National Council of State Boards of Nursing. (Last accessed 7.11.2011).

www.nursingworld.org: American Nurses Association. (Last accessed 7.7.2011).

www.rn.ca.gov/npa/title16.htm: California Nurse Practice Act. (Last accessed 7.7.2011).

www.nlnac.org: National League for Nursing Accrediting Commission. (Last accessed 7.7.2011).

chapter

9

Critical Thinking and Clinical Judgment in Nursing

● LEARNING OUTCOMES

By the end of this chapter, the student will be able to:

1 Describe the importance of critical thinking in today's society and in registered nursing practice.

2 Describe the relationship of evidence-based research, critical thinking, and clinical judgment in the profession of nursing.

3 Describe the major contributions throughout the 1900s to the evolving definition of critical thinking.

4 Compose a definition of critical thinking.

5 Describe the role played by context in critical thinking.

6 Differentiate between critical thinking and feeling.

7 Identify critical thinking abilities and dispositions.

8 Describe the importance of critical thinking abilities, dispositions, and judgment.

9 Differentiate between critical and creative thinking.

10 Describe the role of critical thinking in the nursing process.

11 Analyze client situations using a variety of critical thinking modes, including problem solving and reasoning.

analysis

background
    assumptions

belief

clinical judgment

context

creative thinking

critical thinking

critical thinking

abilities

critical thinking
    dispositions

deductive reasoning

evidence-based
    practice

inductive reasoning

inference

informal logic

judgment

metacognition

nursing process

reasoning

reflective practitioner

reflective skepticism

self-regulation

synthesis

worldview

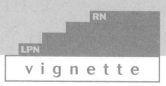

v i g n e t t e

Sally Caruthers is a first-semester LVN returning to school. Tim DeMot is a second-year student.

SALLY: Critical thinking, critical thinking, critical thinking. What is it? We have a quiz every week, a test every month, and now the instructor says we have to take this critical thinking test. How do I prepare for this?

TIM: Boy, I know it sounds like a lot, but you'll be able to do it! This test is not high up there on the ones you need to be concerned about. This critical thinking test is taken in the first semester and again at the end of the program. Once you get the results from the first test, you can tell what your critical thinking level is when you enter the program. These values are also critical to the faculty. You know how they're always talking about "SLOs" for accreditation? Well, they told me that they use the information from the two test results for the National League for Nursing (NLN), and to assess the student learning outcomes (SLOs) upon program completion as evidence that students have developed these skills within the program. It's kind of like all that "evidence-based practice" the nursing faculty talk about in class. In other words, evidence that we've developed our critical thinking skills throughout the program.

SALLY: I guess all that complaining was needless. I think I need to listen better in class. Even though the test results aren't part of our grade, I can see now why they are doing it. Thanks.

TIM: The faculty compares our critical thinking entry scores with the ones on the test we will take right before we graduate. Through the assignments given, such as group projects, case studies, computer-assisted learning tools, and many other learning activities, our critical thinking skills should increase as we go through the program. The faculty also needs the information to make necessary changes in the program curriculum for continuous improvement.

SALLY: OK, that all makes sense. I'll just concentrate and do my best and not worry about it then.

TIM: The tools the instructors use help us prepare to do the complex thinking, problem solving, analysis, and creative thinking required of a nurse. So, even though we don't get graded, it's all part of the big picture to prepare us professionally. The class content on critical thinking will be coming up with the nursing care planning process in about 2 weeks, if I remember correctly. Do you want to go over my notes from last year? It may help you understand more about what is going on.

SALLY: Not right now. I have to study for my psychology test. But can we have lunch together in the student center this afternoon? You've stimulated my curiosity. It helps me to know what is included in the big picture.

TIM: Great. Yeah, I'll see you this afternoon then for lunch.

● THE NEED FOR CRITICAL THINKING

What is critical thinking? When is thinking critical rather than just thinking? Why is there such a need for critical thinking in today's world?

Smith (1990) described the role critical thinking plays in shaping and reframing values and cultural beliefs:

> Why do some cultures elevate the role of women and others demean it? Why do different groups take differing views on abortion, sex, child labor, material wealth, education, and respect for all people, for all animals, for the entire world? Economics or power may have been at the beginning of some or all of these attitudes, but they are perpetuated by stories. They are believed, and held to be natural and right, simply because they make sense to people; it is what they think.

> The great problems of the world today—political, environmental, social, and economic—are not due to lack of facts, and probably not to lack of thought either. They reflect the values of people and governments, the stories they believe. There will be no solutions if we constantly wait for new skills and knowledge; what is required is an ability to recognize and understand the stories that are currently being played out, their consequences, and how they might be changed, in ourselves and others. (p. 132)

As the structure and concept of church, family, community, and civic responsibility have undergone rapid, extensive change, the importance of critical thinking has intensified.

Craven and Hirnle (2007) stated that "simple memorization-style thinking is insufficient to complement the nurse's tasks of sorting, organizing, and identifying relevant information for efficient, effective use. The growing complexity of healthcare demands the use of critical thinking for effective, creative and efficient nursing care." Norris (1985) noted the following:

> Critical thinking is not just another educational option. Rather it is an indispensable part of education, because being able to think critically is a necessary condition for being educated, and because teaching with the spirit of critical thinking is the only way to satisfy the moral injunction of respect for individuals, which must apply to students as well as to anyone else. According to this reasoning, students have a moral right to teaching that embodies the spirit of critical thinking and a moral right to be taught how to think critically. Thus, to abide by the moral principle of respect for person, teachers must recognize the student's right to question, to challenge, and to demand reasons and justifications for what is being taught (Siegel, 1980, p. 14)?.... In addition, there is a responsibility to teach them to do these things well, because in the end students must choose for themselves: there is no escaping this truth (p. 40).

Munnich (1990) noted that oftentimes curricula in schools are based on the "tradition" of white, male Western dominance. She advocated including the "different display **9.1** **The Spirit of Critical Thinking**

"Critical thinkers have confidence in their ability to figure out the logic of anything they choose. They continually look for order, system and interrelationships."

From Elder, L., & Paul, R. (2003). *Analytic thinking: How to take thinking apart and what to look for when you do* (2nd ed.). Dillon Beach, CA: Foundation for Critical Thinking.

voice" (described by Gilligan, 1982) of women and various cultures and races in structuring curricula, writing texts, and designing learning activities. Critical thinking during the creating and reshaping of background assumptions can occur only in an environment of such "alternative traditions" (Display 9.1).

thinking critically

Can you think of any learning activities in which you were involved in which the teacher's assignment or exercise caused you to see things differently? What techniques were used that assisted you in seeing things through a new lens? What were your reactions to the exercise?

Failure to develop thinking skills impedes lifelong learning as one enters the workforce, experiences new situations, and is confronted with new articles, media coverage, and ethical dilemmas. According to Adams and Hamm (1990), "Critical thinking involves the ability to raise powerful questions about what's being read, viewed or listened to" (p. 39). They stressed the need for critical thinking and collaboration in a democratic society to balance reason, individualism, and community. The lifelong tasks of thinking and learning are especially critical in the global positioning of countries in an era of international competition, continuous and rapid technological and sociologic change, and the increasing ethical dilemmas posed by these changes.

thinking critically

Recall a time in your nursing experience when you were able to solve a problem, answer a question, or work through a situation for which you had not been taught the information. How were you able to do this? What thinking tools had you learned that you were able to modify or adapt and use in this new situation? How did your own culture and values come into play in your analysis?

● CRITICAL THINKING IN NURSING

The need for critical thinking in nursing has never been greater. As we embark on health care reform and changes in the health care industry, encounter rapid technological change, experience great demographic shifts, and confront difficult ethical dilemmas, RNs must bring with them the critical thinking skills to make wise decisions and collaborate on change that will have a positive impact on future generations. Also, as the opening vignette shows, many schools have opted to test critical thinking skills before students enter or exit the program. So, LPN/LVNs who are returning to school need to know more about critical thinking. Bandman and Bandman (1988) described the need for critical thinking in graduates entering registered nursing practice at this time of tension in the discipline:

> By defining the conditions under which sound and valid conclusions are drawn, critical thinking facilitates the use of the nursing process. Critical thinking is a liberating force in all human thoughtful activity, but especially to nurses?.... Nursing is in a state of change; activity in defining its theory, practice, and social mandate and critical toward its current status. The nursing profession is experiencing distress and pressure from within and without regarding its purposes, educational preparation, practice, roles, theory, research, and in its relation to medicine. This is, therefore, an auspicious time in which to use canons of critical thinking and logic to inquire openly into the assumptions, beliefs, goals, and values that characterize nursing. (pp. 1–2)

This is still true today. Wilkinson (1996, 2001) noted the challenges for nursing brought about by scientific and technological advances in a rapidly changing care environment.

LeStorti et al. (1999) described the evolving role of the professional nurse from the traditional role of being task oriented (eg, reporting and recording and executing physician's orders) to one of being role oriented, including being a problem solver, decision maker, educator, and change agent. Alfaro-LeFevre (2009, 2011) emphasizes the need for critical thinking and clinical judgment as nurses examine outcomes for quality care, engage in evidence-based practice, prioritize, and incorporate multiple facets of knowledge to move from novice to expert thinking. Benner and Hooper-Kyriakidis (2010) expand on Benner's theme of "novice to expert" as they examine the development of clinical reasoning skills in nurses who become more skilled at recognizing patterns and themes in patients, reflect on these, think critically, and use judgment to provide a more highly skilled clinical practice.

As we entered the 21st Century, the National League for Nursing (NLN, 2000), in its review of the practice of professional nursing, identified clinical decision making as one of eight core components of nursing practice for entry-level RNs. In addition, the NLN delineated 51 assumptions about the future environment in which the RN educated in an ADN program will practice. One of these assumptions was that "critical thinking skills will be essential." Over the past decade, ADN programs have integrated critical thinking skills into the curriculum. Accrediting associations examine nursing curriculum for the presence of critical thinking skills, and the NCLEX-RN has incorporated such skills as well.

The National Council of State Boards of Nursing (NCSBN) is responsible for developing the test plan for the NCLEX-RN. Every 3 years, the NCSBN conducts a comprehensive workplace analysis of Registered Nursing to ensure that the test plan for the NCLEX-RN is current with the demands of today's practice of nursing. The most recent 2010 NCLEX-RN detailed test plan states, "Nursing is a dynamic, continually evolving discipline that employs critical thinking to integrate increasingly complex knowledge, skills, technologies and client care activities into evidence-based nursing practice" (NCSBN, 2010).

• CRITICAL THINKING DEFINED

Critical thinking as a concept has a rich history, has been defined a number of ways, and has continued to evolve over time. In the early 1900s, critical thinking was viewed as problem solving, creative thinking, or what Dewey (1933) termed "reflective thinking." He used this term to refer to "the kind of thinking that consists in turning a subject over in the mind and giving it serious consecutive consideration." He also used such terms as "suspended judgment" and "healthy skepticism" when speaking of what we now call critical thinking.

In the mid-1900s, attempts were made to define critical thinking in a more concrete way. Ennis (1962) developed what he believed to be a comprehensive yet simple approach to the concept. He defined critical thinking as "the correct assessing of statements" and outlined 12 aspects of critical thinking, including grasping the meaning of statements and making judgments about them.

Lists of critical thinking skills (also termed proficiencies or abilities) appeared during the next two decades with the following frequently appearing: "identifying assumptions, both stated and unstated, both one's own and others; clarifying, focusing, and staying relevant to the topic; understanding logic (including inference, deduction, and induction); and judging sources, their reliability and credibility" (Idol & Jones, 1991, p. 14). Snook (1974) took exception to this approach, stating, "To imagine that thinking can be broken down into its component parts which are then programmed is to misunderstand the nature of thinking" (p. 154).

The third quarter of the century brought about contributions from the disciplines of mathematics, science, and engineering, with "problem solving" receiving much attention. Polya (1971) outlined a four-stage approach: understanding the problem, devising a plan, carrying out the plan, and looking back. Woods, Wright, Hoffman, Swartmen, and Doig (1975) described an adaptation of Polya's approach, adding a "think about it" step before planning for their engineering students.

Continued research in the areas of reasoning and problem solving by scientists, psychologists, and philosophers provided multiple facets to the evolving concept of critical thinking. Guilford (1967) described "creative problem-solving" in an attempt to merge the two concepts, and also incorporated the step of "incubation" into Polya's method to allow for what he called "intuitive leaps."

The 1960s saw an intense focus on feelings, challenging beliefs, and using drugs to escape reality and to refute mores of "the establishment." It was a time to "do your own thing" and "go your own way." Ruggiero (1984) noted, "The result of that extremism was the neglect of thinking." However, an important contribution was made to the development of the concept of critical thinking. Creativity, challenging background assumptions, and exploring alternatives became important elements in the discussion of critical thinking during the 1970s. Such discussion also gave rise to the importance of dispositions of the thinker. To think critically, one must not only possess the skills and abilities to reason, problem solve, and explore alternatives but also be inclined to do so and have the desire to engage in such activity.

The 1980s witnessed a renewed fervor of discussion about critical thinking. More fuel was added to the fire in the debate regarding whether critical thinking skills could be learned out of context (ie, on their own, separate from a specific discipline of subject matter). In addition, an emphasis on metacognition (thinking about thinking) emerged as authors examined the thinking process, as well as how one assesses and regulates one's thinking process.

Current literature explores the relationships among the concepts of problem solving, reasoning, critical thinking, creative thinking, and metacognition, and how we teach these. Does critical thinking incorporate the others? Are they distinct but interrelated concepts? Can they be taught, and if so, how can they be taught in and out of context? Do our current teaching methods teach them?

Katz, Carter, Bishop, and Kravits (2001) described critical thinking for nurses as important thinking that requires essential questioning. They noted, "Using critical thinking, you question established ideas, create new ideas, turn information into tools to solve problems and make decisions, and take the long-term view as well as the day-to-day view" (p. 114).

Raingruber and Haffer (2001) also emphasized the power of questioning for nurses: Learning to ask "what else?" and "what if?" They defined critical thinking as "a multi-faceted process that includes logical, rhetorical, and humanistic skills and attitudes that promote the ability to determine what one should believe and do. Critical thinking requires one to actively process and evaluate information, to validate existing knowledge, and to create new knowledge. It involves reflective thinking" (p. 3).

Critical thinking is sometimes referred to as "reflective thinking." According to Marquis and Huston (2006, 2008, 2011), critical thinking components include insight, intuition, the willingness to take action, and empathy. They also advocate intuitive decision making by nurses, using emotional intelligence, and considering the ethical and cultural issues involved. Table 9.1 provides a review of cognitive

table
9-1 COGNITIVE SKILLS USED IN CRITICAL THINKING

Skill	Definition	Application to Nursing
Interpretation	Clarifying the meaning Clustering relevant data	Identifying a nursing diagnosis
Analysis	Examining ideas and analyzing arguments	Making informed decisions based on data and not on assumptions
Evaluation	Looking at the outcomes of one's actions	Determining the outcomes based on nursing actions
Inference	Interpretations or conclusions should logically follow from the evidence Looking for alternatives	Looking at relationships between findings and coming up with meaning and relevancy
Explanation	Reasoning behind one's actions based on data presented	Using knowledge and strategies to support your conclusions
Self-regulation	Looking at one's personal professional practice needs	Reflecting on your own performance and experiences Identifying whether you need to get advanced certification or to go back to school

Adapted from Ignatavicius, D. D. (2001). 6 Critical thinking skills for at-the-bedside success: Key ways to practice, nurture, and reinforce staff members' cognitive skills. *Nursing Management, 32*(1), 37–39; Facione, P. (1990) *Critical thinking: A statement of expert consensus for purposes of educational assessment and instruction. The Delphi report: Research findings and recommendations prepared for the American Philosophical Association* [ERIC Doc No. ED 315-423.] Washington, DC: Educational Resources Information Center.

skills used by nurses in critical thinking. Scriven and Paul (2007) defined critical thinking as "the intellectually disciplined process of actively and skillfully conceptualizing, applying, analyzing, synthesizing, and/or evaluating information gathered from, or generated by, observation, experience, reflection, reasoning, or communication as a guide to belief and action." It is based on "clarity, accuracy, precision, consistency, relevance, sound evidence, good reasons, depth, breadth, and fairness."

● CRITICAL THINKING VERSUS FEELING

When developing critical thinking skills and abilities, and when thinking critically in context, we cannot avoid confronting issues through our own "lenses." We each carry with us our own "world view," which is composed of our age- and gender-related, cultural, ethnic, religious, and sociologic viewpoints. We rely on feelings, intuitions, and experiential knowledge when posing and selecting solutions for new problems and when confronting issues that arise. Bar-Levav (1988) wrote:

> We hold on to our rationalizations tenaciously, since our view of ourselves as rational beings depends on their validity.... Man still tends to hide even from himself the fact that many of his life's most important choices and decisions are made on the basis of feelings, not rationally. (p. 343)

He further added:

> Feelings commonly camouflage themselves as thoughts.... But much thinking is circular and ruminative and leads to conclusions already arrived at by our feelings.... Learning to really think requires first that we make room for it by diminishing the domain of feelings.... Notions from our infantile past in the form of feelings commonly persist as guideposts in adult living. (p. 34)

O'Neill (1985) stressed that the major concept in critical thinking is the ability to distinguish bias from reason and fact from opinion. This is difficult, at best, as Brookfield (1987) described, because critical thinking is not seen as a wholly rational, mechanized activity. It involves such emotive aspects as feelings, intuition, and sensing. As Bar-Levav (1988) pointed out,

> Feelings are the residues of our lifelong individual experiences.... Rather than reflecting current reality, feelings express our expectations based on what we already know from before. They are therefore totally unreliable as a guide to actions in the present. (p. 116)

When transitioning to the RN role, the LPN/LVN, to practice independently, is challenged daily to identify feelings and to discriminate between fact and opinion. She or he, when thinking critically, notes personal beliefs and "brackets" (or sets aside) these feelings and background assumptions to confront issues and approach and solve problems in an unbiased, nonjudgmental manner.

thinking critically

Can you remember some occasions when your own beliefs and background assumptions have prevented you from seeing alternative solutions to problems or additional facets of some issues?

NCLEX-RN *Might Ask* 9.1

The nursing instructor is explaining critical thinking to a new LVN student. The instructor knows the student needs further clarification when the student incorrectly states the following:

   A. "Critical thinking is acting on how I am feeling about the situation."
   B. "Critical thinking is looking at all possible options."
   C. "Critical thinking involves using new technologies to solve problems."
   D. "Part of critical thinking involves looking at how age, culture, and backgrounds influence how nurses think."

• *See Appendix A for correct answer and rationale.*

The NLN (2000) described the need for critical thinking in entry-level RNs in order to make decisions and exercise clinical judgment. The NLN stated:

> Clinical decision making encompasses the performance of accurate assessments, the use of multiple methods to access information, and the analysis and integration of knowledge and information to formulate clinical judgments. Effective clinical decision making results in finding solutions, individualizing care, and assuring the delivery of accurate, safe care that moves the client and support person(s) toward positive outcomes. Evidence based practice and the use of critical thinking provide the foundation for appropriate clinical decision making. (p. 8)

• CRITICAL THINKING AND CREATIVE THINKING

Although controversy exists regarding the relationship of creative thinking to critical thinking (namely whether one encompasses the other or if they are distinct, discrete forms of thinking), there is agreement that they work synergistically to produce "good thinkers."

Dale (1972) noted the need for creativity in society, stating that imitating the past yields death. Only a creative society can survive. Dale stated, "To be creative is to be thoughtfully involved, to be a concerned and active participant, not a disengaged spectator." Perkins (1984) pointed out that the ultimate criterion of creativity is output. He described creative thinking as "thinking patterned in a way that tends to lead to creative results.... We call a person creative when that person consistently gets creative results, meaning, roughly speaking, original and otherwise appropriate results by the criteria of the domain in question" (pp. 18–19).

As in descriptions of critical thinking, a common theme is the emphasis on attitudes or dispositions of the thinker. Ruggiero (1988) suggested, "Creative ideas often come from associating things not commonly associated or from actively bringing together antithetical elements" (pp. 24–25). He also attributed the "disposition to be curious, to wonder, to inquire" as the "trigger mechanism for creative thinking" and notes that the "production of ideas is stimulated by deferring judgments" (pp. 25–26).

The interrelatedness of critical thinking and creative thinking is readily apparent. As Marzano (1991) pointed out, "Creative thinking is closely related to critical thinking, however, the emphasis is more on the generation of new and unique ways of conceiving information than on the thoughtful analysis of information" (p. 427).

He said the following dispositions, taken from his list of thinking dispositions, form the basics for creative thought:

- Engaging intensely in tasks even when answers or solutions are not immediately apparent
- Pushing the limits of one's knowledge and abilities to keep improving one's knowledge and skills
- Generating, trusting, and maintaining one's own standards of evaluation
- Generating new ways of viewing a situation outside the boundaries of standard conventions (p. 426)

Egan (1986) and Brookfield (1987) also noted the presence of risk taking as a characteristic of creative thinkers, along with such characteristics as "optimism, confidence, acceptance of ambiguity and uncertainty, a wide range of interests, flexibility, tolerance of complexity, curiosity, persistence, and independence" (Brookfield, 1987, p. 115). Brookfield further noted commonalities among creative thinkers:

- Creative thinkers reject standardized formats for problem solving.
- They have interests in a wide range of related and divergent fields.
- They can take multiple perspectives on a problem.
- They view the world as relative and contextual, rather than universal and absolute.
- They frequently use trial-and-error methods in their experimentation with alternative approaches.
- They have a future orientation; change is embraced optimistically as a valuable developmental possibility.
- They have self-confidence and trust in their own judgment. (pp. 115–116)

Brookfield summarized that "developing these capacities is a major task of those helping adults to think critically" (p. 116).

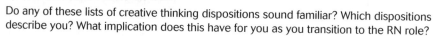

thinking critically

Do any of these lists of creative thinking dispositions sound familiar? Which dispositions describe you? What implication does this have for you as you transition to the RN role?

Smith (1990) provided a detailed account of the concept of creative thinking:

Most people who talk about creative thinking want something more than imaginativeness. There are usually three other requirements: the thinking (or, rather, its observable consequence) must reach *high standards*, it must be *original*, and it must be the result of *intention* rather than chance (p. 13).

● MODES OF CRITICAL THINKING

After reading and thinking about the nature of critical thinking, you now have not only a greater understanding of the concept but also a greater appreciation of the need for critical thinking in nursing. You may be wondering if, given the need for critical thinking at the RN level, the ADN educational program will be different from your prior education at the LPN/LVN level.

As discussed, the higher-order thinking skills of analysis, synthesis, and evaluation are integral to the practice of registered nursing and beyond what is required of the LPN/LVN. Although the NCLEX-RN test plan includes questions to test knowledge, comprehension, application, and analysis, most of the questions test at the levels of application and analysis. These higher-order thinking skills are included in the ADN curriculum and are developed through four modes of critical thinking: problem solving (using the nursing process); reasoning and informal logic; reflection, challenging beliefs, and imagining alternatives; and metacognition and self-regulation. The following sections explore each of these four modes of critical thinking and learning activities within each mode that foster critical thinking.

Problem Solving

Problem solving as a mode of critical thinking has received a great deal of attention throughout the years in the areas of science and mathematics. Polya (1971) outlined a four-stage approach to problem solving: understand the problem, devise a plan, carry out the plan, and look back. In an effort to incorporate more reasoning and reflection, Guilford (1967) included an incubation step, and Woods et al. (1975) added a "think about it" step before planning. Bransford and Stein's (1984) IDEAL problem-solving method was a further adaptation: identify the problem, define the problem, explore alternative approaches, act on a plan, and look at the effects.

Nursing as a science-based discipline also embraced a problem-solving method. The American Nurses Association (ANA, 1973) *Standards of Nursing Practice* adopted a five-step nursing process model of assessment, analysis, planning, implementation, and evaluation. This model has evolved since then with the incorporation of nursing diagnosis as a core concept in the model. The use of nursing diagnosis reflects the increased independent and interdependent (collaborative) nature of registered nursing practice. At its roots, nursing process as a science-based problem-solving model is a linear model. Higher-order thinking skills (eg, analysis, synthesis, evaluation) are incorporated, and reasoning and informal logic can be applied.

LeStorti et al. (1999) combined the concepts of problem solving and creative thinking to formulate "creative problem solving." They defined this as "thinking directed toward the achievement of a goal by means of a novel and appropriate idea of product" (p. 63). Nursing today requires creative problem solving in new roles such as patient advocacy and case management. In addition, as noted by Silverman and Casazza (2000), some of us think and learn in a linear analytic manner, whereas others use a more holistic, visual approach.

Registered nursing programs use nursing process extensively for developing thinking skills in students. A study by Harrington (1992) of nursing faculty in 70 ADN programs in the state of California revealed that 40% of respondents defined critical thinking as problem solving and the use of nursing process. An additional 25% described critical thinking as using analysis, synthesis, and evaluation. Nearly all schools (98%) reported using case studies involving problem solving and nursing process as a learning activity and found them highly effective in fostering critical thinking skills in students.

Reasoning and Informal Logic

Reasoning and informal logic as modes for critical thinking have also received a lot of attention. Focusing on reasoning as a description of critical thinking, Glasman, Koff, and Spiers (1984) outlined four areas of activity:

1. The ability to identify and formulate problems, as well as the ability to propose and evaluate ways to solve them
2. The ability to recognize and use inductive and deductive reasoning and to recognize fallacies in reasoning
3. The ability to draw reasonable conclusions from information found in various sources (written, spoken, tables, graphs), and to defend one's conclusions rationally
4. The ability to distinguish between fact and opinion (p. 467) (Table 9.1)

Authors often equate critical thinking with reasoning and informal logic. In the discipline of nursing, an important contribution was made by Bandman and Bandman (1988), who stressed the need for reasoning and informal logic in registered nursing practice. The purpose of their text *Critical Thinking in Nursing* was "to identify and strengthen the critical thinking skills of nurses by demonstrating the role of scientific reasoning, logic, and philosophy in increasing the effectiveness of the nursing process, and every-day nursing decisions" (p. xi).

Such learning activities as inductive and deductive reasoning exercises and formal debates foster reasoning skills. In the Harrington (1992) study, inductive and deductive reasoning activities were used widely, whereas formal debates had been used by only 19% of those surveyed.

Reflecting, Challenging Beliefs, and Imagining Alternatives

Many authors have cited limitations to the informal logic and problem-solving approaches to critical thinking. Subject matter knowledge, the role played by background assumptions, and the need to take an active role in modifying beliefs have emerged as important elements of critical thinking. Meyers (1986) noted serious limitations to the general logic and problem-solving approaches, including concern that skills taught separate from subject matter have shown little carry over to the disciplines and that these approaches do not support "a central element in critical thinking [which] is the ability to raise relevant questions and critique solutions without necessarily posing alternatives" (p. 5).

Further describing this reflective thought, Brookfield (1987) wrote that thinking critically is "reflecting on the assumptions underlying our and others' ideas and actions, and contemplating alternative ways of thinking and living" (p. x). He further stated that critical thinking "involves calling into question the assumptions underlying our customary, habitual ways of thinking and acting and then being ready to think and act differently on the basis of this critical questioning" (p. 1). Brookfield (1987) also noted nine important critical thinking themes. The first five themes deal with recognizing critical thinking, whereas the last four are components of critical thinking:

1. Critical thinking is a productive and positive activity.
2. Critical thinking is a process, not an outcome.
3. Manifestations of critical thinking vary according to the contexts in which it occurs.
4. Critical thinking is triggered by positive and negative events.
5. Critical thinking is emotive as well as rational.
6. Identifying and challenging assumptions is central to critical thinking.
7. Challenging the importance of context is crucial to critical thinking.
8. Critical thinkers try to imagine and explore alternatives.
9. Imagining and exploring alternatives lead to reflective skepticism. (p. 5)

The role played by background assumptions in impeding critical thinking and the necessity for the critical thinker to modify these as needed was also addressed by experts in the 1980s. Brookfield (1987) emphasized that although critical thinking involves identifying and challenging assumptions and exploring and imagining alternatives, it is not a passive process. Rather, it is a "praxis of alternating analysis and action" (p. 23) as you refute new ideas or integrate them, modifying current beliefs. Paul's (1992) strong sense definition of critical thinking, in which multilogical issues are examined from a variety of perspectives, challenging values and beliefs, is consistent with Brookfield's notion of "critical thinking praxis." As Brookfield (1987) noted, "the ability to imagine alternatives to one's current ways of thinking and living is one that often entails a deliberate break with rational modes of thought in order to prompt forward leaps in 'creativity'" (p. 12).

It is often difficult to set aside our biases and challenge our beliefs. It is only through reflection and empathic listening that we can imagine alternatives. In registered nursing practice, making accurate nursing diagnoses and designing a plan of care with a client demand that such multiple perspectives be used. Learning activities in the affective domain and case studies in which problems arise and the nurse is confronted with multifaceted issues foster critical thinking skills in this mode.

Raingruber and Haffer (2001) suggested four critical thinking approaches that nurses can use: reading and reflecting on narratives, asking questions consistent with Stephen Brookfield's critical thinking processes, using "mind maps," and using a reflective journal.

Metacognition and Self-Regulation

Most authors who have written in the area of critical thinking have discussed the importance of "thinking about thinking," or metacognition. Beyer (1987) and others emphasized the synergy among critical thinking skills, dispositions, and metacognition. Beyer described the importance of "helping students become independent thinkers, proficient at self-initiated and self-directed thinking.... The teaching of thinking consists of teaching students to think about their own thinking, consciously and deliberately, while engaged in thinking for functional purposes" (p. 191). Some authors include the concept of metacognition as part of the critical thinking process, whereas others clearly distinguish it as a discrete thinking process that is essential to being a critical thinker.

Beyer (1987) concurred with the concept of self-regulation, delineating three major metacognitive operations: planning, monitoring, and assessing. He noted that "although these operations may appear to be sequential, in practice they are not strictly linear but recursive" (p. 192) and that these metacognitive operations (in addition to thinking skills and dispositions) are vital to effective thinking or critical thinking.

Burton (2000) described the necessity of "reflective practice" in today's nursing profession. Such self-regulation is important to the nurse's ability to think critically, considering unique patient/client needs. Reflection allows the nurse to check her or his own background assumptions and biases to be more objective in individualizing care.

Costa (1984) defined metacognition as the "ability to know what we know and what we don't know ... to plan a strategy for producing what information is needed, to be conscious of our own steps and strategies during the act of problem solving, and to reflect on and evaluate the productivity of our own thinking" (p. 57). He differentiated this from mere "inner language," which begins in most children around the age of 5 years, noting that metacognition, a formal thought operation, does not develop until about 11 years. He further stated, "Probably the major component of metacognition is developing a plan of action and then maintaining that plan in mind over time" (p. 58).

Marzano (1991) equated metacognition with self-regulation. He explained that metacognition, like critical and creative thinking, is dispositionally based, noting that an "individual is behaving in a self-regulated, metacognitive manner when he or she plans, is sensitive to feedback, evaluates progress, and uses available resources" (p. 427).

In nursing school, your ability to think about your thinking, why you developed a nursing care plan a certain way, or why you took specific actions in caring for a client will be valuable to your learning. Raingruber and Haffer (2001) suggested using mind maps or a journal to "track" your thinking process. This is an example of metacognition.

Appearing more recently in the literature has been an emerging redefinition of the concept of metacognition to include aspects of motivation and initiative in the learner. Idol, Jones, and Mayer (1991) wrote that metacognition refers to two dimensions of learning: self-appraisal and self-regulation. They commented on metacognition's newly defined relation to motivation, stating, "In the past, metacognition was defined largely as an individual behavior and was not initially linked to motivation. Now, it is defined as shared behavior (thinking aloud), and it includes the learner's beliefs, judgments, attitudes, motivation, and self-concept" (p. 73).

As you embark on the ADN program, you may encounter learning activities that cause you to think about your thinking patterns and process. You may be asked to keep a journal, record verbatim communications you have had in the clinical area, or draw cognitive maps (mind maps) representing your thinking process. Teacher role modeling of thinking patterns and processes also assists students in understanding metacognition and self-regulation.

NCLEX-RN *Might Ask*   9.2

> A senior nursing student is being evaluated on critical thinking during client care. Which of the following statements by the student would show the need for additional **education** on the subject?
>
>   A. "It is important to find out if the client is telling me the truth."
>   B. "It is important to verify evidence to support what the client is saying."
>   C. "I have a feeling that this is the right thing to do."
>   D. "I am making this decision based on the facts I have found."
>
> · *See Appendix A for correct answer and rationale.*

● CRITICAL THINKING AND THE TEACHING–LEARNING PROCESS

Many teaching strategies have been developed in the past few decades to foster critical thinking in students. If it has been some time since you were in school, you may find the classroom setting quite different. There may be many times where you feel uncomfortable that the teacher is not "telling you what to memorize," but rather leaving you to that role. You will likely be asked to much more active in the teaching and learning process than you have previously experienced as a student. And, you may even be asked to take a lead role in "teaching role" for a case study or ethical debate, with the teacher serving as a "guide on the side." The need for teachers to employ critical thinking methods in the curriculum has never been greater, and yet the challenge has also never been greater. Today's teaching and learning environment exists in an era of increasing diversity among students, larger class sizes, and economic pressures causing both faculty and students to have less time and fewer resources to engage in these new methods.

Further complicating the above is the fact that methods used for critical thinking often vary from discipline to discipline. However, several authors have described techniques that can be used across multiple disciplines. Raths, Wassermann, Jonas, and Rothstein (1986) stated, "Thinking activities ... are open-ended, in that no single, 'correct' answers are being sought.... Many answers are acceptable and appropriate. Each activity calls for the exercise of one or more higher-order mental functions" (p. 47). Dale (1972) suggested that the role of the teacher is to give the student just enough help to avoid frustration but not too much, or the student becomes dependent and is robbed of the joys and risks of independent thinking. He described that the teacher's role is not to provide knowledge on which the student makes choices, but rather to stimulate the student to think independently about choices and their consequences and to develop values: "To be creative is to be thoughtfully involved, to be a concerned and active participant, not a disengaged spectator." See Display 9.2 for more ideas for promoting critical thinking.

Teaching strategies for critical thinking often involve reading and writing techniques. Paul (1992) described the important role of critical reading:

> *Critical reading is an active, intellectually engaged process* [italics added] in which the reader participates in an inner dialogue with the writer. Most people read uncritically and so miss some part of what is expressed while distorting other parts. A critical

display **9.2**   **The Spirit of Critical Thinking**

- Group work
- Noting patterns
- Building outlines or models
- Bringing dissimilar ideas or opposing views together
- Modeling
- Mind mapping
- Case studies
- Position papers
- Computerized instructive scenarios

reader realizes the way in which reading, by its very nature, means entering into a point of view other than our own, the point of view of the writer. A critical reader actively looks for assumptions, key concepts and ideas, reasons and justifications, key concepts and experiences, implications and consequences, and any other structural features of the written text, to interpret and assess it accurately and fairly. (p. 642)

Paul also provided a discussion of critical writing:

To express oneself in language requires that one arrange ideas in some relationship to each other. When accuracy and truth are at issue, then we must understand what our thesis is, how we can support it, how we can elaborate it to make it intelligible to others, what objections can be raised to it from other points of view, what the limitations are to point of view, and so forth. *Disciplined writing requires disciplined thinking; disciplined thinking is achieved through disciplined writing* [italics added]. (pp. 643–644)

Jones, Tinzmann, Friedman, and Walker (1987) used the term "strategic teaching," meaning the use of teaching strategies to decrease teacher direction so students take responsibility for their own learning. The teacher must assist the learner in constructing meaning so that the "learner is strategic, working actively to link the new information to prior knowledge and drawing on a repertoire of thinking strategies."

Teaching strategies whereby students assimilate and group information, note patterns, or build models are useful in fostering critical thinking. Jones et al. (1987) suggested that students use organizational patterns and graphic outlining or mapping. Drawing diagrams, building visual models, and using cards or computer models to classify ideas, create groupings, and bring dissimilar ideas together can all be helpful tools for thinking critically about the material. In addition, the student must think about thinking through systematic critique as described earlier. This includes reading between the lines for implications and reading beyond the lines for application. Ruggiero (1988) concurred with this, suggesting that faculty encourage students to be curious and ask questions, such as "How will it be when applied?" and "How will different people react to it?"

There is increasing support in the literature for modeling and the use of exemplars. Critical thinking is an abstract concept that is both difficult to describe and to operationally define. Often, the learner can best learn its use through modeling and effective use of exemplars. Paul (1985) stressed that the teacher must raise opposing views, explore background assumptions, and examine inconsistencies. To facilitate this process in students, the teacher must be able to model these behaviors.

Adams and Hamm (1990) advocated the use of collaborative teaching strategies, citing debates, role play, composition of letters to newspapers and the media, and other collaborative processes as means for developing critical thinking skills. Interdisciplinary small group projects are also effective teaching strategies in the cooperative learning approach. Adams and Hamm also advocated the use of computers to stimulate interaction, thinking, and collaboration.

Heyman and Daly (1992) suggested a number of teaching strategies for occupational programs, including visualization techniques, literature, case studies and oral communications, and problem solving and models. Miller and Malcolm (1990) advocated critical thinking in nursing:

> Changes could be made whereby students could engage in more problem-solving activities, case study analysis, more discussion and reflection, and position papers rather than passively listening to lectures.... Nursing educators can foster critical thinking in students by reinforcing the spirit of inquiry and independent critical thought. (p. 73)

They also stressed the need for nurse educators to consider not only the students' cognitive levels but also their learning styles. Using a variety of methods will address the diversity of learning styles of students and thereby promote greater student success in developing critical thinking skills. Use of collaborative work groups, writing reflective responses to questions posed, brainstorming, mind-mapping, journaling, and analyzing both written case studies and computer simulations individually and in groups are all helpful tools for the varied learning styles of students. Harrington (1992) provided numerous examples of teaching strategies used in ADN programs to foster critical thinking in students.

Teaching strategies to foster critical thinking in clinical practice proposed by Persaud, Leedom, and Land (1986) included the use of feedback lectures, with students divided into groups and given problems to solve; clinical simulations using a decision-making model; computer-assisted video instruction; and case studies integrating medical–surgical and maternal–child content areas. Chau (2001) advocated the use of videotaped vignettes to enhance students' critical thinking abilities. Kirkpatrick, Ford, and Castelloe (1997) noted the role of storytelling by nurses as a means for thinking critically about the actual experiences of others. Benner, Tanner, and Chesla (1996) concurred, noting the need for nurse "experts" to serve as role models for those who are at a novice level. Gambrill (1990) suggested that clinical practitioners strive to improve their accuracy of judgments and decisions about clients by learning more about sources of error. Teaching strategies such as role modeling and critiquing case studies allow for such learning, especially among students who have experience at a novice level in clinical practice.

In addition to the critical thinking activities already described, advances in technology have been especially supportive of developing critical thinking skills in student in the field of nursing. Today's computer simulations, as well as advanced technology in manikins used in skills laboratory settings, provide students with interactive learning activities that allow them to learn not only from the case studies themselves but also from their errors in nursing actions taken.

● CONCLUSION

The concept of critical thinking has had a lengthy history. Defining critical thinking, distinguishing it from feeling, examining its relationship with creative thinking, and understanding the need for it in education have all been important as one then applies these to the discipline of nursing. In transitioning from the LPN/LVN to RN role, you will find critical thinking skills essential to your practice. Additionally, with constantly advancing technologies, and the accompanying ethical dilemmas the nurse faces, the application of critical thinking skills to evidence-based practice becomes imperative for enriching the art and science of nursing for high-quality care.

As you participate in the ADN program, you will likely encounter many new teaching strategies and learning activities to foster critical thinking. View these as an opportunity for growth as you transition to the more autonomous practice of the RN.

student exercises

1. Set a timer for 10 minutes. Write as many words or phrases as you can that come to mind when you hear the words "critical thinking."

2. Using the words or phrases you listed, compose your own definition of critical thinking.

3. Describe a situation in nursing when you took inappropriate or incomplete actions. What aspect of critical thinking could you have used to strengthen or correct your actions? (Suggestions: bracketing feelings or background assumptions; using reasoning and judgment skills; using analysis, synthesis, and evaluation better; challenging assumptions or exploring alternatives; applying metacognitive or self-regulatory processes)

References

Adams, D. M., & Hamm, M. E. (1990). *Cooperative learning: Critical thinking and collaboration across the curriculum*. Springfield, IL: Charles C. Thomas.

Alfaro-LeFevre, R. (2009). *Critical thinking and clinical judgment: A practical approach to outcome-focused thinking* (4th ed.). Philadelphia, PA: Saunders.

Alfaro-LeFevre, R. (2011). *Critical thinking, clinical reasoning, and clinical judgment: A practical approach* (5th ed.). Philadelphia, PA: Saunders.

American Nurses Association. (1973). *Standards of nursing practice*. Kansas City, MO: Author.

Bandman, E. L., & Bandman, B. (1988). *Critical thinking in nursing*. Norwalk, CT: Appleton & Lange.

Bar-Levav, R. (1988). *Thinking in the shadow of feelings*. New York, NY: Simon & Schuster.

Benner, P., & Hooper-Kyriakidis, P. (2010). *Clinical wisdom and interventions in acute and critical care: A thinking-in-action approach* (2nd ed.). New York, NY: Springer.

Benner, P., Tanner, C., & Chesla, C. (1996). *Expertise in nursing practice: Caring, clinical judgment, and ethics*. New York, NY: Springer.

Beyer, B. K. (1987). *Practical strategies for the teaching of thinking*. Boston, MA: Allyn & Bacon.

Bransford, J., & Stein, B. S. (1984). *The IDEAL problem solver: A guide for improving thinking, learning, and creativity*. New York, NY: W.H. Freeman.

Brookfield, S. D. (1987). *Developing critical thinkers: Challenging adults to explore alternative ways of thinking and acting*. San Francisco, CA: Jossey-Bass.

Burton, A. J. (2000). Reflection: Nursing's practice and education panacea? *Journal of Advanced Nursing, 31*(5), 1009–1017.

Chau, J. P. C. (2001). Effects of using videotaped vignettes on enhancing students' critical thinking abilities in a baccalaureate nursing program. *Journal of Advanced Nursing, 36*(1), 112–119.

Costa, A. L. (1984). Mediating the metacognitive. *Educational Leadership, 4*(3), 57–62.

Craven, R., & Hirnle, C. (2007). *Fundamentals of nursing: Human health and function* (5th ed.). Philadelphia, PA: Lippincott Williams & Wilkins.

Dale, E. (1972). *Building a learning environment*. Bloomington, IN: Phi Delta Kappa.

Dewey, J. (1933). *How we think*. Boston, MA: DC Health.

Egan, G. (1986). *The skilled helper: A systematic approach to effective helping*. Monterey, CA: Brooks Cole.

Elder, L., & Paul, R. (2003). *Analytic thinking: How to take thinking apart and what to look for when you do* (2nd ed.). Dillon Beach, CA: Foundation for Critical Thinking.

Ennis, R. H. (1962). A concept of critical thinking. *Harvard Educational Review, 32*(1), 81–111.

Facione, P. (1990) *Critical thinking: A statement of expert consensus for purposes of educational assessment and instruction. The Delphi report: Research findings and recommendations prepared for the American Philosophical Association.* [ERIC Doc No. ED 315-423.] Washington, DC: Educational Resources Information Center.

Gambrill, E. (1990). *Critical thinking in clinical practice: Improving the accuracy of judgments and decisions about clients*. San Francisco, CA: Jossey-Bass.

Gilligan, C. (1982). *In a different voice*. Cambridge, MA: Harvard University Press.

Glasman, N., Koff, R., & Spiers, H. (1984). Preface. *Review of Educational Research, 54*, 461–471.

Guilford, J. P. (1967). Problem solving and creative production. In J. P. Guilford (Ed.), *The nature of human intelligence*. New York, NY: McGraw-Hill.

Harrington, N. (1992). *A survey of teaching strategies used in California community college nursing programs to foster critical thinking*. Unpublished doctoral dissertation; University of San Diego, San Diego, California.

Heyman, G. A., & Daly, E. R. (1992). Teaching critical thinking in vocational-technical and occupational classes. In C. A. Barnes (Ed.), *Critical thinking: Educational imperative, new directions for community colleges* (No. 77). San Francisco, CA: Jossey-Bass.

Idol, L., & Jones, B. F. (Eds.). (1991). *Educational values and cognitive instruction: Implications for reform*. Hillsdale, NJ: Erlbaum.

Idol, L., Jones, B. F., & Mayer, R. E. (1991). Classroom instruction: The teaching of thinking. In L. Idol & B. F. Jones (Eds.), *Educational values and cognitive instruction: Implications for reform*. Hillsdale, NJ: Erlbaum.

Ignatavicius, D. D. (2001). 6 Critical thinking skills for at-the-bedside success: Key ways to practice, nurture, and reinforce staff members' cognitive skills. *Nursing Management, 32*(1), 37–39.

Jones, B. F., Tinzmann, M. B., Friedman, L. B., & Walker, B. B. (1987). *Teaching thinking skills: English/language arts*. Washington, DC: National Education Association of the United States.

Katz, J. R., Carter, C., Bishop, J., & Kravits, S. L. (2001). *Keys to nursing success*. Upper Saddle River, NJ: Prentice-Hall.

Kirkpatrick, M. K., Ford, S., & Castelloe, B. P. (1997). Storytelling: An approach to client-centered care. *Nurse Educator, 22*(2), 38–40.

LeStorti, A. J., et al. (1999). Creative thinking in nursing education: Preparing for tomorrow's challenge. *Nursing Outlook, 47*(2), 62–66.

Marquis, B., & Huston, C. (2006). *Leadership role and management functions in nursing: Theory and application*. Philadelphia, PA: Lippincott Williams & Wilkins.

Marquis, B., & Huston, C. (2008). *Leadership role and management functions in nursing: Theory and application* (6th ed.). Philadelphia, PA: Lippincott Williams & Wilkins.

Marquis, B., & Huston, C. (2011). *Leadership role and management functions in nursing: Theory and application* (7th ed.). Philadelphia, PA: Lippincott Williams & Wilkins.

Marzano, R. J. (1991). Creating an educational paradigm centered on learning through teacher-directed, naturalistic inquiry. In L. Idol & B. F. Jones (Eds.), *Educational values and cognitive instruction: Implications for reform* (pp. 411–442). Hillsdale, NJ: Erlbaum.

Meyers, C. (1986). *Teaching students to think critically: A guide for faculty in all disciplines*. San Francisco: Jossey-Bass.

Miller, M. A., & Malcolm, N. S. (1990). Critical thinking in the nursing curriculum. *Nursing and Health Care, 11*(2), 67–73.

Munnich, E. K. (1990). *Transforming knowledge*. Philadelphia, PA: Temple University Press.

National Council of State Boards of Nursing. (2010). *National Council of State Boards of Nursing 2010 NCLEX-RN detailed test plan*. Chicago, IL: Author.

National League for Nursing. (2000). *Educational competencies for graduates of associate degree nursing programs.* Sudbury, MA: Jones and Bartlett.

Norris, S. P. (1985). Synthesis of research on critical thinking. *Educational Leadership, 42*(8), 40–45.

O'Neill, T. (1985). *Censorship-opposing views.* St. Paul, MN: Greenhaven Press.

Paul, R. W. (1985). Bloom's taxonomy and critical thinking instruction. *Educational Leadership, 43*(2), 36–45.

Paul, R. W. (1992). *Critical thinking: What every person needs to survive in a rapidly changing world.* Rohnert Park, CA: Center for Critical Thinking and Moral Critique, Sonoma State University.

Perkins, D. N. (1984). Creativity by design. *Educational Leadership, 42,* 18–25.

Persaud, D., Leedom, C., & Land, L. (1986). Facilitating critical thinking in clinical practice. In *Thinking across the disciplines: Proceedings of the fifteenth annual conference of the International Society for Individualized Instruction* (pp. 1–10). Atlanta, GA: International Society for Individualized Instruction.

Polya, G. (1971). *How to solve it.* Princeton, NJ: Princeton University Press.

Raingruber, B., & Haffer, A. (2001). *Using your head to land on your feet: A beginning nurse's guide to critical thinking.* Philadelphia, PA: F.A. Davis.

Raths, L. E., Wassermann, S., Jonas, A., & Rothstein, A. (1986). *Teaching for thinking: Theory, strategies, and activities for the classroom.* New York, NY: Teachers College Press.

Ruggiero, V. R. (1984). *Beyond feelings: A guide to critical thinking* (2nd ed.). Mountain View, CA: Mayfield.

Ruggiero, V. R. (1988). *The art of thinking: A guide to critical and creative thought* (2nd ed.). New York, NY: Harper & Row.

Scriven, M., & Paul, R. (2007). *Defining critical thinking.* Dillon Beach, CA: Foundation for Critical Thinking. Retrieved July 1, 2007, from http://www.criticalthinking.org/page.cfm?PageID=410&CategoryID=51

Siegel, H. (1980). Critical thinking as an educational ideal. *Educational Forum, 45*(1), 7–23.

Silverman, S. L., & Casazza, M. E. (2000). *Learning and development: Making connections to enhance teaching.* San Francisco, CA: Jossey-Bass.

Smith, F. (1990). *To think.* New York, NY: Teachers College Press.

Snook, I. A. (1974). Teaching pupils to think. *Studies in Philosophy and Education, 8*(3), 154–155.

Wilkinson, J. M. (1996). *Nursing process: A critical thinking approach.* Menlo Park, CA: Addison-Wesley.

Wilkinson, J. M. (2001). *Nursing process and critical thinking* (3rd ed.). Upper Saddle River, NJ: Prentice-Hall.

Woods, D. R., Wright, J. D., Hoffman, T. W., Swartmen, R. K., & Doig, I. D. (1975). Teaching problem-solving skills. *Engineering Education, 66*(3), 238–243.

Suggested Reading

Benner, P. (1984). *From novice to expert: Excellence and power in clinical nursing practice.* Menlo Park, CA: Addison-Wesley.

Bloom, B. S. (Ed.). (1974). *The taxonomy of educational objectives: Affective and cognitive domains.* New York, NY: David McKay.

Burns, S., & Bulman, C. (2000). *Reflective practice in nursing: The growth of the professional practitioner* (2nd ed.). London, UK: Blackwell Science.

Carr, E. C. J. (1996). Reflecting on clinical practice: Hectoring talk or reality? *Journal of Clinical Nursing, 5,* 289–298.

Ennis, R. H. (1987a). A taxonomy of critical thinking dispositions and abilities. In J. B. Baron & R. J. Sternberg (Eds.), *Teaching thinking skills: Theory and practice* (pp. 9–26). New York, NY: Freeman.

Ennis, R. H. (1987b). Critical thinking and the curriculum. In M. Heiman & J. Slomianko (Eds.), *Thinking skills instruction: Concepts and techniques.* Washington, DC: National Education Association of the United States.

Ennis, R. H. (1989). Critical thinking and subject specificity: Clarification and needed research. *Educational Researcher, 18*(3), 4–10.

Green, C. (2000). *Critical thinking in nursing: Case studies across the curriculum.* Upper Saddle River, NJ: Prentice-Hall.

McPeck, J. E. (1990). *Teaching critical thinking.* New York, NY: Routledge, Chapman & Hall.

Vanetzian, E. V. (2001). *Critical thinking: An interactive tool for learning medical–surgical nursing.* Philadelphia, PA: F.A. Davis.

www.criticalthinking.org: The Foundation for Critical Thinking Web site . (Last accessed 7.21.2011).

www.ncsbn.org: National Council of State Boards of Nursing. (Last accessed 7.21.2011).

www.nln.org: National League for Nursing. (Last accessed 7.21.2011).

www.nursingworld.org: American Nursing Association. (Last accessed 7.21.2011).

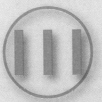
Role Concepts Essential for RN Practice

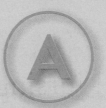

Provider of Care

10

The Nursing Process: Assessment and Caring Interventions

● **LEARNING OUTCOMES**

By the end of this chapter, the student will be able to:

1 Discuss the historical development of the nursing process.

2 Explain the reasons the nursing process was developed.

3 Discuss the importance of the nursing process in guiding nursing practice.

4 Describe the five components of the nursing process.

5 Formulate an actual nursing diagnostic statement using the PES format.

6 Write a measurable expected outcome using a case study.

7 Describe the difference between expected outcomes, interventions, and evaluation.

8 Discuss the role of evidence-based research in the nursing process.

● KEY TERMS

American Nurses Association

analysis

assessment

collaborative problem

cues

data

diagnosis

evaluation

evidence-based research

focused assessment

goals/expected outcomes

holistic approach

implementation

Joint Commission on Accreditation of Healthcare Organizations (JCAHO)

measurable need

National Council of State Boards of Nursing

North American Nursing Diagnosis Association International (NANDA-I)

nursing diagnosis

Nursing Interventions

Classifications (NIC)

Nursing Outcomes Classifications (NOC)

nursing process

objective data

outcome criteria

planning

primary source

problem

secondary source

subjective data

taxonomy

validation

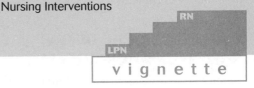

vignette

Jane Smith, LPN, and Enrique Martinez, RN, are taking a coffee break at Paterno Medical Center. Jane is a first-semester student at State Community College. Yesterday, she had her first classroom lesson in planning nursing care.

JANE: Boy, we just had a really difficult class on the nursing process.

ENRIQUE: Oh, yes. I remember the days in school where we had to do those monster 20-page care plans.

JANE: Well, we don't have to do that this semester. We have a care plan due in a week on our clients. It sure is a time-consuming process to do the research and to follow the plan through.

ENRIQUE: Yes, and although the hospital doesn't require care plans like you do them in school, we use the nursing process in a hospital to guide our patient care. Care plans become useful when there is a change from the usual things that you do for the client; or a change from the critical pathway established by our institution. That is something that needs to be communicated to everyone. If it weren't for care plans, everything I know about a client would be here! [He points to his head.] And I work twelve-hour shifts so I'm not here everyday. Verbal exchange of information isn't good enough anymore! It needs to be in writing so all RNs know the plan.

JANE: I know. Our instructor says it's a way to learn a disciplined approach so I don't overlook anything. She also says that care plans are a way to communicate the client's many complex problems. But you are right; care plans are also a learning tool to help me think critically. And besides … I need all the help I can get learning how to put it all in here! [She points to her head and giggles.]

FROM LICENSED PRACTICAL NURSE TO PROFESSIONAL NURSING PRACTICE

In the vignette, Jane Smith and Enrique Martinez are discussing learning and using the nursing process in clinical practice. If you had LPN training during the past 30 years, you probably learned about the nursing process and are using it at work to assess and evaluate client care. However, if you were trained since the early 1990s, the nursing process may have been covered but not emphasized. You probably had little to no time looking at this planning and communication tool with any detail. Perhaps you are practicing where you read the nursing plans of care but do not write them. It is quite different when you must develop the plan of care.

Practicing LPNs continue to perform and have input into many vital functions in the nursing process. As an RN, you will be designing, implementing, and evaluating the entire process. You will be involved in the process from beginning to end, and thus, as Jane stated, will be using a disciplined approach to think critically and solve complex problems.

AN HISTORICAL OVERVIEW OF THE NURSING PROCESS

Nursing as a profession is in its infancy. Although nursing in various forms has existed throughout history, it was not until the profession defined what nurses were and what nursing did that the nursing process was first established. Many of the interventions that nurses did in the past were based on trial and error, intuitive problem solving, and scientific methods. Although Hall first used the term nursing process in 1955, it was not until 1967 that Yura and Walsh first published what they described as the steps in the nursing process (Taylor, Lillis, LeMone, & Lynn, 2011). In the beginning, the steps of the nursing process were assessment, planning, intervention, and evaluation. In 1974, Gebbie and Lavin established nursing diagnosis as a step in the process.

In 1973, the first national conference on nursing diagnosis was held, and, in 1982, the North American Nursing Diagnosis Association (NANDA) was born. Every 3 years, the NANDA meets to contribute to growing knowledge and to revise nursing diagnosis terminology. Because the NANDA has provided a common language that has been adopted by nurses in many nations, the NANDA was renamed North American Nursing Diagnosis Association International, or NANDA-I, in 2003. Currently, there are almost 200 diagnostic statements, and NANDA-I continues to accept and test new and existing nursing diagnoses.

Other nursing organizations have continued working on taxonomies that are based on the NANDA-I nursing process. A taxonomy is a scientific classification system. It is similar to the numeric classification system learned in biology that includes kingdom, phylum, class, order, family, genus, and species. Nursing interventions and outcomes are being researched and organized by two associations closely linked with NANDA-I. These organizations are called the Nursing Interventions Classification (NIC) and the Nursing Outcomes Classification (NOC) groups. The nursing profession has needed an organizing structure to facilitate communication, enhance standardization, help teach new nurses, develop curricula, promote research, use nursing information systems, and promote a reimbursement system.

Many nursing organizations have espoused the nursing process as the organizer of nursing care. The American Nurses Association (ANA, 1998) addressed the steps of the nursing process in their *Standards of Clinical Nursing Practice*, and the National League for Nursing requires that all educational programs incorporate the steps of the nursing process into the curriculum. The National Council of State Boards of Nursing has rewritten the NCLEX-RN in terms of the nursing process.

Other health care organizations also use the nursing process. The Joint Commission on Accreditation of Healthcare Organizations (JCAHO) mandates that documentation must be according to the nursing process. Thus, the nursing process is used widely throughout nursing and other health care arenas. So, what is the nursing process?

● THE NURSING PROCESS: OVERVIEW AND STEPS

The nursing process is a systematic problem-solving method that guides nurses in giving client-centered, goal-oriented care in an effective and efficient manner. The process is systematic, and it consists of sequential steps or phases similar to the steps of the scientific method used in laboratory studies and the general problem-solving process. Table 10.1 shows a comparison of these three processes.

The nursing process is circular, dynamic, and flexible, with a great deal of interaction and overlap, as depicted in Figure 10.1. In uncomplicated situations, the nursing process can be followed sequentially, with each step relying on the accuracy of the one preceding it and influencing the one that follows it. In complicated or emergency situations, all five phases may occur simultaneously. In any event, the various elements of the process enable the nurse to do the following:

- Collect client data
- Think critically about the data
- Identify client strengths and needs or problems
- Establish priorities and expected outcomes

table
10-1   COMPARISON OF THE SCIENTIFIC METHOD, PROBLEM-SOLVING METHOD, AND NURSING PROCESS

Scientific Method	Problem-Solving Method	Nursing Process
1. Define problem.	1. Encounter problem.	1. Assess
2. Collect data.	2. Collect data.	2. Diagnose
3. Formulate hypothesis.	3. Analyze data to specify problem.	3. Plan
4. Design plan to test hypothesis.	4. Determine plan of action to resolve problem.	4. Implement
		5. Evaluate
5. Test hypothesis.	5. Execute action plan.	
6. Interpret results.	6. Evaluate plan for effectiveness in problem resolution.	
7. Evaluate for study conclusion or revision.		

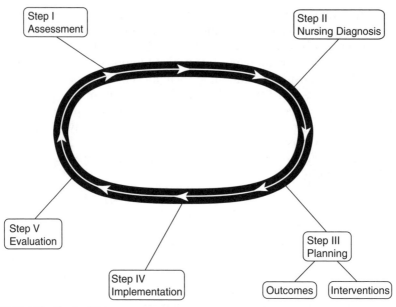

FIGURE 10.1 The Nursing Process.

- Develop an individualized plan of care based writing interventions on evidence-based research
- Provide client-centered individual care
- Evaluate the effectiveness of care and attainment of client expected outcomes

Table 10.2 shows the steps and activities of the nursing process.

The nursing process is recognized as client-centered because it involves the nurse and client interacting in each phase to ensure that an individualized plan is

table
10-2
STEPS AND ACTIVITIES OF THE NURSING PROCESS

Assessment	Diagnosis	Planning	Implementation	Evaluation
Collect data	Identify patterns	Establish priorities	Reassess	Review outcomes
Validate data	Validate diagnosis	Establish outcomes	Set priorities	Collect data
Organize data	Formulate nursing diagnostic statement	Plan nursing care	Perform or delegate nursing care	Determine goal attainment
Report data		Write plan of care	Document actions	Terminate or modify plan of care Evaluate quality of care provided

developed. The plan focuses on client strengths and specifies the client's desired expected outcomes with nursing actions needed to meet those outcomes. If the client is unable to participate in the process because of age or health condition, a family member or support person participates in the process.

Although the primary purpose of the nursing process is to help the nurse manage client care, as mentioned in the beginning of the chapter, the process has gained acceptance in use for documenting client care, writing nursing care plans, defining professional standards of clinical practice, and testing nursing knowledge and abilities for licensure. The nursing process also provides a means for conducting research to improve the quality of care. This research is called evidence-based research.

Reviewing client expected outcomes and evaluating the extent to which a client has achieved outcomes could help identify factors that positively or negatively influence quality care. Identification of nursing interventions that affect expected outcome attainment can guide self-improvement (eg, better handwashing in an individual nurse's practice or change in hospital policy for central line redressing) and nursing in-service programs. Recognition of needed system changes, such as a more timely medication delivery system, can lead to development of more efficient institutional practices, policies, and procedures.

The nursing process consists of five essential steps or phases: assessment, diagnosis, planning, implementation, and evaluation (Fig. 10.1). Following these steps helps the nurse identify and handle a client's problems in an orderly and systematic way.

Assessment

The first phase of the nursing process, assessment, is the continuous and systematic collection, validation, and communication of client data. During the assessment phase, the nurse establishes and develops a comprehensive database by observing, interviewing, and examining the client, with the objective to gain insight and information about the client's condition/situation. As an LPN, you have probably been asked to help with data collection, such as obtaining vital signs or weight. The RN then used that information to make sound clinical nursing judgments in the diagnostic and planning phases.

NCLEX–RN *Might Ask*   10.1

> The primary nurse is providing orientation to a new nurse. Together they are reviewing the nursing plan of care for an elderly client. The primary nurse knows that the new nurse needs additional help with the nursing process when the new nurse states the nursing process is
>
>   Ⓐ. an extension of the medical plan.
>   B. developed with the client.
>   C. comprehensive.
>   D. a systematic problem-solving method.
>
> * See Appendix A for correct answer and rationale.

Assessment activities that are necessary for greater understanding of the client's situation are:

* Collect data: Gather client information.
* Validate data: Determine accuracy of information.
* Organize data: Cluster cues into related groups that show illness or health patterns.
* Report data: Document and report findings.

COLLECTING DATA

Because nursing is a holistic profession, data collection involves gathering information about the client, family, or even the community. Information is gathered about physiological, psychosocial, cultural, developmental, spiritual, and environmental aspects of the client.

When it comes to an individual client, data collection involves making general observations, obtaining a health history or admission nursing database, reviewing diagnostic studies, and performing a physical examination. The nurse must keep in mind that the single most important source of information is the interview with the patient. The significant others are also excellent sources, but because of privacy laws (HIPAA), the patient should always be consulted when others are used as a data source (see Chapter 16). Additional information can be gained from secondary sources, such as reviewing client records and consulting with the client's family members and other health care professionals.

The focus of a nursing assessment is getting to know the person. Nurses should attempt to gain as much information as possible directly from the client. The client is considered the primary source of information. Secondary sources, such as medical records and other health care providers, are useful for supplementing and validating the information obtained from the client. Good interviewing skills are essential to obtaining the required client data and communicating concern for the client (see Chapter 11). The physical examination should be accomplished in a thorough and organized way using a consistent and systematic approach, such as head to toe or body systems.

The nurse should use evidence-based assessment techniques and instruments in collecting data (Ierardi, 2010; Stillwell, Fineout-Overholt, Melnyk, & Williamson, 2010). In emergency situations, the nurse may base her or his interventions on a partial assessment. But as soon as the emergency has passed, the nurse should finish that assessment or delegate it to a nurse continuing with the care of the client. As an LPN you assisted the RN with assessments and learned much by observing nurses and physicians' perform physical assessment. As the RN student nurse, you will be learning to conduct a more in-depth physical assessment and will be adding to that skill throughout your nursing career. The history/database and physical assessment should be obtained as soon as possible after a client presents for care (hospital admission, home health visit, or clinic appointment).

EVIDENCE-BASED RESEARCH

Communication to physicians is paramount in today's fast-paced nursing world. Evidence-based research proves that communication tools help communicate assessments and improve quality care. One of these tools is SBAR. Situation,

Background, Assessment, and Recommendation is a tool that "can ease tensions and promote quality care by ensuring the clear concise reporting of patient issues" (Ierardi, 2010, p. 33).

The nursing assessment should be comprehensive and include data concerning all aspects of the client's health. Most health care facilities and nursing schools have developed assessment tools (forms) to collect and report assessment data (Display 10.1).

Use of an assessment tool helps prevent omissions in data collection and improves data analysis in the diagnostic phase. Tools are extremely important during data collection, but it takes practice and experience to focus and follow cues on areas of need that are particularly troubling.

---

display 10.1   **Body Systems Assessment Tool (Quick Physical Assessment Tool)**

Appearance Overall	Head/Neck	Thorax/Lungs	Heart/Vascular
Demeanor	Eyes	Respiratory pattern and regularity	Heart sounds
Grooming	Symmetry	Tracheal midline	Pulses
Posture	Speech	Symmetry of chest wall movement	Capillary refilling Edema
Response to nurse	Mouth/lips (dry moist/color)	Breath sounds Clubbing Retractions	JVD

VS	Skin	Abdomen	Equipment/ Invasive Lines
T: ____	Color	Configuration	IV type, drip rate
P: ____	Temperature	Bowel sounds	O_2 type, flow
R: ____	Texture	Percussion	Foley catheter
BP: ____	Turgor	Palpation	Drainage tubes
			Tube feedings
SaO$_2$: ____	Pressure ulcers	Pulsations	Dressings

Neurologic	Extremities	Safety	Psychosocial
Orientation	Strength	Bed position	Strengths
GCS	Symmetry Positioning	Call bell Bed rails	Needs Family
Follows commands		Bed check	Religion
Cranial nerve check		Assistance	Coping skills
Pupils/direct/		OOB order	Education level
consensual		Level of activity	

JVD, jugular venous distension; VS, vital signs/temperature, pulse, respirations; BP, blood pressure; SaO$_2$, peripheral oxygenation; O$_2$, oxygen; GCS, Glasgow Coma Scale; OOB, out of bed.

display 10.2	Subjective Data Associated With Objective Data*
Subjective	**Objective**
"I have pain." "I'm not hungry." "I have difficulty urinating."	Pulse 120/min, respiration 36/min; sweating profusely Absent bowel sounds; abdomen distended; eats less than 25% of breakfast tray contents Urine foul smelling, cloudy; urinary output 100 mL in 8 h

*Objective data are what the nurse observes; subjective data are what the client says.

A comprehensive database should include subjective (client's and family verbal information) and objective (observable, measurable data) information about the client (Display 10.2).

The depth and breadth of data collected in assessment depend on the purpose for the assessment as determined by the client's developmental stage, nursing care needs, and urgency of the situation. Once the nurse establishes a comprehensive database determining priorities for ongoing assessment, a more focused assessment can be used to update and evaluate specific problems or needs that have been identified. A focused assessment is done to concentrate on one area, specifically the patient's primary problem gathering as much information as possible in this area. A comprehensive assessment is obtained during initial contact with the client (admission to hospital, home health, or clinic). To strengthen and update the information, an ongoing focused assessment of the client's problem areas is conducted during each client–nurse contact.

VALIDATING DATA

"Validation is the act of confirming or verifying" (p. 237) (Taylor et al., 2011) Incomplete or inaccurate assessment data might lead to false assumptions. Data should be validated always with the client or another source. Validation ensures that information is accurate and complete. The nurse must confirm subjective data by asking more questions, eliciting confirmation from a secondary source, or confirming the data with objective information. For example, a nurse might infer that a child is not hungry because he did not eat the pork chop and squash served at dinner. However, seeking validation of the observed behavior by asking, "You did not eat much. Aren't you hungry tonight?" can lead the nurse to discover that the child just did not like the food. Inconsistency in a client's behavior and verbal responses should always be double-checked to avoid misunderstandings or incorrect inferences. Using inaccurate or incomplete information can result in errors of problem identification in the diagnostic phase of the nursing process. Validating data prevents missing information, misunderstanding situations, jumping to conclusions, and focusing in the wrong direction (Berman, Snyder, & McKinney, 2011).

The nurse collects and validates subjective and objective data (Display 10.2). Subjective data are what the client says; for example, he or she indicates "I have pain," "I'm not hungry," or "I have difficulty urinating." Objective data are information the nurse gathers on what is felt, smelled, seen, or heard. It is also something that can be confirmed by another nurse.

ORGANIZING DATA

It is necessary to organize collected data to identify problems and formulate nursing diagnoses. "Just as putting similar puzzle pieces together helps you get a beginning idea of what the puzzle will look like when its finished, clustering related health data together helps you get a beginning picture of various aspects of health status" (Alfaro-LeFevre, 2010). Use of an assessment tool facilitates some organization of the data during collection, but it does not always bring related information together for a more holistic view of the client. Clustering relevant data into established categories for interpretation can produce a better clinical picture of the client's strengths and problems. A nursing model is more effective for establishing nursing diagnoses because it reveals the functional health or human response patterns that nursing interventions are most effective in managing. Other models may be helpful at times. For example, in an emergency situation, using the airway, breathing, circulation (ABC) model approach, rather than the functional health patterns, helps the nurse set priorities (Display 10.3). Nurses may cluster data according to body systems. The nurse who thinks critically may want to look at a particular healthcare problem by using one model and look at the same problem by using a different model. Each one may give him or her a different perspective and therefore different patterns.

In 2002, NANDA-I approved of Taxonomy II, which has 12 nursing domains that link nursing diagnoses. Display 10.3 looks at data from the following case study using this system. As a student, it is important to find and follow the model or system used by the school you are attending or the institution where you are caring for clients. When you become comfortable with this system, you may want to try others under guidance from an instructor or clinical mentor.

REPORTING AND DOCUMENTING DATA

The final activities in the assessment phase are reporting abnormalities to expedite treatment and documenting all collected data in a clear, concise, and timely manner to facilitate continuity of care by other members of the health care team. Record specific objective observations of client status and avoid use of nonspecific terms, such as good, average, normal, and poor, which are subject to interpretation. Documented information should be written legibly and according to legal and professional standards. Many institutions have implemented electronic nursing plans of care and documentation in standardized computerized forms. If these have been implemented, there should still be space for the nurse to individualize and tailor-make the plan of care to the client.

Read the following case study. Then, look at Display 10.3. The client data on Bill Akins is organized according to Gordon's (2007) functional health patterns. We ask questions throughout this chapter about the story of Bill and Roy Akins and their nurse, Gloria Linquist.

display 10.3 Data Organization According to Gordon's Functional Health Patterns

CLIENT DATA BILL AKINS

1. 69-year-old male
2. Widowed 2 years: two children
3. Occupation: retired economics professor
4. Religion: Baptist
5. Height: 5 ft, 11 in.; weight 170 lb
6. Temperature: 98°F; pulse: 62/min, irregular; respiratory rate: 16/min
7. Blood pressure: 112/64 mm Hg
8. Alert and oriented
9. Swims 4 days a week at college pool
10. Walks a 3-mi. course 3 days a week
11. Smoked cigars and pipe for 30 years; quit 8 years ago
12. Lungs clear
13. Episodic mild–moderate chest pain, activity controlled with nitroglycerin SL
14. Voiding clear urine; 250–300 mL every 3–4 h
15. No bowel movement in 3 days
16. Son states hospitals terrify him
17. Son asks many questions about father's condition
18. Son and daughter visit frequently
19. Allergic to ampicillin
20. Patient states he likes to take care of himself; does not want to be a burden to children
21. Awakens frequently during night
22. Wants to know what kind of activity restrictions he will have
23. Likes to barbecue and picnic in summer with family members
24. Intermittent headaches relieved with Tylenol
25. Abdominal cramping; passing gas
26. Bed rest

DATA ORGANIZATION BY FUNCTIONAL HEALTH PATTERNS

Health perception–health management pattern: 9, 10, 20
Nutritional metabolic pattern: 5, 6, 7, 11, 12, 14, 15, 19, 23, 25
Elimination pattern: 14, 15, 24, 25, 26
Activity–exercise pattern: 9, 10, 13, 22, 23,26
Cognitive–perceptual pattern: 8
Sleep–rest pattern: 13, 21, 24
Self-perception–self-concept pattern: 20
Role–relationship pattern: 1, 2, 3, 4, 17, 18
Sexuality–reproductive pattern: 2
Coping–stress tolerance pattern: 11, 13, 22, 24
Value–belief pattern: 4, 20

DATA ORGANIZATION BY NANDA TAXONOMY II DOMAINS

Domain I	Health Perception–Health Management Pattern	9, 10, 11
Domain II	Nutritional–Metabolic Pattern	5, 6
Domain III	Elimination Pattern	12, 14, 15, 25, 26

Domain IV	Activity/Exercise Pattern	13, 21, 22, 26
Domain V	Sleep–Rest Pattern	13,21, 24
Domain VI*	Cognitive–Perceptual Pattern	8
Domain VII	Self-Perception–Self-Concept Pattern	20
Domain VIII	Role and Relationship Pattern	3, 22,23
Domain IX	Sexuality Reproductive	2
Domain X	Coping–Stress–Tolerance Pattern	20, 23, 24
Domain XI	Value–Belief Pattern	4,20

*Domain IV is further explored in Display 10.11.

From North American Nursing Diagnosis Association International. (2008). *Nursing diagnosis: Definitions and classification, 2009–2011*. Philadelphia, PA: Wiley-Blackwell.

• CASE STUDY OF BILL AKINS •

Roy Akins, age 35 years, enters his father's room at Seaview Medical Center to visit for the first time since Bill Akins, age 69 years, was admitted after experiencing a heart attack 3 days earlier. Gloria Linquist, RN, is standing at the bedside talking to Bill about the heart medications he had just taken for the first time. As Roy quickly and briefly touches his father's outstretched hand, he looks nervously at the IV bottles, monitors, and oxygen tubing attached to his father's nose.

Roy: How's it going, Dad?

Bill: Not too well. They say I've had a heart attack.

  Gloria notices Roy's pale color, shaky voice, and trembling hands and offers him a chair.

Gloria: Your father has had a heart attack but his condition is stabilizing.

Roy: How long does he have to stay here? I'd like to take him home as soon as possible.

Gloria: A few days. As soon as we get his medications regulated and his condition remains stable.

Bill: Could you help me get comfortable in this bed, Gloria? This is the hardest mattress I've ever laid on. I could use some fresh air and something to drink.

Gloria: Sure thing.

  Gloria assists Bill to turn, arranges the pillow more comfortably under his head and shoulders, turns up the air conditioning, and asks the nurse's aid to retrieve some juice from the unit kitchen.

Gloria: You two relax and visit for a while. I'll go see about getting a foam mattress pad for your bed. We'll go for a short walk in about an hour, Bill. Ring if you need anything.

  Later, Roy comes to the nurses' station to speak with Gloria.

Roy: I'd like to leave the phone number of my motel so that you can get in touch with me if necessary. I'm glad my Dad's OK. I sure was scared when my sister called and told me he had a heart attack. I wasn't sure I could come visit him. I do appreciate all those things you are doing for him.

thinking critically

1. List the subjective data the nurse would obtain from Bill and Roy.
2. What objective data would Gloria be collecting about Bill and Roy?

Diagnosis

When the nurse has completed the collection, validation, and organization of client data, it is time to begin the second phase of the nursing process to analyze and synthesize the data to determine what the client needs. The purpose of the second phase is to determine the actual problems, that is, the human response condition for which the client is at risk.

The use of the nursing diagnosis to describe what nurses can do for clients experiencing a human response to injury or illness is still somewhat controversial and inconsistently applied in clinical nursing practice. Resistance may arise from reluctance to devote the time it takes to develop a nursing diagnosis, confusion about the difference between nursing and medical diagnoses, or confusion about the changing terminology proposed by NANDA-I.

NURSING DIAGNOSIS DEFINED

As defined by NANDA-I, the nursing diagnosis is a clinical judgment about individual, family, or community responses to actual or potential health problems or life process. Nursing diagnoses "provide the basis for the selection of nursing interventions to achieve outcomes for which the nurse is accountable" (NANDA-I, 2008, p. 277).

The activities in the diagnostic phase include the following:

* Identifying patterns or clustering data
* Validating diagnosis
* Formulating diagnostic statements

IDENTIFYING PATTERNS

The interrelationship of the assessment phase and the diagnosis phase occurs when the nurse analyzes data obtained in the assessment and identifies patterns to determine the client's nursing diagnosis.

The ability to cluster data intuitively and to identify problems develops with experience (Benner, 2001). Nursing students and beginning practitioners should expect to follow guides and use resources to accomplish this diagnostic activity. Caution should be taken to avoid making decisions about client strengths and problems with insufficient, inaccurate, or inconsistent information. If cues do not match or seem inadequate for the category, additional information should be gathered (focused assessment) to validate the diagnosis. Display 10.4 provides an example of data analysis for the clinical example of Bill Akins.

VALIDATING DIAGNOSIS

When the client's information has been analyzed and a nursing diagnosis selected, it needs to be validated with the client and/or family. Validation provides an opportunity to examine the client's perception of the problem and determine whether there is a willingness to participate in its resolution. Through validation, the client's motivation and desires regarding care can be realized. Some clients are not ready or motivated to resolve problems that are clearly evident to health care providers. Use of client validation allows the client to be an informed and willing participant in his or her care.

FORMULATING DIAGNOSTIC STATEMENTS

When you have completed the assessment phase clustering the data, it is time to determine whether the client's situation is normal, altered, or at risk for altered functioning and to name the problem by using the NANDA-I label that most closely matches your patient's cues. Patients can have four types of nursing problems: actual, risk for, possible, and wellness diagnoses (Display 10.5).

---

display 10.4 **Data Analysis for Clinical Example of Bill Akins**

Gloria has a concern about Bill Akins' level of rest and reviews the clustered cues for his sleep–rest pattern category:

1. Episodic mild–moderate chest pain with activity; controlled with nitroglycerin SL
2. Awakens frequently during night
3. Intermittent headaches relieved with Tylenol

Before drawing any conclusions about Bill's inability to achieve a restful sleep at night, Gloria questions the completeness and accuracy of the existing information and conducts a focused assessment. Although she knows that he awakens frequently during the night, no information indicates the reason for this. Gloria further evaluates the physiological, psychological, and environmental factors that might be contributing to Bill's inability to get a good night's rest.
Gloria's focused assessment includes the following:

1. Frequency of voiding secondary to increase in diuretics
2. His tolerance for unit noise, lights, and presence of staff in the room; noise and activities concerning other patients in the unit
3. Bill's concern over his condition, fear of dying, and lifestyle changes after discharge
4. Bill's level of comfort and frequency of chest pain during the night
5. Bill's ability to obtain rest during other periods during the day

---

If the client has signs or symptoms of an acute illness, you will be formulating an actual nursing diagnostic statement. Such a statement has three parts. Because it is an actual problem, this is the only nursing diagnostic statement that has three parts. A list of nursing diagnostic labels (with their definitions) has been developed by NANDA-I for clinical use and testing (s ee Appendix B). The list is reviewed and updated every 2 years. Each NANDA-I nursing diagnostic label (a problem statement) is accompanied by a list of defining characteristics (a cluster of signs and symptoms commonly associated with the diagnosis) and related causes or etiologies (factors that cause or contribute to the problem). A nurse formulating a nursing diagnosis must pick from this list and not create her or his own, unless they are researching a new diagnosis.

display 10.5	Types of Nursing Diagnostic Statements

Actual: Three-part nursing diagnostic statement
Risk for: Two-part nursing statement
Possible: Two-part nursing statement
Wellness: One-part nursing statement

When writing diagnostic statements, use the proper components of the PES format, as outlined in Display 10.6.

Link the NANDA-I diagnostic label (problem) and etiology (cause) with the words "related to" (RT), and state the signs/symptoms (defining characteristics) that support the diagnosis with the phrase "as evidenced by" (AEB).

Here is an example of an actual nursing diagnostic statement that might be applied to Bill Akins. Because it is an "actual" nursing diagnostic statement, it has three parts.

- Constipation (problem) related to bed rest and lack of exercise (etiology), as evidenced by decreased frequency of bowel movements, headache, abdominal cramping, and passing flatus (signs and symptoms).

RISK DIAGNOSIS Risk for diagnostic labels are used when the client's database shows no evidence of defining characteristics. The following is an example:

- Risk for decreased cardiac output (problem) related to irregular heart contractions (etiology).

Risk or potential nursing diagnostic statements are extremely important in a health care environment that has shifted to predicting, preventing, and managing. As an LPN/LVN, an advantage you bring is your background knowledge and experience of seeing complications in your previous care.

SYNDROME DIAGNOSIS A syndrome diagnosis is formulated when the nurse has a cluster or group of symptoms that alert the nurse to a complex set of conditions requiring expert assessment and interventions. There are five syndrome–nursing diagnoses in the NANDA diagnostic labels. These diagnoses only have one part, the diagnostic label itself. For Bill Akins, a possible one could be disuse syndrome.

WELLNESS DIAGNOSIS A wellness diagnosis is formulated when a healthy client wants to attain a higher level of function in a specific area. Wellness diagnoses are written as one-part statements using the phrase "readiness for enhanced," followed by the listed problem label. The following are examples:

- Readiness for enhanced fluid balance and
- Readiness for enhanced communication.

display 10.6	PES Format for Writing Actual Nursing Diagnostic Statements

P = Problem statement (NANDA stem)
E = Etiology or causes/risk factors
S = Signs/symptoms: defining characteristics

Syndrome and wellness diagnoses may not be used frequently or as commonly as the other two types, so the student new to nursing diagnoses will most likely concentrate on risk or actual nursing problems.

---

thinking critically

Review the database for Bill Akins in Display 10.3, and write actual and risk nursing diagnoses, not used in the previous examples, using the PES format.

1. Actual nursing diagnosis
   NANDA stem: _____
   Etiology (RT): _____
   Signs/symptoms (AEB): _____

2. Risk nursing diagnosis
   NANDA stem: _____
   Etiology (RT): _____

MEDICAL VERSUS NURSING DIAGNOSES

Medical diagnoses and nursing diagnoses differ in several ways. Medical diagnoses identify disease and organ dysfunctions, whereas nursing diagnoses describe the client's response to actual or potential health problems or conditions. A second major difference is that medical diagnoses do not change as long as the disease is present, whereas nursing diagnoses can change from day to day as the client's response to illness changes. Most significantly, medical diagnoses require medical intervention and treatment, whereas nursing diagnoses are within the legal scope of independent nursing practice. The use of medical diagnoses in nursing diagnostic statements should be avoided when possible (see Table 10.3).

Planning

The planning phase of the nursing process involves developing strategies to resolve the client's identified problems and help the client achieve an optimal level of functioning. When possible, client strengths identified in the diagnostic phase should

---

NCLEX–RN *Might Ask*   (10.2)

The nurse is formulating a nursing diagnostic statement for a client with an *actual* health care problem. Which of the following statements is *correct* regarding an actual nursing problem?

   A. Ineffective airway clearance RT thick sputum
   B. Risk for fall RT weakness and orthostatic hypotension
   C. Sleep pattern disturbance RT death of spouse AEB inability to get to sleep and excess sleepiness during the day
   D. Decreased cardiac output RT ineffective heart pumping and death of myocardial tissue

· See Appendix A for correct answer and rationale.

table
....
10-3

COMPARISON OF NURSING VERSUS MEDICAL DIAGNOSIS FOR BILL AKINS

Medical Diagnosis	Nursing Diagnosis
Myocardial infarction	Decreased cardiac output
Bowel obstruction	Constipation
Anxiety	Disturbed sleep pattern
Anxiety	Risk for ineffective individual coping

be used to resolve problems. Planning and implementation activities often occur concurrently in simple or complex situations. The written plan of care is a major outcome for this step in the nursing process. Planning phase activities include the following:

- Establishing priorities
- Establishing client expected outcomes
- Planning nursing interventions
- Writing an individualized plan of care

ESTABLISHING PRIORITIES

The initial step in developing a nursing care plan is to examine the identified needs and set priorities. The ABCs of cardiopulmonary resuscitation can be used when setting priorities because they allow quick and easy screening for problems that require immediate. Maslow's (1968) hierarchy of needs may be used with problems that are not life threatening (mobility, pain, nutrition), need referral to others (diet consultation), or require ongoing attention (wound care, counseling). Priorities are set by considering the severity of the situation (life-threatening conditions take priority over personal enrichment) and recognizing the differences between clients. A plan is tailored to meet the client's individualized needs. One client may be ready and willing to perform his or her own dressing change after watching the nurse one or two times, whereas another may need a supportive family member to do it. Display 10.7 shows a few suggestions on how to establish priorities for client nursing diagnoses.

display 10.7   **Establishing Priorities for Nursing Diagnoses:**
Questions the RN Should Ask

1. Does it involve the ABCs of emergency care?
2. Can you use Maslow's hierarchy of needs?
3. How many symptoms does the client exhibit?
4. Do the symptoms appear in clusters?
5. What priority does the client place on the problem?
6. Is there a simple solution that can be performed immediately?

NCLEX–RN *Might Ask*   (10.3)

> The nurse has identified the following problems list for a client who has been admitted to a long-term care facility. Which of the following would be a *top* priority nursing diagnosis?
>
>   A. Self-esteem, low, situational
>   B. Activity intolerance
>   C. Risk for decreased cardiac output
>   (D) Ineffective airway clearance
>
> · *See Appendix A for correct answer and rationale.*

ESTABLISHING EXPECTED OUTCOMES

The terms goals, objectives, and expected outcomes are often used interchangeably in practice, references, and educational situations. In the 1990s, the NOC group initiated the use of outcomes to determine the effectiveness of nursing actions (Moorhead, Johnson, & Maas, 2004). The NOC has developed a list of 542 research-based interventions that encompass nursing activities for each intervention (Doenges, Moorhourse, & Murr, 2010). A nurse may develop an expected outcome on his or her own, or may use an NOC evidence-based one.

Client-expected outcomes are written statements of specific, measurable, realistic, and timed statements of goal attainment. Because they are behavioral statements describing the action to be seen or heard, they should begin with action verbs (Carpenito-Moyet, 2008). They present information that facilitates evaluation. Expected outcomes help all nurses involved in a client's care know specifically what the planned care is trying to accomplish. (See Table 10.4 for some examples of appropriate action verbs to use.)

Problem: Risk for self-esteem disturbance related to perceived effects on sexuality

Expected outcome: Client will state changes in body structure and function by 2 days postop.

The ANA's (1998) *Standards of Clinical Nursing Practice* specifically states that expected outcomes need to be individually tailored to clients. The standards address six criteria that planning outcomes must achieve. Display 10.8 lists the ANA's criteria for measurable outcomes.

---

display 10.8   Measurable Outcome Criteria According to the ANA

1. Expected outcomes must be related to the nursing diagnosis.
2. When appropriate, expected outcomes must be formulated with the target population (ie, patient, family, community).
3. Expected outcomes must address current and potential capabilities of the client and be culturally sensitive.
4. Expected outcomes need to take into consideration the resources available to the client.
5. Expected outcomes need to provide continuity of care.
6. Expected outcomes must be documented as measurable goals.

table
....
10-4 ACTION VERBS

Measurable	Unmeasurable
List	Know
Describe	Understand
Explain	Feel
Discuss	Experience
Assemble	Accept
Report	

Alfaro-LeFevre (2010) recommended a five-part outcome statement: subject (client), verb (will walk), condition (with walker), criteria (50 ft), and specific time (three times a day). If the subject is assumed to be the client for whom the nursing care plan is written, the outcome statement begins with the verb. The following are examples using Bill Akins.

1. Nursing diagnostic label: Risk for decreased cardiac output related to irregular heart rhythm
   i. Expected outcome: (Client) will state that he has no chest pain for the next 24 hours.
2. Nursing diagnostic label: Constipation related to bed rest as manifested by decreased frequency of bowel movements, abdominal distention, and passing flatus
   Expected outcome: (Client) will report the passage of soft, formed stool within 1 day.

Verbs used in outcome statements should be behavioral, measurable, and specific. Choose action verbs that measure success. Verbs such as know, understand, think, accept, and feel should be avoided.

Expected outcomes may be short or long term, depending on the specific problem being addressed. Short-term outcomes can have target dates that can be achieved in a few hours, a day, or a week. Long-term outcomes require more time, perhaps several weeks or months (Carpenito-Moyet, 2008). "Target dates can be realistically established by paying attention to the usual progress and prognosis connected with

NCLEX–RN *Might Ask*

10.4

The nurse is designing expected outcomes for a client with the nursing diagnosis of excess fluid volume RT excess oral fluid intake AEB S3 heart sounds and crackles in the lungs. Which of the following would be a properly written expected outcome for this client?

    A. The client will list foods high in cholesterol.
    B. The client will have clear lung sounds within the next 4 hours.
    C. The client will lose 5 lb within the next week.
    D. The client will have his or her lung sounds assessed every 4 hours.

• See Appendix A for correct answer and rationale.

the patient's medical and nursing diagnoses" (Cox, Hinz, Newfield, & Scott-Tilley, 2007). Care should be taken to sequence large objectives into smaller increments to prevent discouragement and ensure reasonable attainment of the care plan. For example, a client who wants to lose 150 lb may become discouraged when facing a weight-reduction outcome of such magnitude. A more realistic approach may be an outcome of 5 lb per month.

---

thinking critically

Write goal or client outcome statements for the nursing diagnoses you developed for Bill Akins in the previous Thinking Critically activity.

PLANNING NURSING INTERVENTIONS

In the planning phase, it is important to identify specific nursing measures that can resolve the issues and problems identified in the diagnostic phase. Nursing interventions are treatments based on evidence-based research and clinical judgment that a nurse performs to create a successful outcome. They consist of nursing ongoing assessments for possible complications, teaching, counseling, consulting, giving referrals, and performing direct client care tasks, such as bathing, dressing, toileting, and ambulating. Sometimes intervention activities may be referred to as the "AMT method." Display 10.9 gives the components of the AMT method of writing nursing interventions.

To further contribute to the science of nursing, the nursing interventions selected should be evidence based. "Evidence-based practice is nursing is a problem-solving approach to making clinical decisions, using the best evidence available" (Taylor et al., 2011) (Display 10.10). Evidence-based research is key for nursing growth because it translates nursing research into improved delivery of care. Resource materials that a nurse could use include the NIC system, research-based nursing literature, and texts.

The NIC system was developed in Iowa to standardize nursing interventions. The NIC has developed 514 interventions, and each has a label name, a definition, and a list of activities. Display 10.11 lists some acute cardiac care interventions from the NIC that a nurse could use in Bill Akin's case.

Nurses must develop both collaborative and independent actions. Collaborative actions are nursing interventions that engage other health care providers such as physicians, social workers, dieticians, pharmacists, and physical therapists. The nurse must also use time wisely and delegate interventions when appropriate.

---

display 10.9   **Nursing Interventions: The AMT Method**

A = Assessments: What ongoing assessments do I need to perform?
M = Measures: What nursing actions (measures) or physical tasks do I need to do?
T = Teaching: What kinds of teaching do I need to do with this client?

---

d i s p l a y   10.10   **How to Use Evidence-Based Research**

---

1. Identify the problem or issue from the client, family, or community.
2. Search the literature for data supporting the problem or issue.
3. Evaluate the research using the scientific method.
4. Choose interventions justified by the evidence.
5. Evaluate the outcome: Is it the same, improved, or worsened?
6. If the change is positive, incorporate it into practice.

Standardized planning guides are usually available in nursing schools and clinical practice settings to make the work of planning care easier. However, these plans are guides that need to be adapted and individualized to each client situation. In using standard plans, such as computerized plans, standard care plans, and critical pathways, it is important to screen the material and apply information that applies only to a particular client. Not all information given in a standard plan is applicable to every client. In addition, the nurse must use scientific rationale for the selected interventions, as well as be creative and willing to add alternative activities and actions so that nothing is missed. When used correctly by nursing students and clinical nurses, standard plans can provide valuable direction for developing an individualized nursing care plan. If used incorrectly or excessively relied on without

---

d i s p l a y   10.11   **NOC/NIC Taxonomy Applied to Bill Akins**

00029 Domain 4: Activity/rest
Class 4: Cardiovascular/pulmonary responses
　Nursing diagnostic label: risk for decreased cardiac output

　NOC Outcomes
　Cardiac pump effectiveness, circulation status
　Tissue perfusion, vital signs status

　NIC Interventions
　4044 Cardiac. Care Acute Interventions
　Assess chest pain (I)
　Provide immediate and continuous assess to nurse (I)
　Monitor heart rate and rhythm (I)
　Auscultate lung sounds (I)
　Administration of IV fluids (P)
　Select best EKG lead for monitoring (I)
　Determine cardiac enzyme levels (P)

　Non-NIC Interventions
　Monitor chest radiograph (P)
　Perform daily weight (D)
　Assess daily weight (I)
　Check urinary output (D)
　Teach use of BP- and cholesterol-lowering medications (I, C)
　Consult nutritionist for low-cholesterol diet (C)

Actions are independent (I), physician generated (P), collaborative (C), and can be delegated to appropriately trained personnel (D).

changing them, they can block professional growth, decrease critical communication, and may bring harm to a client.

WRITTEN PLAN OF CARE

Once the interventions are identified, it is time to write a nursing care plan (nursing orders) so that all nursing personnel involved in the client's care have clear direction for implementing the plan of care. The written plan needs to include the nursing orders, which clearly reflect the three intervention types that organize nursing interventions assessment, measures (acting), and teaching. In Display 10.12, the nursing orders include these types of interventions.

Written nursing orders should be specific, clear, and always contain the date the order was written, the action to be performed, who is to do it, and a descriptive phrase that includes the specifics needed for the activity (how, when, where, how much, how long). For example, 4/2/95: Assist Kate to walk to the end of hall with walker 10 AM, 1 PM, 4 PM, and 7 PM daily. M. Wilson, RN.

Written nursing care plans come in a variety of designs, including portable cards, Kardex, multiple-page forms, or computer-generated documents. Despite the differences in forms, the basic components for written care plans are the nursing diagnosis, client-centered outcomes, and specific nursing interventions. Nurses and nursing students need to become competent in the use of whatever type is required in their own clinical practice or educational program settings to implement and document a client's care properly.

---

thinking critically

Write nursing interventions for the expected outcomes you developed for Bill Akins in the previous Thinking Critically activity. Be sure to include the three intervention types appropriate for ongoing assessment, measures (actions), and teaching activities of nursing care.

Implementation

Implementation is the action phase of the nursing process. During this phase, the written nursing care plan is followed, and the nursing orders are executed to move the client toward achievement of his or her established goals. Implementation activities include the following:

- Reassess
- Set priorities
- Perform or delegate nursing interventions
- Document actions

REASSESSING

Implementation requires more that just doing; it requires revisiting some of the activities used in previous phases to ensure that new events and changes in the client's situation are constantly being identified and incorporated into the client's care. In each client encounter, the nurse gathers information on the client's condition to identify

---

display 10.12 **Sample Individualization of Standard Nursing Care Plan**

NURSING DIAGNOSIS: Risk of ineffective thermoregulation related to limited metabolic compensatory regulation secondary to age (neonate)

CLIENT-CENTERED OUTCOMES:

1. Infant will maintain temperature between 36.4°C and 37°C (target date).
2. Parents will explain/demonstrate techniques that keep infant's temperature stable/ normal (add target date).

Standardized Care Plan	Individualized Care Plan
1. Monitor infant's temperature.	1. Assess axillary temperature every hour until stable after birth; check once per shift thereafter.
2. Teach parents how to protect infant from hypothermia and hyperthermia.	2. Show parents how to dress and bundle infant for home and out-ings, and how to conserve heat dur-ing bathing. Explain how to protect infant from drafts and heat loss in the environment.
3. Reduce/eliminate sources of heat loss; prevent hyperthermia.	3. Wrap infant in one or two blankets; use that and booties if appropriate to keep temperature between 37.4°C and 37°C; protect from dampness, drafts, and cold surfaces. Keep room temper-ature at 70°F. Place infant in crib away from windows, doors, and walls.
4. Make referrals to community resources for infant care.	4. Offer free public health/neonatal nursing home visit(s) after discharge. Give name, address, telephone num-ber, or appointment to well-baby clinic or pediatrician.

---

changing problems. The data obtained are used to document the client's condition and evaluate whether nursing interventions are effective and client outcomes are being met.

SETTING PRIORITIES

Just as priorities were established during the diagnostic phase, priorities need to be reestablished on a daily and sometimes hourly basis to ensure that the client's immediate needs are met.

---

display 10.13 **Evaluation of the Expected Outcome**

Expected outcomes are evaluated.
Interventions are not evaluated.

PERFORMING OR DELEGATING NURSING INTERVENTIONS

The RN carries the primary authority and responsibility for directing client care in institutional and community settings. When implementing the plan, the nurse either performs the interventions personally or delegates them to another member of the nursing team (nursing assistant or LPN). Chapter 11 goes into more detail on delegation. When a group of clients is under the care of a nurse, she or he is responsible for assessing and reviewing the plan of care with each client and communicating the needs and schedule of planned interventions with the other members of the nursing care team. The nurse generally reserves direct performance of nursing interventions for educating, communicating, and providing complex technical skills and procedures.

Evaluation

Evaluation is the final step in the nursing process. It is recognized as a separate, distinct phase and an ongoing process (Alfaro-LeFevre, 2010). Evaluation might be described as using nursing process within nursing the process. Activities include reassessment, rediagnosis, replanning, and, in some situations, reimplementation. The expected outcome, not each intervention, should be evaluated (Display 10.13). When possible, the client and family, with the consent of the client, should participate in the evaluation of the outcome.

Nurses begin evaluation by reviewing client goals/expected outcomes to determine whether they were measurable, realistic, and appropriate for resolving the client's problems. It is then necessary to collect data about the client's condition, being alert for changes and unknown factors that have positively or negatively influenced goal achievement.

Barriers and facilitators to outcome achievement may be unknown factors, such as client reactions, worsening condition, cultural beliefs, moral values, and religious beliefs of the family. Reviewing how the nursing team applied the interventions is equally important when developing a comprehensive database on which to make a judgment about goal attainment.

After collecting subjective and objective data, the nurse analyzes the information to formulate a conclusion about the client's behavioral responses to the nursing interventions used. Some nursing diagnoses will be resolved, whereas others will be completely or partially unmet. It is also possible for new problems and new diagnoses to develop simultaneously. If the nursing diagnosis is resolved, it can be eliminated from the plan. Partially met nursing diagnoses should be additionally assessed, and necessary modifications should be made to the plan of care. If new problems have developed, new nursing diagnoses should be identified and a new plan of treatment written.

● CONCLUSION

The nurse uses the nursing process in a variety of settings with clients of all ages to identify actual and potential health issues and problems, as well as to design strategies for resolving them.

This chapter provides a brief review of the five basic steps of the process and explores its application in meeting the expected outcomes of nursing care. By providing individualized care through a combination of independent and collaborative actions, nurses are valued contributors to the health care system in providing holistic, comprehensive care.

References

Alfaro-LeFevre, R. (2010). *Applying nursing process: A tool for critical thinking* (7th ed.). Philadelphia, PA: Lippincott Williams & Wilkins.

American Nurses Association. (1998). *Standards of clinical nursing practice* (2nd ed.). Washington, DC: Author.

Benner, P. (2001). *From nurse to expert: Excellence and power in clinical nursing practice, Commemorative Edition.* Upper Saddle River, NJ: Prentice-Hall Health.

Berman, A., Snyder, S., & McKinney, D. (2011). *Nursing basics for clinical practice.* Upper Saddle River, NJ: Pearson Education.

Carpenito-Moyet, L. (2008). *Nursing diagnosis: Application to clinical practice* (12th ed.). Philadelphia, PA: Lippincott Williams & Wilkins.

Cox, H., Hinz, M., Newfield, S., & Scott-Tilley, D. (2007). *Cox's clinical applications of nursing diagnosis* (5th ed.). Philadelphia, PA: F.A. Davis.

Doenges, M., Moorhouse, M., & Murr, A. (2010*). Nursing diagnosis manual: Planning individualizing and documenting client care* (3rd ed.). Philadelphia, PA: F.A. Davis.

Gordon, M. (2007). *Manual of nursing diagnosis* (11th ed.). Boston, MA: Jones and Bartlett.

Ierardi, J. (2010). "Back in the day" What we learned from outdated nursing practices. *Nursing, 40*(4), 32–33.

Maslow, A. (1968). *Toward a psychology of being* (2nd ed.). New York: Van Nostrand Reinhold.

Moorhead, S., Johnson, M., & Maas, M. (2004). *Nursing Outcomes Classification (NOC)* (3rd ed.). St. Louis, MO: Mosby.

Newfield, S., Hinz, M., Tilley, D., Sridaromont, K., & Maramba, P. (2007). *Cox's clinical applications of nursing diagnosis.* Philadelphia, PA: F.A. Davis.

North American Nursing Diagnosis Association International. (2008). *Nursing diagnosis: Definitions and classification, 2009–2011.* Philadelphia, PA: Wiley-Blackwell.

Stillwell, S., Fineout-Overholt, E., Melnyk, B., & Williamson, K. (2010). Search for evidence: Strategies to help you conduct a successful search. *American Journal of Nursing, 110*(5), 41–47.

Taylor, C., Lillis, C., LeMone, P., & Lynn, P. (2011). *Fundamentals of nursing: The art and science of nursing care* (7th ed.). Philadelphia, PA: Lippincott Williams & Wilkins.

Suggested Reading

Ackley, B., & Ladwig, G. (2011). *Nursing diagnosis handbook: A guide to planning care* (9th ed.). St. Louis, MO: Mosby.

DiCenso, A., Guyatt, G., & Ciliska, D. (2005). *Evidence-based nursing.* Philadelphia, PA: Elsevier.

Lunney, M. (2010). Use of critical thinking in the diagnostic process. *International Journal of Nursing Terminologies and Classification, 21*(2), 82–88.

McEacheron, I. (2007). *Nurse management demystified.* New York: McGraw-Hill.

Wilkinson, J. M. (2008). *Nursing process diagnostic handbook with NIC interventions and NOC outcomes* (9th ed.). Upper Saddle River, NJ: Pearson Prentice-Hall.

On the (WEB) *www.ahrq.gov/about/nursing/nrsevbr.htm:* Link to the "Evidence-based Resources for Nurses" article on the Agency for Healthcare Research and Quality Web site (Last accessed 3.1.2011)

www.AlfaroTeachSmart.com: Rosalinda Alfaro-LeFevre, RN, MSN. A great reference for critical thinking and care planning (Last accessed 3.1.2011)

www.allhealthnet.com/Nursing/Nursing&Research: A database that lists nursing research journals (Last accessed 3.2.2011)

www.careplans.com: Provides sample care plans (Last accessed 3.2.2011)

http://www.nanda.org/: North American Nursing Diagnosis Association International (Last accessed 3.3.2011)

www.rncentral.com: RNCentral; contains a lot of information on care plans and nursing (Last accessed 3.1.2011)

http://www.nursingworld.org/EspeciallyForYou/StudentNurses/ Thenursingprocess.aspx: ANA Web site for the nursing process (Last accessed 3.2.2011)

http://www.youtube.com/watch?v=6TO51_hFKzk: The nursing action in process—2008 (30 minutes) (Last accessed 3.3.2011)

11

The Nurse as Communicator

● **LEARNING OUTCOMES**

By the end of this chapter, the student will be able to:

1 Describe the importance of effective communication to quality nursing care.

2 Distinguish between therapeutic, social, and collegial relationships.

3 Describe the characteristics of effective therapeutic, caring nurses.

4 List ways a nurse can judiciously use communication skills to prevent a malpractice claim.

5 Discuss the two types (forms) of communication.

6 Identify factors promoting effective communication.

7 Describe blocks to communication.

8 Discuss the effective communication techniques used in therapeutic communication.

9 Evaluate therapeutic communications by using a checklist or process recording.

10 Describe effective communication techniques applicable across the life span.

11 Identify key factors that enhance or detract from collegial communication.

12 Recognize communication patterns by self and others.

13 List the five rights of delegation according to the NCBSN.

KEY TERMS

accountability
active listening
assertiveness
blending
blocks in
   communication
caring behaviors
clarification
collaboration
collegial
   communication
cultural sensitivity
decoding
delegation
empathy
encoding

false assurance
feedback
general leads
nonverbal
   communication
paralanguage
privileged
   communication
problem solving
process recording
responsibility
restating
SBAR (situation-
   background-
   assessment-
   recommendation)

self-awareness
silence
social relationships
summarization
sympathy
synergy
therapeutic
   communication
therapeutic humor
trust
verbal communication
   blocks

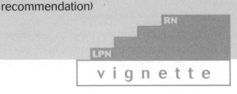

vignette

James Clancy, a 68-year-old, retired Irish-American firefighter, has severe bilateral arterial occlusive disease. Conservative treatment for his disease with diet, exercise, and medication has failed. Tomorrow, he will be admitted to the hospital for bilateral above-the-knee amputations. Nurse Charles Seymour, RN, and student nurse Marie Laurent, LPN, are entering Mr. Clancy's room for his morning assessment.

Mr. Clancy is disheveled and unshaven, with puffy eyes. He is difficult to wake.

MARIE: Hello, Mr. Clancy. My name is Marie Laurent. I am a student nurse and will be doing your care today.

MR. CLANCY: Why do you always have to be doing something with me? Leave me alone. I just want to sleep.

MARIE: Mr. Clancy, you look tired. Did you sleep well last night?

Mr. Clancy's legs are painful at the slightest movement and he grimaces when moving them back and forth in an agitated manner. He states in a much louder voice, "What do you think? I'm losing my legs tomorrow. Why don't you just let me die? I'm no good to anyone this way."

Marie looks at Charles with a helpless look on her face and backs away from Mr. Clancy. She remains silent but sad and thoughtful-looking.

CHARLES: Was it pain in your legs that caused you to lose sleep last night or worrying about the surgery?

MR. CLANCY: Both! What do you think? You are always doing things with me. Don't you understand how much pain I'm in? I'm in agony when I move the tiniest bit, now I hear I need to go for more tests today. I'm in agony when I get on and off that stretcher.

CHARLES: (Moves closer to Mr. Clancy, drops to his level, pauses, and looks directly at him.) I can give you something stronger for the pain, and we can use your bed to transport you.

261

MR. CLANCY: All I'm asking is for someone to meet me halfway. I really don't want to have this surgery, and I'm in more pain when I'm moved.

CHARLES: I realize that this is a difficult decision for you. (Charles pauses, stays close to Mr. Clancy, and has a look of genuine concern on his face but remains silent.)

MR. CLANCY: I don't want this. What will I do with the rest of my life? How will I get anywhere without help?

CHARLES: (Responds in a dramatically quieter voice.) It sounds as if you have not made up your mind completely yet about this surgery.

MR. CLANCY: I still think my legs can get better.

CHARLES: Let's talk about what the doctor said yesterday and review the information some of those tests are telling us. Then, we can call Dr. Marin and ask if he can spend some time with you …. However, this is your decision, and you have the right to refuse surgery.

Later, Charles and Marie are discussing Mr. Clancy's case.

MARIE: I never know what to say when patients get angry and upset. The same approach doesn't work with everyone.

CHARLES: It's hard to know what to say when someone is so upset and writhing in pain. But there are some good principles of communication that I always remember. First, don't get so caught up in emotions that you can't think straight. Second, talk less and listen more. Third, be human and try to get at the root of the problem from the client's perspective. Then, I also review what has worked well and what hasn't.

MARIE: Yes, I remember some of those skills from my LPN training. I remember starting off wanting to give patients that kind of attention. It takes ongoing education and working on it … doesn't it?

CHARLES: Yes, no one knows everything about communication. Concerned health care professionals go to seminars to enhance their skills. With reminders and education, everyone listens better. The patient is happier, the staff feels satisfaction, and the quality of care is better.

● EFFECTIVE COMMUNICATION

Scenarios such as the one involving Charles, Marie, and their patient Mr. Clancy are repeated everyday in health care settings. To be effective in delivering nursing care, nurses not only need to be good communicators but also need to be able to skillfully defuse situations such as Mr. Clancy's. Communication is the key to human relationships and the glue of human interaction; it is an essential need of humans, a universal characteristic of life and living. Students of human communication have attempted to determine what is helpful or not helpful, what is detrimental, what promotes growth and satisfaction, and what blocks understanding. Continuing education and working at it is key to improving communication.

The skill of communication was introduced in your previous nursing studies. It is one you continue to use in your clinical practice and everyday life. Many seasoned nurses say that they, like Marie, feel helpless in certain circumstances. Like Charles, the entire health care system is realizing the need to brush up on good communication, study exemplary mentors, and practice for better client outcomes. This chapter is divided into two sections. The first section reviews concepts of communication (verbal and nonverbal) and caring and provides for effective communication with clients. The second section approaches the subjects of effective team building, assertiveness skills, and delegation.

● BASIC COMMUNICATION REVISITED

The process of communication is not a simple one. It is helpful to review the simple two-person communication model developed by Berlo (1960) (Fig. 11.1). This model involves many variables that affect the sender, the message, and the receiver. It all begins with a message and the sender's desire to be understood. The sender communicates the message by encoding verbal and nonverbal signals to the receiver. The receiver decodes the message, that is, tries to understand the meaning of the message. Feedback is given to the sender from the receiver, and the process continues. There are many preexisting factors that influence communication, including the physiological, biological, cultural, and gender-specific characteristics of the participants. These variables can also alter the clarity of communication. Anywhere in this model, a breakdown in the message can occur, causing miscommunication or an inaccurate message to be conveyed between the two participants.

● TWO FORMS OF COMMUNICATION: NONVERBAL AND VERBAL

In the model of communication (Fig. 11.1), the sender and receiver impart both nonverbal and verbal messages (or cues), which are exquisitely interrelated. Nonverbal behaviors support, emphasize, confuse, or contradict what the verbal part of the message implies. Although the predominant cultures of the United

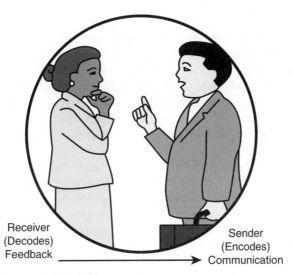

Receiver
(Decodes)
Feedback

Sender
(Encodes)
Communication

FIGURE 11.1 The Communication Model.

Factors That Promote Nonverbal Communication

Focus undivided attention on active listening skills.
Sit down to listen whenever possible.
Use silence judiciously.
Moderate the voice tone and pace.
Use good eye contact.
Minimize gesturing.
Smile appropriately.
Simplify the language.
Use proper touching techniques.
Respect cultural diversity.
Try to "blend" with the client's nonverbals.
Identify and explore inconsistencies/contradictions.

States emphasize and consciously recognize verbal communication as most important, most communication is nonverbal. There needs to be congruency and consistency between the verbal message the nurse is trying to express and the nonverbal communication cues, or trust in the nurse may not be established. Techniques that can be successful in promoting effective communication include active listening, judicious use of silence, speaking clearly and distinctly, maintenance of eye contact and open body gestures, simplicity of word use, and a caring touch (Display 11.1). Nurses are usually aware of their verbal statements but may be unaware of what they "telegraph" or tell the client with nonverbal cues.

Nonverbal Communication

ACTIVE LISTENING

Effective communication occurs when you "listen for feelings as well as words" (Alfaro-LeFevre, 2010, p. 65). Active listening helps establish and maintain the trust and genuineness necessary in the helping relationship. It is the most therapeutic technique a nurse can use. The nurse's attitude is paramount for active listening. The nurse needs to convey readiness to hear and understand what the client wants to say without argument, judgment, or interruption. Although silence is passive, active listening is not. As the name implies, it requires intense action and concentration on the part of the nurse. Nonverbal and verbal information are processed and understood. Listening behaviors can be observed while learning from a seasoned nurse mentor but must be actively practiced to work effectively within the nurse's practice.

Behaviors a nurse can perform to enhance attentive listening are called the "posture of involvement." The nurse should turn toward the client and lean slightly forward. To convey an open and less threatening position, the nurse should make an attempt to be at the client's eye level when possible. This will make the client feel less like he or she is being talked "down to" or being "talked at" and more like an equal partner in the communication. Moving closer to the client without violating his or her body space will help lessen the distance from formal to therapeutic. Sit down whenever possible even if it's only for a moment. This communicates that you are taking the time to listen, and the patient thinks that you are actually there for longer than usual.

Timing is critical with active listening. Every effort should be made to decrease interruptions at this time. In the home setting, it may mean turning off televisions or radios (with the patient's permission). In the hospital, it may mean drawing the curtain and pulling up a chair momentarily. Decreasing interruptions allows both nurse and client to focus on emotions, facts, and problem solving. As a rule, listen twice as much as you speak.

SILENCE

Silence can be both a verbal technique and a nonverbal technique of enhancing quality discussion. Silence on the nurse's part allows full concentration on the client. The proper use of silence decreases the pace, allowing the nurse to observe and interpret the client's meaning. The nurse may miss valuable information and cues if the sometimes uncomfortable void of silence is full of meaningless conversation. Be patient and don't fill in the words for the client.

PARALANGUAGE

Clarity, quality, pitch, tone, and tempo of the spoken word are called paralanguages. Paralanguage deals with "how" a word or words are said, independent of "what" is said. Speak to the client in a clear, moderate voice at a medium rate of speed. Mumbled, indistinct, fast communication can be misinterpreted, even in clients without special needs. It may also contradict caring behaviors that the nurse wants to foster. Speaking clearly presents a clear message. Use verbal checks—such as asking the client whether you are speaking clearly enough or speaking too fast—periodically throughout the conversation to determine whether your intentions have been clear to the client.

EYE CONTACT, BODY POSTURES, AND GESTURES

Eye contact and moderate body gestures can enhance the quality of effective nurse–patient interaction. Friendly, open eye contact by the nurse promotes interest and caring. Comfortable eye contact does not include glancing, darting, shifting, or fixed gazes. An inability by the nurse or patient to maintain eye contact may convey anger, mistrust, or even suspicion.

The nurse must be culturally sensitive when using eye contact. In Asian and Hispanic cultures, direct eye contact can indicate disrespect. Patients from these cultures may not look at the nurse directly and may give the impression that they are not sincere or not listening. The nurse needs to be culturally sensitive when dealing with nonverbal messages from other cultures. Chapter 13 contains more information on cultural sensitivity.

Although eye contact is dictated by cultural norms, facial expressions are not. Charles Darwin (1872) noted that facial expressions have universal meanings. Laughing, smiling, frowning, and crying convey similar emotions transculturally.

The nurse needs to initially adopt a friendly, open facial expression. The nurse who frowns or nervously paces the room indicates nonverbally that she or he has terminated the interaction. Warmth and caring can be displayed by a relaxed stance and posture, with shoulders level and flexible and hands unclenched.

Gestures are motions made with the body and hands that have culturally defined meanings. Although uplifted hands with the head cocked may mean the communicator is not sure in one culture, it may mean something vastly differently in another. As a rule of thumb, the nurse should use a minimum of gestures if he or she is not sure of the audience's cultural heritage. Avoid crossing arms and legs. These are sometimes interpreted as closed postures and do not convey openness (Pagana, 2009).

APPEARANCE

Clients and nurses can communicate much about grooming, hygiene, and emotional and mental status by their appearance. There is an adage relevant to this situation: "Looks can be deceiving." A nurse needs to question further and not make snap judgments about a client's status based on appearance alone. A client who enters a community clinic with untrimmed hair and dressed in worn clothes but who is essentially clean and has no body odor may, at first glance, convey the impression of being homeless. However, the nurse may find this client is employed but barely making ends meet or is well-off but lives alone.

The nurse also needs to be acutely aware of her or his own nonverbal cues. Self-awareness includes the need for the nurse to be conscious of her dress and behavior and how it affects those around him or her. A nurse who has clean, neatly tailored and pressed clothes, neatly manicured nails, and a prominently worn name badge conveys a strong professional self-concept as he or she enters the room. Evidence-based research indicates clients also want to see who is caring for them, and the name tag with the nurse's professional status (RN, LPN) should be prominently displayed (Windle, Halbert, Dumont, Tagnesi, & Johnson, 2008).

TOUCH

Although touch is listed last, it is an important nonverbal communication because it involves sensory input from the body's largest organ—the skin. Touch can be a powerful communicator of caring, respect, and acceptance. "Nursing has always been a high-touch profession" (Schuster & Nykolyn, 2010). Touch is a basic human need and part of every nursing procedure. How the nurse performs a vital signs assessment, gives a bed bath, or administers medication conveys the nurse's basic philosophy about those in his or her care. Touch, like humor, should be used in small amounts with close observation paid to the client's verbal and nonverbal reactions. If the nurse invades the client's "safety zone," the nurse needs to step back, increasing physical distance to restore respect and comfort. This client has clearly conveyed that more conversation needs to take place before physical care can be done.

thinking critically

Referring to the example of the vignette, visualize Mr. Clancy and the nurses. Write down the nonverbal communication Mr. Clancy is conveying to the nurses.

According to Brinkman and Kirshner (2002), people in trusting relationships need to emphasize their similar nature in order to change from conflict to cooperation. They use a term called "blending." "Blending is any behavior by which you reduce the differences between you and another in order to meet them where they are and move to common ground" (p. 36). To increase blending in the previous situation, the nurse would try to subtly mimic a facial expression and body posture of the client. In doing this, the nurse is imitating nonverbal behaviors that two people getting along would demonstrate. It is important that the person does not take offense or feel that he or she is being mocked. Thus, this takes some skillful practice and self-awareness.

Verbal Communication

Verbal communication deals with the content of "what" is said during a therapeutic interaction. Although there are many different techniques and you have been introduced to some in your previous training, as a nurse, you need to revisit the basics and refine them periodically to enhance your professional effectiveness. Verbal communication is a lifelong learning skill. The nurse may use general leads, open-ended questions, shared observations, restatement, clarification, silence, and summarization in promoting effective interaction (Williams, 2008). A summary of these techniques is included in Table 11.1.

SIMPLICITY

Nurse–client relationships require a client to interpret and understand words that have taken the nurse many years of study to understand. In the medical setting, clients are not unlike strangers in a land where a foreign language is being spoken. It is the nurse's role as the advocate and as the health care worker with the most patient contact to explain words and medical problems in a way that the client, family, or community can understand. Use of complex words to describe treatment, medications, or complications can confuse the client, leading to feelings of anger and frustration. The nurse should use simple terms or concrete layman's examples when describing the more complex medical protocols.

GENERAL LEADS

General leads are brief words or phrases to tell the listener that reception is occurring; these leads encourage the client to communicate further. Phrases such as "I see," "Oh, then what happened," "Tell me more," and "I follow what you are saying" are useful when trying to promote more information exchange.

OPEN-ENDED RELEVANT QUESTIONS

Open-ended questions encourage the client to elaborate on a subject. They do not require a "yes" or "no" answer. They may be useful in situations in which the client is guarded or resistant to talking. Questions may begin with "who," "what," "when," or "where." "Why" questions are usually avoided because they tend to place the client on the defensive. Open-ended questions add depth and relevance to the communication.

table
·················
11-1
SUMMARY OF VERBAL THERAPEUTIC COMMUNICATION TECHNIQUES

Technique	Examples
1. General leads	"I see ..." "Go on ..." "I hear what you are saying."
2. Open-ended relevant questions	"Where would you like to begin?" "Tell me more about what happened to you." "Can you describe what you were feeling?"
3. Sharing observations	"Are you uncomfortable when you ...?" "I noticed that you have a hard time when you ..." "You seem to be in more pain today ..."
4. Restating	*Client*: "I'm sorry about doing that." *Nurse*: "You're sorry." *Client*: "I'm angry about taking all of these pills!" *Nurse*: "You're angry about taking pills."
5. Clarification	"I'm not sure I understood ..." "I didn't follow that part about ..." "Did I understand you to say ..." "Could you give me an example of how this affects you?"
6. Silence	*Client*: "I'm afraid of losing both of my legs." *Nurse*: Stops, sits down in a chair by the bed, leans close to the client, and takes an offered hand.
7. Summarization	"So far we have talked about ..." "I think the main ideas you have told me are ..." "Have I got this straight about your problem with ..."

SHARING AN OBSERVATION

To perform this technique, the nurse needs to observe behaviors in the client. Some examples of this include "I haven't seen you drink anything today. Am I wrong?" or "You seem sleepier today." Such questions are neutral and allow the client to confirm or deny the nurse's observation. They can often be used to initiate a conversation.

RESTATING

When restating what a client has said, the nurse uses a verbatim segment of what the client has said. An example is as follows:

Patient: "I'm afraid to do this dressing here at home."
Nurse: "You are afraid to do this at home?"

As with general leads, this technique lets the client know that the nurse is following the intent of the interaction. This technique should not be relied on frequently because the client may start to believe that the nurse is mocking or making fun of him or her.

CLARIFICATION

Clarification is essential to ensure effective communication. An individual may make a statement that is unclear to the interviewer; in such a situation, the interviewer must clarify the meaning of the statement. Leads such as "I don't quite understand," "Could you explain that again?" and "I think what you are saying is …. Am I wrong?" are examples of clarification. It is tempting for the novice interviewer to believe it is best to pretend to understand and hope the meaning will become clear later in the interaction. However, such an approach is usually not effective.

SUMMARIZATION

A helpful way to conclude an interview or a therapeutic interaction is to summarize the ideas developed, clarify expected outcomes, and list the actions to be taken by the individual (summarization). Mutually acceptable outcomes are important in some situations. In other circumstances, the helping person must be able to accept client actions and decisions with which he or she does not agree. An example of the closure this places on the communication would be "Taking everything we talked about under consideration, I believe what we have agreed on is …" or "We have discussed …. Are there any other concerns you have before we move forward?"

NCLEX–RN *Might Ask* (11.1)

The nurse is interviewing a client. The most effective therapeutic technique a nurse can use in the communication process is

  A. general leads.
  B. active listening.
  C. using open-ended questions.
  D. a professional appearance.

• See Appendix A for correct answer and rationale.

Verbal Communication Blocks

Verbal blocks in communication are words spoken by the nurse, which decrease the ability of the nurse to get at the heart of the client's needs. They are words or phrases that are frequently used in the social setting and may be used out of sympathy. Blocks in communication include providing false assurance, giving advice, being moralistic, and changing the subject.

FALSE ASSURANCES

One of the most frequently used blocks in therapeutic communication is providing false assurance to the client. "It's okay; everyone feels that way" and "You'll see, everything will be just fine" are phrases the nurse might say after a client reveals a major problem or concern. Unintentionally, the nurse has belittled the individuality of the client's experience. The client may perceive that the nurse does not take him or her seriously, because these statements trivialize what the client is experiencing. Each client is unique and wants the nurse to recognize his or her experience as such.

Instead of false assurances, the nurse should respond with neutral statements, such as "Tell me more about ..." or "You sound worried or fearful about ...."

GIVING ADVICE

Although clients frequently ask the nurse what he or she would do, giving advice may prematurely end the interaction with the client. Clients are really not asking for advice; they are working through the decision-making process. The client may believe that the nurse is controlling the client by telling him or her what to do. Giving advice also fosters a feeling of dependency and leads the client to believe that the nurse knows what is best for him or her. Statements that indicate advice-giving include "The best thing for you to do is ...," "Why don't you ...," and "If I were you, I'd ...."

The best way to eliminate this behavior by the nurse is self-awareness that it is occurring. Another technique a student could use is asking for feedback from the clinical instructor. Alternatives to giving advice include "I wonder if you've considered ..." and "Maybe we should look at .... Let's talk about all of the options you might have." In this way the nurse, instead of imposing his or her will, is asking the client to explore options.

BEING MORALISTIC

When a nurse responds with a moralistic statement, he or she is adopting a judgmental attitude. Similar to giving advice, it negates the client's right to choose and belittles the feelings the client may express. The nurse needs to be aware of personal values and how they can affect client interaction. Transcending these values will allow the client the respect and right to choose what he or she wants. Moralistic statements, such as "I'm glad you've come to your senses" and "You should never feel that way," should be revised to be more neutral in tone—for example, "You sound upset" or "Tell me more about how you feel."

CHANGING THE SUBJECT

Changing the subject involves introducing an unrelated topic into the discussion. This diverts the client from revealing intended feelings and thoughts.

The nurse may react by changing the subject when the content is sudden and surprising or when the subject is too painful for the nurse to discuss. This block in communication tells the client that the nurse is no longer listening, and it is a quick way to end the interaction. A sample of this block would be as follows:

Client: "I want to kill myself right now."
Nurse: "Did you have any visitors today?"

One of the easiest ways to deal with surprise revelations is the use of silence. The adage, "If you don't know what to say, don't say anything," may be helpful for the nurse to keep in mind. However, silence cannot be the nurse's only communication tool, or the client will question the nurse's competence.

A summary of types of blocks in communication is included in Table 11.2.

• PROCESS RECORDINGS

Newer technologies provide ways for nurses to practice and improve their therapeutic communications. Interactive videotape, role playing, and computerized learning scenarios can safely simulate the proper use of therapeutic techniques until the student gains comfort. In your class work, you may be asked to video- or audiotape your interaction with another student and analyze that conversation. It may be helpful to use a checklist (Display 11.2) to fine-tune your use of therapeutic techniques.

A common teaching tool used to refine therapeutic communication in nursing programs is a process recording. According to Varcarolis, Carson, & Shoemaker (2006), "process recordings are written records of a segment from

table 11-2 SUMMARY OF BLOCKS IN COMMUNICATION

Technique	Examples
1. False assurances	"Don't worry." "Things will all work out for the best."
2. Giving advice	"I think you should ..." "Everyone I know does this when this happens."
3. Being moralistic	"You should be ashamed of your behavior." "Someone your age should ..."
4. Changing the subject	*Client:* "I have been very depressed for about a week." *Nurse:* "Come, let's play a nice game of checkers." *Client:* "When my baby died, I thought I couldn't go on." *Nurse:* "How many other children do you have?"

---

display **11.2**   **Therapeutic Communications Performance Checklist**

The following checklist can be used by a student to evaluate the use of therapeutic interventions during a client interaction or videotape of a client interaction.

Yes   No

1. Introduces self and states the purpose of the visit.
2. Addresses the client as Ms., Mrs., or Mr. unless permission has been given to use the first name.
3. Identifies expected outcomes for the day and termination time.
4. Maintains eye contact and minimizes gestures.
5. Maintains consistency between verbal and nonverbal communication.
6. Subtly approximates verbal/nonverbal client behaviors.
7. Avoids rushing or forcing the conversation (sits, if possible).
8. Avoids dominating the conversation with personal details.
9. Asks open-ended questions.
10. Promotes expression of client feelings.
11. Clarifies and restates main ideas.
12. Offers alternatives to the plan of care.
13. Avoids the use of blocks in communication.
14. Summarizes the content of the exchange.
15. Terminates the relationship by identifying.

Outcomes accomplished
Needs to work on
Comments

_____
_____
_____

---

the nurse–client session that reflect as closely as possible the verbal and nonverbal behaviors of both the nurse and client." See Display 11.3 for a sample of a process recording.

Once the student has reviewed verbal and nonverbal communication techniques and blocks, the phases of the nurse–patient relationship need to be examined.

• THERAPEUTIC COMMUNICATION

Therapeutic communication is an essential skill for nurses in all areas of health care. "The therapeutic relationship is a close helping relationship based on trust which allows the nurse and client to work together collaboratively" (Mohr, 2006, p. 56). Communication is the medium through which all nursing services are provided. There are three types of communication: therapeutic, social, and collegial. The same basic components of therapeutic communication can be used in all three types of communication.

Characteristics of Therapeutic Communication

"Therapeutic communication is the base of interactive relationships and affords opportunities to establish rapport, understand the client's experiences, formulate

display **11.3**	**Sample Process Recording**

Client initials: _____   Student name: _____

Client diagnosis: _____   Date: _____

Setting: _____   Instructor: _____

Clinical site: _____

Nonverbal and Verbal Data	Thoughts/Feelings	Analysis of Client/Student Communication Techniques

individualized or client-centered interventions and optimize health care resources" (Antai-Otong, 2010, p. 55). There is a difference between the social interaction reinforced by cultural beliefs, such as politeness, and therapeutic communication (Table 11.3). In a social interaction, communicating individuals generally attempt to fulfill their own needs. Often, individuals in a social conversation are not aware of or concerned about others' feelings and needs. Social communication often dwells on factual information, which is usually of a superficial nature, rather than feelings or emotions. When emotions are discussed in a social conversation, the needs of both participants are addressed.

In contrast, therapeutic interaction involves a helping person, such as a nurse, assisting someone in physical or emotional need, to gain a better understanding and satisfaction of that need through verbal and nonverbal techniques. The nurse plans interaction that focuses on the client's needs, rather than the nurse's needs. This interaction is designed to empower the client to meet his or her needs better and thereby change behaviors for more effective and satisfying living. To promote this process, nurses must periodically revisit, strengthen, and update effective caring techniques.

table
11-3   CHARACTERISTICS OF SOCIAL AND THERAPEUTIC RELATIONSHIPS

Social	Therapeutic
Self-serving	Focused on client
Polite	Respectful, sincere, patient
Superficial content	Feelings and emotional content
Sympathy	Empathy
Lacks clarity/validation	Clarity/validation essential
Minimal problem solving	Effective problem solving/coping Outcomes oriented Confidential

NCLEX–RN *Might Ask*

11.2

The use of therapeutic communication by the nurse in patient interaction is *primarily* done to

- A. foster dependence on the nurse.
- B. discuss the client's inner secrets.
- C. allow the client to trust the nurse.
- D. obtain information required for outcome-oriented nursing care.

· See Appendix A for correct answer and rationale.

Characteristics of Effective, Therapeutic, Caring Nurses

Therapeutic relationships are more effective if the nurse demonstrates caring behaviors. These are displayed by the verbal and nonverbal cues that the nurse uses to establish, promote, and terminate the relationship. Table 11.4 lists caring characteristics used by successful nurses to help patients solve problems and contrasts these characteristics with some communication pitfalls to avoid.

TRUST

The nurse must establish trust with the client to be an effective communicator and change agent. Keeping promises, being there, and using therapeutic communications that accept the client's feelings as valid can establish trust. The client needs

table
11-4   CARING CHARACTERISTICS/TIPS TO PREVENT MALPRACTICE

Caring Characteristics	Tips to Prevent Malpractice
Trustworthy Knowledgeable Nonjudgmental Empathetic	Involve the client in the informed consent process.
Genuine Accepting	Be available and accessible to the client.
Warm Patient	Do not make promises you cannot keep.
Authentic Respectful	If you say you're going to do something, then do it.
Understanding Use of humor	Listen and look for cues striving for understanding the emotions.
Confidential	Share information on a "need-to-know" basis.

to trust that what happens to him or her is kept in judicious confidence. The nurse needs to respect the client and show genuineness in his or her treatment. Patience and understanding shown by the nurse can be helpful when the client's verbalization of feelings is often painful and time consuming.

The patient has the right to confidentiality and all of his/her health care information is considered privileged communication; only those involved with care have the right to know about this information (Boyd, 2008; Mohr, 2006). Communicable diseases, child/elder abuse, and gunshot and/or knife wounds are the exception and are reportable under the law. To prevent malpractice against the nurse, physician, and hospital, the nurse should follow tips to prevent malpractice (Table 11.4). The client needs to trust that the nurse will keep all information confidential. With the enactment of HIPAA, all health care providers can share information on a "need-to-know-only" basis. Legalities are explored in more depth in Chapter 16.

EMPATHY

A distinction between sympathy and empathy is helpful. Sympathy, common in social relationships, is described as feeling sorry for a client, reacting to the situation as a friend would under the same circumstance. In contrast, empathy is defined as understanding the client by mentally placing himself or herself in the client's situation (Boyd, 2008). The nurse attempts to avoid projecting emotionalism into the situation and remains objective.

THERAPEUTIC HUMOR

"Humor refers to being amusing, funny or comical to express feelings and thoughts in a manner comfortable with oneself and others" (Antai-Otong, 2010, p. 54). Humor can be a powerful tool, physiologically and psychologically, when used in both patient and staff communication. Done with common sense and in good taste considering the individual, laughter and humor have been known to stimulate the immune system, increase pulmonary volumes, promote coughing, and increase cardiac exercise by increasing the heart rate (Cousins, 1983; McGhee, 1998). Psychologically, well-timed humor can diminish anger and frustration, leading to the release of tension, creating a human connection.

A smile and a relaxed attitude are the easiest to present initially but can be hard to do on a busy day. However, they help set an initial positive tone to the conversation and show care early in the relationship. There are many other ways to enhance humor appropriately. Cartoons, toys and props, joke books, music, and DVDs can be provided to promote therapeutic humor. Many hospitals now encourage the use of clowns and volunteers to cheer clients and provide diversion from pain. Many websites promote the use of professional, therapeutic humor in the workplace.

Negative humor can be harmful or offensive to the client (Pagana, 2009). Display 11.4 lists times when humor and laughter are inappropriate and may

display 11.4	Inappropriate Situations for the Use of Humor

Timing is important for the effect of humor to be a positive experience. The nurse should use caution when engaging in humorous, playful behavior when the client is

- Trying to communicate something important
- Receiving unexpected and unwelcome test/diagnostic results
- In the same room with a patient who is very ill
- New and the nurse has not yet established a trusting relationship
- Offended by content (ie, age, religion, gender, race, politics, and gossip)
- "Put down" by the nurse's use of sarcasm
- Showing nonverbal signs of wanting a more serious relationship
- Experiencing pain from the act of laughter (abdominal or chest sutures)

be perceived as unprofessional. There are no hard, fast rules with laughter and humor, but considering individual variations in taste, humor is best approached in a test-the-waters manner. Go slowly and try a few light comments, noting the verbal and nonverbal reactions in the client. If the client is open to the approach, more techniques may be added but always with observation of the client's reaction.

● COMPETENCE IN COMMUNICATION ACROSS THE LIFE SPAN

The communication skills that have been covered are generalized and useful in communicating with any clients, families, coworkers, or groups. However, there are times when specific techniques are useful, such as when the nursing care of children, adolescents, or older adults is involved.

Infants and children are sensitive to nonverbal communication. Tone of voice and gesture can startle or frighten a small child. Comforting techniques such as cuddling, patting, or rocking in the presence of the primary caregiver are important to adopt. When children are very young, the caregiver may be the only accurate source of needed information. Using simple words and short sentences and talking to the child at eye level are important tips to remember. Toys, games, and dolls or puppets help children relate to situations. They should be used frequently to communicate with this age group. When caring for older children, it is important to talk to the primary caregiver and to the child.

The adolescent stage of development can be a trying time for both the nurse and the caregiver. One of the most important techniques for this age group is to listen first and remain nonjudgmental. A sense of give and take is important and should be maintained with thoughtful, creative, firm limit setting. This will encourage the adolescent to express himself or herself because it shows tolerance and respect for his or her budding individuality. Every effort should be made to give the adolescent a sense of modesty and privacy.

Communication with the older adult presents other challenges for the nurse. Assessment of the client is important. Sensory needs, such as hearing and seeing difficulties, accentuate the need for the nurse to face the client, talk directly to him or her, and use simple nonverbal gestures to help facilitate clear interaction. Establishing priorities for what is necessary for the client to know can assist the client in retaining needed information. The nurse should stick with one topic at a time, allowing time for the client to respond with an answer. Selecting a time in which the client is less fatigued or stressed will help facilitate communication. Knowing the client's previous experiences with health-related issues can help the nurse relate them to what the client is experiencing in the present. Consistent thought and consideration for the dignity of the older client is paramount, so the nurse should address such clients in the manner they request. Include a significant other in the care when permission is granted by the client so that another set of ears and eyes can help.

● COMMUNICATION AS A TEAM MEMBER IN THE HEALTH CARE SETTING

Social and therapeutic communications are important aspects of an RN's practice. Effective communication and collegial teamwork are essential for the delivery of safe, high-quality client care. Because nurses have a pivotal knowledge about clients, they need to have strong working relationships with other health care colleagues, assertiveness skills to act on the client's best interest, and the ability to delegate appropriate tasks clearly and concisely to trained unlicensed assistive personnel (UAPs). As an LPN transiting into the role of an RN, you will need to communicate persuasively as a colleague as your scope of responsibility and accountability broadens. Many of the same communication techniques for therapeutic communication with clients can be applied throughout the workday with coworkers.

Team Building

In the transitional role, the LPN will be moving from a role that might have included some responsibility for UAPs working with him or her to a strong leadership role. The nurse needs to foster collegial communication. Collegial communication is skillful verbal, nonverbal, and written communication that results in enhanced relationships with colleagues, quality care, and better documentation. Communication between colleagues is known as collaboration. Nurses have worked in numerous group situations. They may range from staff meetings and care conferences to project teams and patient support groups.

For groups to work well, there must be a sense of trust, group identity, and synergy (Tuckman, 1965). Synergy is the ability to accomplish more together than the individual members of the group. Similar to therapeutic communication, team members need to be clear and brief in their verbal/written communication. RNs need to

- Use active listening skills
- Know when to speak and when to be silent
- Use positive body language

- Be sensitive to nonverbal communication cues
- Praise in public and give constructive criticism in private

In their mission to provide quality care, a team of colleagues may progress through stages. According to Tuckman (1965), these are forming, storming, norming, and performing. Many of the same attributes for the stages of a therapeutic relationship learned as an LPN are similar to these stages (Table 11.5). A team of colleagues may dissolve in the storming stage if they do not recognize this as a healthy stage in team building. Display 11.5 lists the necessary qualities of an effective team member.

Interaction with Administrators and Physicians

Although nurses are great listeners, they frequently lack the skills to effectively communicate in an interdisciplinary setting. Being a member of the interdisciplinary team begins with respect for a person and his or her role within the team. Sometimes LPNs, RNs, and other health care workers can lose sight of important contributions made by others. Nurses may also have tunnel vision, failing to see the broader aspect of change. Focusing on the small things and not the "bigger picture" can cause physicians and administrators to have a dim view of nurses and their much-needed input into system changes. Change should be viewed as an opportunity rather than an imposition. A third reason nurses fail to connect with powerbrokers within the organization is that they fail to be proactive and tend to react. To counteract these needs, nurses need to

- Suggest solutions for problems
- View themselves as self-confident with high self-esteem
- Be visionary
- Become actively involved

To help achieve these ends and have a voice that is respected, nurses need to learn, practice, and refine assertiveness skills.

table
11-5 STAGES OF TEAM DEVELOPMENT COMPARED TO STAGES OF A THERAPEUTIC RELATIONSHIP

Team Development*	Stages of Therapeutic Relationship
Forming—polite but informal; figuring out players and goals	Preinteraction—gathering patient data and plans for a meeting
Storming—power struggles and conflict occur	Orientation—establishing trust, needs determination; identifying problems and suggested outcomes
Norming—getting organized; figuring out rules and confronting problems	Working—stressors analyzed; resistance behaviors explored
Performing—open, honest confrontation and collaboration; respect and quality work	Termination—reviews outcomes and determines effectiveness

*From Tuckman, B. (1965). Developmental sequences of groups. *Psychology Bulletin, 63,* 384.

| display 11.5 | Qualities of an Effective Team |

Members of an effective team

- Assume responsibility for their actions.
- Respect and trust others.
- Listen completely to others.
- Provide consistent positive and negative feedback (even when tough).
- Commit to the goals of the team.
- Build winning alliances.
- Recognize, support, and reward success.

Miscommunication is often the root cause of patient injury. "SBAR" is quickly becoming an acronym for steps to take in providing immediate action and include specific information. SBAR (pronounced S-BAR) stands for situation, background, assessment, and recommendation.

- **S**ituation: Identify yourself, the client, room number, and change in status
- **B**ackground: Provide relevant background information that relates to the situation
- **A**ssessment: Offer the nurses' analysis of the source of the problem (critical thinking)
- **R**ecommendation: What would help resolve the situation or problem?

Assertiveness in Communication

Assertiveness is defined as "learned behavior that includes standing up for one's rights without violating the rights of others" (Varcarolis et al., 2006). Assertiveness behaviors have many of the same attributes as caring communication. An assertive communication style is open, honest, direct, and confident. Strong assertiveness skills enable the nurse to express emotions, including anger and frustration, in a positive manner that focuses on cooperation and problem resolution.

Aggressive communication focuses more on the selfish needs of an individual. There is an "I want ..." underlying communication. In aggressive communication, there is a winner and a loser. Assertive communication fosters a win/win situation where both parties negotiate for a positive outcome. An aggressive individual dominates the discussion and rarely strives to understand the position or emotions of anyone other than themselves. The end results of aggressive behaviors are angry, hostile, or offended colleagues and coworkers (Table 11.6).

Many nurses do not differentiate between assertive and aggressive behaviors. They look at assertiveness as being pushy or uppity and not as a way to enhance meeting the needs of clients and themselves. Nurses may not realize that assertive behaviors can be learned and do have positive outcomes (Table 11.7). There are few negative results from assertive behaviors in communication. They can be learned through observation of skilled mentors and leaders, workshops, and reading. To promote assertive behaviors in communication, you, as a nurse, can

table
.... AGGRESSIVE AND ASSERTIVE BEHAVIORS
11-6

Aggressive	Assertive
"I want ..."	"We need ..."
"I win, you lose."	"I win, you win."
Dominates the discussion	Listens to others
Says one thing verbally, nonverbally conveys the opposite	Congruency between verbal and nonverbal behaviors
Controlling	Cooperating
Fault finding	Nonaccusatory focus (focuses on behavior, not personality)
Only strives to BE understood	Strives for understanding
Focuses on the "other" person	Focuses on problem resolution

- Describe the specific instance that violated your sense of "fair play"
- Express your feelings
- Specify the action or change needed
- Concentrate on the desired results

Nurses must use all communication skills, team building concepts, and assertiveness when delegating to others in the health care team.

Delegation

Delegation is defined as the transfer of responsibility for the performance of an activity from one individual to another, while retaining accountability for the outcome. Nurses have always used nurse helpers throughout history; therefore, working as a team is not a foreign concept for nurses. However, in today's environment of cost cutting and nurse shortages, the nurse must be able to (a) delegate to the appropriate personnel, (b) delegate tasks that they have been trained to perform, (c) identify routine circumstances for delegation, (d) provide the delegate with appropriate direction and communication regarding the task at hand, and

table
.... BENEFITS OF ASSERTIVE BEHAVIOR
11-7

Benefits	Rationales
Decreases stress and anxiety	Because your needs are openly expressed
Decreases the use of brain power	Because you do not ruminate over problems
Increases respect	Because of the openness of colleagues and
Withdraws the invitation for aggression	other workers in open communication
Increases achievement	Because you are standing up for your needs
Promotes team spirit	Your needs are clear
	You are enhancing win/win situations

(e) provide suitable supervision in accordance with state law. When you examine the steps of delegation, according to the National Council State Boards of Nursing (NCSBN, 1995), they closely resemble the steps of the nursing process (Table 11.8).

The first step in the delegation process is to determine the right person to help the nurse. Depending on the place of employment, the nurse helper can be called a nurse's aide, support technician, or care partner. Common language for this nurse helper has been a problem because it has never been standardized. The ANA, National League for Nursing (NLN), NCSBN, and many other nursing organizations have suggested the use of UAPs. Therefore, this discussion will use UAPs as nurse helpers. Regardless of the terminology used, nursing organizations clearly outline that the UAPs are in place to support the RNs' or LPNs' practice but are not a substitute for their professional scope of practice or judgment.

As an LPN, by law, you are a dependent practitioner supervised by an RN, advanced practice nurse, or other independent health care practitioner. Therefore, you have been subject to delegation. In your role transition, you will be delegating and will remain accountable for the outcomes of the actions of UAPs or other licensed personnel. Therefore, your scope and responsibilities will be much broader, greater, and more complex.

For prudent delegation, the nurse must also link the right person to the right task. In assigning a task, the RN must be aware that it is the task, not the responsibility and accountability for the outcome, that is being delegated (Display 11.6). Matching the right person to the task is critical for quality care. Although some nursing organizations have listed (see the *AACN Delegation Handbook* [Snyder, Medina, Bell, & Wavra, 2004]) commonly performed tasks that can be delegated, it is the nurse that needs to decide when the task falls outside the "routine care" that the UAP has been assigned.

When the nurse creates an assignment, he or she must be sensitive to the needs of the UAP. Using the same principles of communication discussed previously, the RN must take the time to give CLEAR direction to that individual. CLEAR is an acronym that may help you remember the steps for promoting clear communication (Display 11.7).

table
················
11-8   THE NURSING PROCESS AND THE FIVE RIGHTS OF DELEGATION

Nursing Process	Five Rights of Delegation*
Assessment	Person (Who)
Plan	Task (What)
	Circumstance (When)
Implementation	Direction/Communication (Where)
Evaluation	Supervision

*From the National Council State Boards of Nursing. (1995). *Delegation: Concepts and decision-making process.* Chicago, IL: Author.

---

display 11.6   **Terms Associated with Delegation**

Accountability: Taking ownership for the actions and/or lack of actions of oneself and others

Assignment: Task or skill for which a UAP, LPN/LVN, or RN is responsible

Delegation: Assignment of responsibility for a task from one person to another; the delegator is responsible for the outcome of this assignment.

Unlicensed Assisted Personnel (UAP): Any unlicensed person to whom a task is delegated

Responsible: Liable to be called to answer for the actions of oneself or others

Supervision: Directing, watching, evaluating, and correcting the actions of others

---

The nurse may not delegate to a UAP or licensed person who lacks training or the ability to perform a skill safely. This becomes a real concern when there are float personnel or unfamiliar personnel working with the RN. The NCSBN (1995) uses the words "competent individual" in its definition of delegation. So, taking the time to assess the level of training of an individual and having them restate the assignment in their own words is essential. Not all tasks should be delegated. If the task has the potential for harm, involves complex assessments and skills or steps of the nursing process, requires critical thinking or problem solving, and is unpredictable in its outcome, the nurse should perform it. There are circumstances that dictate delegation. The RN can only delegate those tasks that are within the realm of agency policies and job descriptions. Tasks must be routine and must be within the UAP's educational training and experience level. An example of how a circumstance would change a routine task usually delegated to a UAP would be that of a glucose finger stick for a diabetic. Routinely, in many health care institutions, finger sticks are delegated to UAPs. If a reported glucose is below normal, the UAP should report the finding to the RN right away. That RN has a priority assessment and intervention date with the patient right away. He or she should assume the responsibility of troubleshooting the situation, because the circumstances have changed and the situation is no longer routine. UAPs do not have the scope of practice to be assigned tasks that produce unpredictable outcomes. The role of the RN is to assume responsibility for this patient.

The last step in the five elements of delegation is that of supervision. Although the nurse delegates to the right person, in the correct communication style, an appropriate task, it is also the nurse's responsibility to confirm that the task has been

---

display 11.7   **CLEAR Communication**

C: Clearly and simply outline the task.

L: Legally know what is within the UAP's job description.

E: Eagerly accentuate positive behfaviors.

A: Acknowledge that differences will occur and treat them confidentially.

R: Respect the individual's culture, gender, and individuality.

completed and evaluated. If the entire delegation process goes smoothly and tasks are completed safely, in a timely manner, and satisfactorily to everyone involved, the work progresses. If the process does not turn out as predicted, then similar to the nursing process, the delegation process needs to be evaluated from the beginning. The nurse must frequently and periodically ask for feedback from the UAP and/or LPN/LVN. The less experienced and more unfamiliar the UAP is to the nurse, the more frequent is the required feedback. It is important to remember that tasks can be delegated. The responsibility lies in the scope of the RN's practice.

● CONCLUSION

This chapter introduces several concepts essential to the nurse's role as a communicator. The importance of recognizing verbal and nonverbal adjuncts to communication and barriers to communication is discussed. Factors that promote effective communication, including therapeutic communication techniques, are explained. Communication as a team member, team building, assertiveness behaviors, and delegation concepts are explored. Suggestions for the use of communication concepts throughout one's life span are made.

student exercises

SITUATION ONE

Nurse Frederick is caring for Mr. N., a patient who has recently received a diagnosis of multiple sclerosis. As Nurse Frederick enters the room, Mr. N. is sitting on the side of his bed, staring vacantly into space. His bath water is set up on his bedside table, and his washcloth is unused. When she says "Hello," he does not respond. She stands by his bedside looking at the flow sheet on her clipboard. Without looking at Mr. N., she asks, "How's the appetite?" A low "Okay" in a monotone voice is the reply. "Have you had a BM?" The nurse is still not looking at him. "Yes." The low monotone voice and vacant stare continue. Next, Nurse Frederick takes Mr. N.'s vital signs. Quickly glancing at him, she records them on the flow sheet. "Looks good," she says and leaves the room.

1. Identify the nonverbal communication of nurse and patient.

2. Identify the barriers to communication demonstrated by the nurse.

3. Suggest some verbal and nonverbal techniques the nurse could have used to encourage Mr. N. to verbalize his concerns.

SITUATION TWO

Student Nurse Reese reports off duty to her charge nurse. She says, "Mrs. Jones slept a little, stated she had chest pain twice, and ate very little lunch. She received a PRN medication and weighed 110 lb."

1. Discuss some areas the nursing student omitted in her report. Why do you think these areas were omitted?

2. Suggest some therapeutic techniques the nursing student might have used to elicit the needed data from Mrs. Jones.

3. Write the response you would use if you were the charge nurse to help the nursing student elicit the needed information.

SITUATION THREE

You have been working hard on a new cost-cutting measure to reduce lost patient charges on your unit. You have presented many good ideas to the nurse manager. Your nurse manager asks you to volunteer for a new committee forming in the hospital composed of administrators and physicians. She wants you to share your ideas in this committee.

1. You are really afraid of making a fool of yourself but want to share your proposal. Using the information on interactions with administrators, outline a plan of how you will present your proposals.

2. During the meeting, one of the physicians challenges you on your ideas. You feel yourself getting red and angry. How can you change this to a win/win situation with assertiveness techniques?

SITUATION FOUR

A new UAP is assigned to your unit. She has had 3 weeks of hospital orientation and seems shy but eager to learn. You assign her the vital signs for four stable patients, glucose sticks, and morning care. Midway through the morning, she comes to you in tears stating that she wants to "quit" and is having a bad day.

1. Using the five steps of delegation, write how you will make this a "good situation" for this new UAP.

2. Using communication skills, explain how you can find out what is happening to this UAP and suggest ways to help you both manage the day.

References

Alfaro-LeFevre, R. (2010). *Applying the nursing process: A tool for critical thinking* (7th ed.). Philadelphia, PA: Lippincott.
Antai-Otong, D. (2010). *Nurse-client communications: A life span approach*. Sudbury, MA: Jones and Bartlett.
Berlo, D. (1960). *The process of communication: An introduction to theory and practice*. New York, NY: Holt, Reinhart and Winston.
Boyd, M. (2008). *Psychiatric nursing: Contemporary practice* (2nd ed.). Philadelphia, PA: Wolters Kluwer Health.
Brinkman, R., & Kirschner, R. (2002). *Dealing with people you can't stand: How to bring out the best in people at their worst*. New York, NY: McGraw-Hill.
Cousins, N. (1983). *Anatomy of an illness: As perceived by the patient*. New York, NY: Norton.
Darwin, C. (1872). *The expression of emotions in man and animals*. London, UK: John Murray.
McGhee, P. (1998). Rx: Laughter. *RN, 61*(7), 50–53.
Mohr, W. (2006). *Psychiatric-mental health nursing* (6th ed.). Philadelphia, PA: Lippincott Williams & Wilkins.

National Council State Boards of Nursing. (1995). *Delegation: Concepts and decision-making process*. Chicago, IL: Author.

Pagana, K. (2009). 7 tips to improve your professional etiquette. *Nursing, 39*(11), 34–37.

Schuster, P., & Nykolyn, L. (2010). *Communication for nurses: How to prevent harmful events and promote patient safety*. Philadelphia, PA: F. A. Davis.

Snyder, D. A., Medina, J., Bell, L., & Wavra, T. A. (Eds.). (2004). *AACN delegation handbook* (2nd ed.). Aliso Viejo, CA: American Association of Critical-Care Nurses. Retrieved July 2, 2007, from http//www.aacn.org/AACN/practice.nsf/Files/DBEd2/$file/1editedrevisedAACNDelegation Handbook%207-1-2004.pdf

Tuckman, B. (1965). Developmental sequences of groups. *Psychology Bulletin, 63*, 384.

Varcarolis, P., Carson, V., & Schoemaker, N. (2006). *Foundations of psychiatric nursing* (5th ed.). St. Louis, MO: Saunders Elsevier.

Williams, C. (2008). *Therapeutic interaction in nursing* (2nd ed.). Sudbury, MA: Jones and Bartlett.

Windle, L., Halbert, K., Dumont, C., Tagnesi, K., & Johnson, K. (2008). An evidence-based approach to creating a new nursing dress code. *Am Nurse Today, 3*(1):17–19.

Suggested Reading

Chitty, K., & Black, B. (2011). *Professional nursing: Concepts & challenges* (6th ed.). St. Louis, MO: Elsevier.

Corson, V., & Shoemaker, N. (2006). *Foundations of psychiatric mental health nursing* (5th ed). Philadelphia, PA: Elsevier.

Keltner, N., Bostrom, C., & McGuinness, T. (2010). *Psychiatric nursing* (4th ed.). St. Louis, MO: Mosby.

McInnis, L., & Parsons, L. (2009). Thoughtful nursing practice: Reflections on nurse delegation and decision-making. *Nursing Clinics of North America, 44*(4), 461–470.

O'Brian, P., Kennedy, W., & Ballard, K. (2008). *Psychiatric mental health nursing: An introduction to theory and practice*. Sudbury, MA: Jones and Bartlett.

Leiper, J. (2005). Nurse against nurse: How to stop horizontal violence. *Nursing 2005, 35*(3), 44–45.

Riley, J. B. (2004). *Communication in nursing* (5th ed.). St. Louis, MO: Mosby.

Sheldon, L. (2004). *Communication for nurses: Talking with patients*. Thorofare, NJ: Slack.

 On the *http://www.youtube.com/watch?v=Nipj7PwCjTc&feature=related:* 4.5 minutes on talking to patients. (45 minutes) How to talk to patients. (Last accessed 3.2.2011)
http://www.americannursetoday.com/article. *aspx?id=4438&fid=4422:* (Last accessed 9.8.2010)
https://www.ncsbn.org/Working_with_Others.pdf: Aspects of delegation (Last accessed 3.2.2011)

12

The Nurse as Teacher

● **LEARNING OUTCOMES**

By the end of this chapter, the student will be able to:

1 Explain the importance of client education as a nursing responsibility.

2 Describe the differences between teaching and learning.

3 Relate principles of teaching–learning to client education.

4 Describe internal and external influences that affect client learning.

5 Identify teaching methods appropriate for cognitive, affective, and psychomotor learning.

6 Relate the teaching–learning process to the nursing process.

7 List assessment data necessary to determine client learning needs.

8 Formulate nursing diagnoses for identified client learning needs.

9 Outline the essential components of a teaching plan.

10 Describe how to implement client education.

11 Explain how to evaluate client education.

12 Discuss the essential elements of documenting client education.

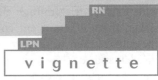

vignette

Mary has been an LVN for 2 years and has just graduated from an ADN program. She is working on a busy medical–surgical unit with another LPN and two UAPs. Mary entered the nursing station at 10 AM and sat down, exasperated.

MARY: How am I going to teach my patients anything when there isn't enough time?

ALICE (HEAD NURSE): What's the problem Mary?

MARY: Mr. Martinez in 203 isn't doing well with his insulin injections because he doesn't speak or understand English well. And he's going home today. Mrs. Duncan is going into surgery in 1 hour, and I haven't taught her how to deep breathe and cough yet. Mr. James is upset about the medication changes Dr. Lotte made and won't take his new heart medications until he knows more about them. Mr. Willis is afraid to take his wife home tomorrow because he can't put her back brace on by himself. I need to change Mrs. Lewis' dressing, but Dr. Craig has ordered a new IV antibiotic and her IV is infiltrated. Some time this morning, I have to irrigate Mr. Martin's colostomy! Writing a teaching plan was one of my strong points in school. Now, I barely have time to explain things to patients as I dash from room to room. My LPN and my UAPs can't help because this is what I have been trained to do, not them.

ALICE: Yes, it does seem like teaching is taking a back seat these days, but I think the importance of teaching is getting greater. Teaching on the run and discharge planning on admission are important, and tools to help everyone communicate are important.

MARY: When will we get those standardized teaching plans everyone has been talking about, Alice? Maybe they would give me some new ideas and reduce the paperwork that's burying me.

ALICE: They should be available in a week or so, but I hope they get used and are not perceived as just busy work.

MARY: Well, I need something. I won't have time to write a teaching plan for all my patients today. I'll just have to hope the nurses on the next shift can figure out what needs to be done based on my charting.

ALICE: You need to teach and chart, Mary. Legally, you have to chart what was taught and how well the patient understood. Come on, I have some time. Mrs. Lewis is your priority. I'll restart her IV. We will get a translator for Mr. Martinez around noon. I believe his wife understands English well and has been involved with his care all along. Mr. Martin will be seeing the stoma nurse, so you can do a reinforcement of her teaching this afternoon.

MARY: Thanks, Alice. I sure appreciate the help.

● THE CHALLENGE OF CLIENT EDUCATION

Mary is right to become concerned about her client teaching. Teaching is such an important legal and professional nursing role that teaching responsibilities are included in most state nurse practice acts and ANA's (1998) *Standards of Clinical Practice*. Nurses who fail to provide proper client education not only increase their risk of civil liability but are also, and more importantly, negligent in their nursing practice. Another challenge to completing competent client education is the downsizing of professional nursing staff positions and the substitution of such positions with UAP staff. Although there is help with the simple physical care, clients are sicker, there is less client contact for assessment, and clients are confused about the roles of their health care providers. Nurses are challenged daily by the increasing demands of the work setting to meet their teaching responsibilities. With the advent of managed care, patients and families are presented with the challenge of managing more complex health problems at home. Learning must now occur in a shorter time, as well as in situations and environments that are not always ideal for learning.

As a result of the nursing shortage and economic downsizing, nurses such as Mary are busier managing larger caseloads with clients who require more complex treatments, teaching regimens, and nursing care. New professionals must have clear communication and documentation skills to make the transition from the health care setting to home safer and more efficient for such clients. In cases such as that of Mr. Martinez, the nurse must be a worldwide citizen who is flexible and open to clients' learning needs, especially needs not previously encountered by the nurse. In addition, nurses are legally bound to protect client confidentiality, so family members of clients who do not speak English should not be used as interpreters unless they have the *consent* of the patient and are caregivers. The nurse is accountable for work that is done by others less skilled in client communication. As an LPN/LVN, you can help with basic assessment skills, but now you are legally, morally, and ethically responsible for the entire process of client education. Teaching is an intangible part of caring. It stays with the client long after the client is discharged.

Research has shown how valuable health teaching is for the health care recipient. Health teaching shortens hospital stays, minimizes complications, and reduces symptoms of illness and surgery (Bastable, 2008). Given a willing client, the extent of client education that can be accomplished is limited only by the depth and breadth of the nurse's knowledge, the constraints of the setting, and the circumstances in which the nurse–client interaction occurs. In each teaching interaction, there is a shared learning experience mostly geared toward and designed for the individual client, but learning also occurs for the nurse.

● TEACHING AND LEARNING DEFINED

"Teaching is a system of activities intended to produce learning" (Berman, Snyder, & McKenney, 2011, p. 277). Client teaching is an ongoing process whereby the nurse organizes experiences in varied ways to facilitate client learning. In the age of the more educated and informed consumer, clients should no longer be viewed as partners in health care but as leaders of their health care team. Empowerment comes when patients can make informed decisions about their care. This increases feelings of control and hopefulness in cases of advanced illness. When appropriately used, client teaching is a powerful means of achieving nursing outcomes to prevent illness, promote or restore health, and facilitate coping with chronic and terminal illness.

Learning is "the process by which a person acquires or increases knowledge or changes behavior in a measurable way as a result of an experience" (Taylor, Lillis, LeMone, & Lynn, 2011, p. 471). To promote learning, the nurse must apply teaching–learning principles. Learning does not help the client alone. With each teaching experience, the nurse enhances his or her own ability to teach, bringing increased satisfaction to the nursing role.

● TEACHING–LEARNING PROCESS: PRINCIPLES OF TEACHING

According to White (2005, p. 226), "the teaching–learning process is a planned interaction that promotes behavioral change that is not a result of maturation or coincidence." Principles of teaching and learning provide basic guidelines for the nurse assuming the role of a teacher. The teaching process and principles closely follow the communication process presented in Chapter 10. These principles are necessary for planning individualized client teaching and selecting teaching materials and methods that best meet client education needs (Display 12.1).

Functional literacy is defined as being able to read well enough to carry out activities of daily living. Health literacy is the ability of someone to read and act upon health information. The Institute of Medicine (IOM) reports a decrease in health literacy is associated with poorer patient outcomes and an increase in health care costs (IOM, 2004).

---

display 12.1   **Principles of Teaching and Learning**

1. Remember why we are teaching: to increase the quality of life.
2. Establish trust.
3. Partner with the learner.
4. Client motivation signifies readiness to learn.
5. Vary teaching style to the client's needs.
6. Individualize strategies and materials.
7. Capitalize on client strengths and resources.
8. Simplify language.
9. Consider developmental stage.
10. Modify the environment.
11. Judiciously use content sequencing.
12. Provide repetition and practice.
13. Relate new learning experiences to client's past.
14. Reinforce newly learned behaviors.

Trust

People learn best when they are accepted, understood, and connected to the health care provider. For the teaching–learning process to succeed, clients must trust their nurse, and nurses must respect the client's ability to learn. Nurses must identify all signs of client frustration and hostility to their instructions. These need to be openly discussed before learning can take place. Client attitudes vary from pleasant and accepting to hostile, bitter, or rejecting. Nurses must also be aware of their own personal biases and how these affect the teaching–learning process (Rankin, Stallings, & London, 2005). Nurses must be sensitive to attitudes and adapt their teaching approach so that learning can occur.

Partnering with the Learner

The teaching–learning process will be more effective and empowering to the client if the client is included in the planning of the learning objectives. Including the client in the teaching–learning process tells the nurse what the client is willing and unwilling to do. Compliance, an older term that pertains to the adherence of the client to his or her health care teaching, has many negative connotations. It implies that the health care provider knows more than the client about his or her health care. "Adherence" or "following the plan of care" might be more appropriate to use, so we will substitute those for compliance. *Adherence* is best attained when the nurse and client agree on outcomes and an action plan. Unless the learning outcomes center around what the client values and is willing to achieve, little learning will take place. It is important to assess the client's understanding of the benefits of treatment, risks for failure to follow health care teaching recommendations, and severity of his or her condition. The use of active listening techniques and clear, simple language go a long way toward establishing trust and understanding.

Motivation

Motivation is the internal desire to learn and is a unique quality of each person (Berman et al., 2011). What motivates one individual may not motivate another. A key concept the nurse must remember is that the best-laid plan may be ineffective if the targeted learner lacks the motivation to learn (Rankin et al., 2005). It helps to enhance motivation if learning is relevant to the client.

If the client believes inapplicable information is being taught, then he or she will have less motivation to learn, seeing less significance of adherence.

The nurse needs to identify emotional, physical, and experiental factors that signal a client is able, motivated, and willing to learn. The emotional state of the client can motivate him or her to learn or inhibit learning. Emotions such as anxiety, depression, denial, and fear can require a great deal of the client's energy and distract him or her from learning. However, anxious parents of a sick child, for example, may be receptive to learning special techniques that allow them to participate in their child's care—the immediate need for this information may override the emotions they are feeling.

Assess for physical barriers to learning, such as pain, acuity of illness, or prognosis of illness. A client who is in pain, weak, or preoccupied with thoughts about illness may be unable to concentrate on instructions and attend to learning.

A client's experiences, background, skills, knowledge, and attitudes regarding a health situation provide the necessary foundation for developing the teaching plan. Learning is more successful if a client builds upon previous knowledge. A client who has cared for a frail elderly relative after a stroke will be better able to cope with a spouse convalescing from a heart attack than a client who has always depended on others to care for ill family members.

NCLEX–RN *Might Ask*   12.1

The nurse is assessing a client's motivation to learn. Which of the following factors could block that client's motivation to learn?

(A) Severe pain
B. Successful past experiences
C. Strong family support system
D. A positive attitude

• See Appendix A for correct answer and rationale

Client attitudes and values can facilitate or inhibit the learning that can be achieved. A client recovering from knee replacement surgery will be more successful in learning to use a walker if he or she values independence and accepts direction and help from others than will a client who wants to be helped and feels safe in a wheelchair.

Learning Style

Learning style is defined by White (2005) as the "manner whereby an individual incorporates new data" (p. 164). The nurse should remember that different people learn differently, and material should be presented in varied ways. Learning is a complex process affected by people's responses to varied sensory input and their orientation to learning. Some individuals learn in a singular mode by performing tasks or by manipulating new information. This is called *kinesthetic learning*. Others learn by hearing new information, which is called *auditory learning*. Many learn better by seeing new ideas or *visual learning*. A combination of modes would address more diverse learning styles. Asking the client how he or she learns best would take into account the diversity of learning. Nurses are more effective teachers if they ask their client learners how they learn best before teaching begins (see Table 12.1).

Regardless of the client's learning style, nurses will be more successful if they vary and combine the different types of sensory input when teaching. Information presented in a variety of ways is understood and remembered better than that which is only seen or heard.

Another aspect of learning style to consider is the client's way of understanding the situation. Some prefer to look at the big picture and then learn about its segments, whereas others like to look at one piece at a time to learn about the whole situation. A client who prefers to see the whole may respond to segmental teaching with the plea, "Would you get to the point; what does all this mean?" A client who

table
············ LEARNING STYLES AND EFFECTIVE METHODS
12-1

Style of Learning	Sense	Example
Kinesthetic	Feeling, touching, and manipulating	Touching ostomy supplies Redressing a wound
Auditory	Listening	Listening to a tape player Listening to a lecture
Visual	Seeing	Reading a booklet or information from the Internet
Auditory and visual	Seeing and listening	Watching a videotape or DVD with commentary

likes to take things segmentally might respond to an explanation of the big picture by saying, "This is very confusing. Can you explain it one step at a time?"

Teaching Materials

Use charts, models, pictures, diagrams, videotapes, television programs, CDs, DVDs, podcasts, and the Internet to enhance learning. Hospitals and ambulatory care settings will increase efficiency and consistency if they use their own commercially packaged educational channels on television for general and specific client education. Self-study modules, along with small group sessions, can be used effectively in the outpatient setting (Lamb, Finlayson, Mathiowetz, & Chen, 2005). However, be careful not to use literature and audiovisuals as a substitute for the nurse–client interaction. With less time and fewer resources available, it is common to see instructional pamphlets or video programs used to teach about medical conditions, such as diabetes, and health education topics, such as breastfeeding. Clients, such as Mr. Martinez in our opening vignette, may not understand written instructions because of language differences, age, or functional illiteracy. Thus, it is important to assess the client's reading ability and fluency in the English language at the onset of a client teaching relationship. There are ways to enhance learning, such as using patient education materials written in other languages.

Illiteracy is common and affects individuals of all races and socioeconomic levels. According to Taylor et al. (2011), about 20% of adults are functionally illiterate, unable to read beyond a fifth-grade reading level. The Workforce Investment Act of 1998 defines literacy as an individual's ability to read, write, and speak English. It also states that literacy means a person should be able to compute and solve problems at levels of proficiency necessary to function on the job, in the family, and in society. In 2003, the results of the National Assessment for Adult Literacy demonstrated that 30 million Americans were below the basic proficient literacy level. They concluded that these adults were not able to do much more than sign a form or search a medical document to determine what they needed to do before a medical test. According to Canobbio (2008), to be effective, teaching materials need to be geared to the sixth- to eighth-grade reading levels. The nurse should always assess the client's literacy level when teaching.

Direct testing is the best method for assessing client literacy but is not practical in clinical settings. Screening tools such as the Newest Vital Sign by Pfizer, Inc., can be tactfully used in about 3 minutes to determine literacy (Weiss et al., 2005) and is available in English and Spanish (Barclay & Vega, 2005). A less accurate but more tactful and expedient method might be to observe and ask clients about their favorite materials for pleasure reading. Assess the client for an inability to focus on reading materials, a tendency to focus on detail, consistent tendency to interpret literature literally, and a lack of ability to concentrate on dominant themes. These are common assessments found in clients who have difficulty reading. In addition, a functionally illiterate client may be slow to interpret information. Careful assessment is the key.

Provide several options (reading, watching, and listening), and then ask simple questions about the content and descriptions of any materials provided. Reduce the amount of reading involved by using gestures, pictures, video- or audiotapes, and diagrams to get across important learning concepts. Use small portable DVD players to augment frequently taught material. Learning sessions should involve small, usable chunks of information. Monitor the client's understanding frequently by return demonstration or questioning him or her.

NCLEX–RN *Might Ask*   12.2

In the home care setting, the nurse is assessing the reading skills of a client with newly diagnosed diabetes. The best way the nurse could assess this skill is by

    A. asking the client to take a literacy test.
    B. checking the client's type of pleasure reading.
    C. making the client read a complex instruction sheet.
    D. asking the client's husband the last year of school the client completed.

• See Appendix A for correct answer and rationale.

Client Learning Strengths and Resources

Determine the client's learning strengths and resources to facilitate learning. Client strengths are the internal physical, psychological, social, and spiritual resources a person mobilizes to cope with problems. See Display 12.2 for examples of strengths that nurses can use to develop a teaching plan.

Resources are external forces such as support systems, housing, income, transportation, and education that influence a person's ability to meet his or her needs. These resources must be considered for teaching to be effective. For example, if Mr. Martinez, our Spanish-speaking client with diabetes, has a language barrier and vision loss, he may never achieve any degree of independence in self-injection unless Mary works to resolve these issues. A hypertensive client such as Mr. James, who has a limited income and lack of housing, may not be able to comply with the medication regimens and diet modifications that would more effectively control the

---

display 12.2   **Examples of Client Strengths**

PHYSICAL STRENGTHS

Maintains good health through daily exercise
Moves about with ease
Maintains skin integrity
Sleeps well
Eats a nutritional diet
Breathes effectively
Stable blood pressure
Independent in activities of daily living

PSYCHOLOGICAL STRENGTHS

Resolves developmental tasks favorably
Demonstrates good problem-solving skills
Verbalizes confidence in philosophy of life
Expresses knowledge about health condition
Has a sense of humor
Shows insight into personal situations
Communicates willingness to learn
Reports ability to cope with health concerns
Verbalizes positive feelings of self-esteem

SPIRITUAL STRENGTHS

Actively participates in church, synagogue, or other organized religious or spiritual
    rituals
Expresses spiritual peace
Verbalizes confidence in religious faith

SOCIAL STRENGTHS

Relates well with spouse, significant other, children, and others
Has a strong support system of family and friends
Uses personal/family resources appropriately
Seeks out appropriate health care resources (eg, insurance, Weight Watchers,
    health club)
Accepts help from family and friends
Is a dedicated employee
Contributes to financial security of family

---

disease. Because discharge planning begins on admission, nurses would be working as a team to meet the needs of most of the clients in our beginning vignette. Mr. Martinez and his wife should have regularly scheduled visits by a diabetes educator and translator. Education may need to be carried into the home setting by a bilingual, culturally sensitive community or parish nurse (see Chapter 13).

thinking critically

Select three clients mentioned in the vignette other than Mr. Martinez. What resources should you identify that would be useful for these clients?

Language and Cultural Background

Take into consideration the client's language, education, socioeconomic background, and cultural factors when deciding what vocabulary to use in teaching. Be sensitive to the client's unfamiliarity with medical terms and jargon.

Simplify terms you normally use, such as "ambulation" to "walk," and try to use terminology with which the client is familiar. If a client does not speak English well, the nurse should obtain a knowledgeable translator to assist with the instruction. All efforts should be made to avoid using the family or a friend as an interpreter unless the patient has given specific permission to do so.

Use analogies, comparisons, examples, and illustrations to promote understanding. Common analogies include comparison of the heart to a pump, the bladder to a reservoir tank, the eyes to a camera lens, a heart valve defect to a leaking washer, and the joints to a hinge.

Developmental Considerations

To individualize teaching and ensure optimum learning, consider the client's developmental level when planning client teaching. *Pedagogy* is the science of teaching children and adolescents. Children and adolescents have varying limitations in attention, concentration, and cognitive and psychomotor skills related to developmental level (Display 12.3).

display 12.3 — Learning Aids for Children, Adolescent, and Adults

Child	Adolescent	Adult
1. Work at the eye level of the child.	1. Earn respect by matching words with actions.	1. Motivated by what is needed to know to function.
2. Check the child's developmental level, which may differ from his or her age.	2. Seek input and opinion, and engage the adolescent in problem solving.	2. Come with experience and knowledge to capitalize upon.
3. Assess self-care abilities.	3. Explore the feelings of the adolescent.	3. Are problem oriented rather than subject oriented.
4. Use dolls, dress-up, or imitation.	4. Assess how health problems affect interactions with peers.	4. Need to know why they are learning something
5. Use video, video games, and computer interactives.	5. Assess and accentuate positive qualities.	5. May like to socialize and learn in groups.
6. Use simple terms.	6. Make language clear and health related.	
7. Use frequent and consistent repetition and reinforcement.	7. Encourage independence and informed choice.	
8. Use short sessions because children have short attention spans.		

Andragogy is the study of how adults learn (Merriam, Caffarella, & Baumgartner, 2007). Adults are generally motivated learners but sometimes lead busy lives and/or lack the self-confidence to try something new. Adults also learn best when they see a clear and immediate need for information to be integrated into their lifestyle.

Health care education needs to be focused on the individual needs of the physically and emotionally challenged. In many cases, learning-disabled nurses have been pioneers in the development of user-friendly health promotional materials. "People with learning disabilities are entitled to the same health opportunities and information as the rest of the population but their level of ability may often contribute to inequities of access" (Dip, Wilkie, McKenzie, & Powell, 2005). For these individuals, using visual aids and gestures, simplifying information, and using short sentences can be helpful. Using family members to carry out more complicated regimens and reinforcement may be necessary. There are also gender-specific differences that might be taken into consideration when planning patient education. There is a need to be more focused on health promotional initiatives when addressing men's health challenges. There are many reasons why men may not access the health care systems as frequently as women. The social stigma of seeking assistance along with the stereotypical male-fostered "man as protector" image may contribute to a lack of important education on subjects such as prostate and testicular cancers and other men's health issues. It is important that health education be accessible yet confidential. An outreach program or clinic may be more successful if conducted at sports events or other traditionally male-attended events.

The process of aging changes many neurosensory body systems. The elderly may have hearing and visual impairments and reduced motor abilities. If the client has difficulty understanding you, shorten the length of the teaching session, establish priorities for teaching the information, and repeat the material as necessary. Display 12.4 gives commonly used techniques for effective learning when teaching the older adult.

Environment

Determine environmental factors that influence client learning. Careful attention should be paid to time constraints, the physical environment, client activity schedules, and client privacy. For example, it may be unrealistic for a nurse to give instructions for self-injection to a patient with diabetes during the morning medication

---

display 12.4   **Tips for Enhanced Learning in the Elderly**

1. Make comfortable.
2. Assess developmental level, motivation, readiness to learn, anxiety, depression, and motor abilities.
3. Present materials slowly.
4. Give frequent feedback.
5. Shorten sentences.
6. Use gestures.
7. Ensure adequate lighting.
8. Decrease distractions.

period, when the nurse is rushed and responsible for administering multiple drugs to several clients or getting clients ready for surgery. It would be better to schedule such teaching in the afternoon or to consult a diabetic nurse educator for help. For clients who do not speak English, the nurse must arrange to have an interpreter present and additional family support. If a client's learning needs can be anticipated, such as relaxation techniques for childbirth or preoperative instructions, arrange for the client to come for more focused instruction in advance of the situation. Perhaps home care visitation can be scheduled at a time when the client is free to meet the care provider, who can then be an additional resource for the client. The nurse uses multiple resources to skillfully enhance teaching and learning.

Sequence

Plan a series of instructions that builds on previous knowledge and lays the groundwork for future learning. Teach from easy to difficult, known to unknown, well to ill, normal to abnormal, and step-by-step for complicated topics.

Instruction in self-injection of insulin and then routine glucose monitoring at home is an example of sequential instruction. Clients are first taught about the insulin, then the steps in preparing the injection, and finally, they are taught the injection technique. When teaching a client to perform blood glucose testing, set up a sequence that begins with the purpose of testing, then progresses through equipment operation and maintenance, the testing procedure, and finally, quality assurance and troubleshooting problems. Not unlike your training as a student, such sequencing of complex procedural steps leads to optimal learning. Having standardized teaching plans that can be adapted for uniqueness, such as the one Mary's unit will be implementing, will help the Marys of the world clearly document progress and communicate with everyone on the health care team.

Repetition and Practice

Repeat, summarize, and ask questions after each segment of instruction. Reviewing material covered in previous teaching sessions or an earlier segment of the teaching period reinforces the learning, rewards the client, and helps the nurse evaluate learning. To provide motivation and enhance incentive, reinforce small successes, especially with the challenging learner.

Provide frequent and repeated opportunities to practice new skills, especially with adults, because adult learners learn by doing. Generally, several practice sessions spaced over a period of time are more effective than one long practice session, during which client fatigue may impede performance. Also, having alternative self-paced modules or booklets will not replace nursing education but can make learning more effective.

Past Experiences

Keep in mind that, at all developmental levels, new learning is contingent on a client's previous life experiences. Use the knowledge of the client or family as a base on which to build. For example, you may use a garden hose as an analogy for blood pressure if the client is a gardener, or the analogy of flushing a radiator to describe how to prime an intravenous line if the client works on cars. Be alert for the client with a previous "bad" experience in the health care setting. In this event, the entire team will have to work harder to win trust and accomplish outcomes.

Reinforcement

Behavioral learning theorists consider rewarding the learner for making the desired response to be the primary basis for learning. The nurse should praise, compliment, or provide a tangible reward when the client achieves the desired learning objective. The type of reward should be appropriate to the client and immediately follow the desired behavioral response. For example, providing a favorite computer game might be effective for a diabetic child, whereas verbal praise and a smile would be more appropriate for an elderly diabetic client who correctly self-administers an insulin injection.

---

thinking critically

Apply the previous principles of teaching if you were the nurse caring for the clients in the vignette. Compare and contrast your application of these principles with those of your classmates and formulate an ideal approach for these clients.

• TEACHING INTERVENTIONS

The nurse can use a variety of teaching strategies to meet the client's learning needs (Display 12.5). Choosing the right strategy, based on a thorough assessment and mutually acceptable goals, will make the experience enjoyable and effective. The method or strategy chosen depends not only on the setting in which teaching

---

display 12.5 **Teaching Strategies for the Clinical Setting**

COGNITIVE (KNOWLEDGE)

Lecture
Discussion
Simulation (apply knowledge in different contexts)
Independent study (reading, video viewing, self-paced modules)

PSYCHOMOTOR (SKILL)

Demonstration/Return demonstration
Guided practice
Independent practice

AFFECTIVE (VALUES)

Discussion
Values clarification
Role playing
Role modeling
Simulation

will occur but also the type of learning that needs to take place (affective, cognitive, or psychomotor). If one approach is unsuccessful, changing or combining modalities, such as seeing, doing, and hearing, may achieve the desired learning outcome.

Lecture

Lectures are an effective and efficient way to teach several people at once. The lecture approach works well with groups who are seeking information on common health care issues, such as diabetes management, prenatal care, and parenting classes. Lectures can capitalize on the diversity of other members of the health care team, lending different perspectives and interest for the listener. One of the problems inherent with the lecture format is that it does not usually promote active participation. The nurse should not confuse telling with learning. When using the lecture technique, the nurse cannot be sure that learning is taking place unless he or she actively engages or evaluates the learner. Lectures are less effective for affective and psychomotor learning or in most acute care hospital settings, where the ill client needs shorter and more individualized instruction.

Discussion

Discussion works well for the cognitive and affective domains of learning. This approach is useful for individual or group instruction in classroom, home, community, or bedside situations. Teacher and learner discussions more commonly involve the exchange of information, ideas, and feelings during brief encounters, such as while preparing a patient for a diagnostic procedure or when the nurse administers medications. Nurses involved with family support groups and organizations such as stroke and ostomy clubs also frequently use this approach.

---

thinking critically

Explain how the clients in the vignette might benefit most from a discussion approach versus a lecture approach in meeting their learning needs.

Simulation

The simulation strategy teaches and evaluates client learning. Because of its interactive nature, simulation promotes partnership in the learning process. The application of information in different scenarios gives the client experience with the subject and lets the nurse evaluate what was learned. For example, a nurse could teach and evaluate how well a hypertensive client learned dietary modifications by providing a sample menu and asking the client to order a meal that best meets sodium and fat restrictions. Computer simulations and Internet resources for clients are becoming more readily available. Reinforcement would be provided if the client chooses correctly, or instruction could continue if an incorrect choice was made.

Independent Study

Many adults are independent learners and prefer self-paced learning through independent study of printed, audiovisual, or online resource materials. A newer trend in health care education is the use of the Internet using handheld mobile devices as a resource for health information. Independent study should not be used in isolation but as a stimulus or precursor to a nurse–client learning interaction. Allowing a client to view a program on breastfeeding before a discussion or the nurse-directed experience of feeding a newborn can spark client questions and make the nurse–client interaction more successful. Careful assessment of client literacy, language, and health care resources should always be considered when using independent study materials.

As with preprinted materials, screening of the Internet resources is critical. Only recently are guidelines for finding reliable resources being developed. Advise the client to look for the Health On the Net Foundation (HON) symbol when surfing for health-related information (Lorenz, 2005). The nurse should be familiar with available resources in his/her area of expertise and can be helpful in showing the client where those sources may be obtained (Display 12.6).

Demonstration/Return Demonstration

Demonstration is the ideal way of teaching procedures, techniques, exercises, and the use of special equipment. Models of body parts, medical practice models, and teaching simulators—such as resuscitation dolls, breast models, and injection mannequins—are available to help clients learn independent health care practices. Providing step-by-step instructions in short, sequential teaching sessions usually works best for complex procedures such as ostomy care or self-injection of insulin. Return demonstration by the client provides opportunities to evaluate and correct problems, praise the client's learning, and make plans for further reinforcement and follow-through, if necessary.

Practice

Client practice—guided, then independent—should always be considered in conjunction with the demonstration strategy for psychomotor learning. After explaining and demonstrating a skill, sufficient time should be planned for the nurse to direct or guide the client through each step of a procedure, such as changing sterile dressings or operating a glucose monitor. Additional independent practice with and without the nurse present will help the client move to more independent functioning. Written materials, videotapes, CDs, DVDs, and podcasts should be given to provide the client with resources for review.

---

display 12.6   **Effective Internet Use for Patient Education**

1. Look for the HON symbol indicating a reliable source.
2. Emphasize that not all online resources are current or accurate.
3. Encourage the client/family to print resources and use them as a basis of discussion with the health care educator.
4. Counsel to use reputable Internet sources in comparison with other resources prior to making informed decisions.

thinking critically

In the vignette, Mr. Martinez was having difficulty with learning self-injection. Assuming that the nurse was using demonstration and practice as teaching strategies, what principle of learning needs emphasis in revising Mr. Martinez's teaching plan so he can be more successful?

Self-Disclosure

Seeing a nurse who has overcome health challenges can help the client change attitudes and values associated with health issues. A nurse who has struggled with a weight issue, given up an addiction to tobacco, or overcome a learning disability may be able to share personal insights that are helpful to a client. Nurses who were former smokers have been excellent role models for clients who are trying to quit smoking to improve their health. Nurses with learning-disabled children can help by sharing beneficial learning strategies and successful outcomes.

Role Playing

Acting out feelings or behaviors gives the learner a chance to experience, relive, or anticipate a situation. Role playing emphasizes the cognitive and affective domains of learning. The client can experiment with different responses to a situation, while the nurse offers guidance and feedback.

Play with puppets and dolls has proven effective in preparing young children for procedures and helping them express negative feelings about hospitalization. Role playing in prenatal class is effective and necessary to help couples get through transition in childbirth. One disadvantage of using role play with adults is that they may feel uncomfortable when using this process. Every effort should be made to help them feel safe to explore feelings and assure them that the exercise will be helpful in meeting their learning needs.

Values Clarification

Encouraging clients to explore and identify their values about health, sickness, and health care issues helps remove barriers to learning new or different approaches to managing health and illness. Identification of values in different aspects of a client's life might serve as a stimulus for changing behaviors in health care practices. A nurse might help a client see the importance of routine follow-up visits for hypertension by comparing it to routine maintenance of a classic car or health maintenance of a pet, depending on the client's interests. Such transference of a common value is an important achievement regarding personal health.

● STEPS IN THE TEACHING–LEARNING PROCESS

Client teaching is most effective when approached through the nursing process, as outlined in Table 12.2. Rather than think of client education as a separate

table

············ NURSING PROCESS VERSUS TEACHING–LEARNING PROCESS

12-2

Nursing Process	Teaching–Learning Process
Assessing	Determine learning needs
Diagnosing	Identify learning needs Nursing diagnoses of learning needs

Planning	Specify learning objectives
	Select teaching method
	    Informal teaching
	    Formal teaching
	    Standardized teaching plans
	Select teaching strategies

Implementing	Implement teaching plan. Prepare materials. Structure teaching sessions Control environment
Evaluating	Evaluate teaching Evaluate learning

and unique nursing function, nurses must integrate client education into their general approach to client care and address learning needs in every aspect of the nursing process. The nurse should be aware that all client interactions are teaching ones. In some situations, the nurse can anticipate a whole series of learning needs, such as the standardized preoperative teaching topics needed by Mrs. Duncan in the vignette, whereas other situations are incidental to ongoing nursing care, such as teaching the purpose and side effects of a newly prescribed drug, as was needed by Mr. James in the vignette before administration of the medication. The wise nurse teaches "on the go" and makes every contact a potential teaching one.

Assessment

An organized and thorough assessment is the first and most essential step for effective learning (Lawton & Carrol, 2005). When a client's situation is assessed, prioritize what the client or family needs to know or learn. A basic educational assessment should include motivation level, comprehension ability, current knowledge level, attitudes about health, and factors that will affect teaching, such as sensory, physical, and mental abilities and language. Ideally, this information should be obtained on admission or during early periods of client contact, when the nurse interviews the client for the nursing database. In addition, the nurse should remain vigilant about obtaining information about the client's learning needs, as revealed through the client's questions and behaviors when the nurse is giving care.

A basic educational assessment can be accomplished by answering the following questions during client interactions:

- What does the client know?
- What does the client think is happening and why?

| display **12.7** | Case Studies |

MR. MARTINEZ—HISPANIC, INSULIN-DEPENDENT DIABETIC CLIENT

In preparation for Mr. Martinez's discharge, Mary visits him, arranging for a hospital interpreter to be present during the sessions. Mary concentrates on speaking to Mr. Martinez, not the interpreter. She learns that Mr. Martinez's mother is knowledgeable about diabetic diet management because she also has diabetes. His mother is also a respected curandira or local healer. Mary arranges for Mr. Martinez's mother to be included in the teaching and for the afternoon nurse to carry on training in the evening. Mary learns that Mr. Martinez is knowledgeable about the signs and symptoms of hypoglycemia and hyperglycemia but has difficulty mixing and preparing his insulins. Part of the problem is that he cannot see well. Because of this, Mary contacts the local Visiting Nurses Association (VNA) for follow-up teaching at home and refers him to the walk-in clinic for vision testing for presbyopia.

MRS. WALLIS—CLIENT UNDERGOING POSTOPERATIVE LAMINECTOMY

Mary's visit to Mrs. Wallis is equally revealing. Mr. Wallis has never had to be responsible for an ill family member. Mrs. Wallis has always cared for their children when they were ill, "nursed" his invalid mother for 5 years after a stroke until her death 2 years ago, and has cared for him after five major surgeries during the past year, including his colostomy care. Mr. Wallis can explain the principles, purpose, and instructions for applying his wife's brace but has avoided handling the brace or practicing its application before Mrs. Wallis' surgery. Mary asks for his assistance in applying the brace so Mrs. Wallis can get up to the bathroom. Mr. Wallis' manipulative skill in arranging the brace for application is good, but he becomes extremely shaky and clumsy when attempting to apply the brace on his wife. Mr. Wallis expresses fear of hurting his wife or not being "a good nurse" like she was during his recovery from surgery. Mary arranges several more supervised practice sessions before discharge and consults physical therapy (PT). These sessions include a lot of praise from both the nurses, PT, and Mrs. Wallis. Eventually, Mr. Wallis becomes the preferred "nurse" in managing the brace because of his consistent and tender approach. Mary also consults VNA for support for Mr. and Mrs. Wallis at home.

- What does the client need to know?
- What worries the client most?
- What does the client want to know?
- How does the client feel about managing the situation independently?

Answers to these questions in Display 12.7 help the nurses discover why Mr. Martinez was having difficulty mastering his insulin injections and exactly what Mr. Wallis needed to be less afraid to take his wife home.

Diagnosis

After collecting the necessary data, the nurse analyzes the information and identifies the nursing diagnosis that most clearly describes the client's learning needs. According to the guidelines of the North American Nursing Diagnosis Association International (NANDA-I, 2009), there are two approaches to diagnosing learning needs. If the learning need is keeping the client from functioning optimally, the problem statement "deficient knowledge" can be used with additional clarification and etiology, as in the following examples:

Mr. Wallis: Deficient knowledge (application of orthopedic brace) related to inexperience and concern about home care management

Mrs. Duncan: Deficient knowledge (postoperative exercises) related to lack of information about postoperative care

Mr. Martin: Deficient knowledge (ostomy care) related to unfamiliarity with home management of colostomy

Deficient knowledge may also be the etiology of the health care problem in other NANDA-I taxonomy categories of human response patterns, such as ineffective health maintenance, anxiety, risk for infection, ineffective coping, and noncompliance. Thus, lack of knowledge, knowledge deficit, lack of understanding, or insufficient information may be used as the etiology of the nursing diagnosis, as in the following examples:

Mr. James: Ineffective health maintenance related to lack of understanding about the disease process, treatment regimen, and home care management

Mr. Martin: Delayed surgical recovery related to insufficient knowledge of colostomy irrigation, peristomal skin care, and incorporation of ostomy care into activities of daily living

When deficient knowledge is used as the problem in the nursing diagnostic statement, the nurse supports the belief that giving information can change behavior. This approach directs nursing care to resolve cognitive learning needs but does not necessarily focus on a client's affective learning needs. However, when the learning need "deficient knowledge" or lack of understanding is used as the etiology, nursing care can be directed toward the affective factors that block the client's ability to maintain health and manage self-care (Carpenito-Moyet, 2008). For example, Mr. Martinez's care plan needed to develop his confidence in mixing insulin correctly, rather than merely providing additional information about insulin injections.

One of the newer nursing diagnostic statements involves receptivity to learning. Readiness for enhanced knowledge is used when a client has "cognitive information related to a specific topic for meeting health related goals and that can be strengthened" (NANDA-I, 2009). This is a wellness diagnosis and might be more appropriate in the recovery, clinic, or home care setting (Wilkinson, 2009).

The nurse must choose a style of diagnosis. However, regardless of which style the nurse uses, both approaches give direction to nursing care and education interventions. To comply with legal and professional nursing standards, every nursing care plan must include at least one nursing diagnosis addressing client education.

Although the term "noncompliance" is a widely accepted nursing diagnosis, it has a negative connotation in the eyes of the client. It can imply that the health care worker has made a judgment about the client, negating the client's choice. The nurse may want to consider substituting the other terms, such as "difference of opinion" or "different values," when talking about the client's learning needs, especially in public.

Planning

Writing a teaching plan or emphasizing the teaching component of the client's general nursing care plan is a major nursing responsibility. When the client's learning needs are identified and presented in a diagnostic statement, the nurse (in collaboration with the client) develops a client-centered teaching plan that establishes outcomes and appropriate interventions. The nurse may develop an individualized teaching plan or individualize a standardized (or model) teaching plan with stated outcomes (learning objectives) and nursing interventions (teaching strategies) that reflect the individuality of the client.

INDIVIDUALIZED PLANS

Individualized teaching plans are generally a component of the client's overall nursing care plan. Educational outcome criteria and teaching interventions are included as one of three approaches (diagnostic, therapeutic, and educational) to resolve an identified human response pattern problem. This type of plan requires more composing and writing time for nurses, but this is the preferred method for ensuring that the unique needs of clients will be addressed.

STANDARDIZED TEACHING PLAN

Standardized teaching plans or model teaching plans have evolved in clinical settings in which teaching situations frequently recur. The standardized preoperative teaching plan is one of the most common plans. Specialty areas such as prenatal clinics, maternity centers, emergency rooms, outpatient ambulatory care centers, and client education clinics are developing other teaching plans to lessen the nurse's work and make client education documentation easier.

Standardized teaching plans are available in books or preprinted guides. They usually include checklists, blank lines, or empty spaces for the nurse to individualize outcomes and nursing interventions and to document the teaching provided. This type of plan should be used as a guide because it does not address the client's individual needs and can cause the nurse to focus only on predictable problems and miss cues to unique client problems.

Nurses must always assess the client's knowledge level first to determine if all the information included in the model plan is needed and then individualize the plan to meet the client's specific needs. Most nursing care planning guides include teaching outcomes and interventions in a general abbreviated form, and nurses need to personalize the teaching plan in more detail for specific clients (Display 12.8).

---

display 12.8   Nursing Care Plan for Postoperative Laminectomy

ASSESSMENT FOR MRS. WALLIS:

Before using the standardized model teaching plan, Mary carefully assessed what Mr. and Mrs. Wallis knew and were able to do regarding positioning, activity precautions, and back brace management. In her assessment, she found Mrs. Wallis could independently log roll when changing position in bed and maintained proper body alignment while lying in bed, sitting, and standing with her walker. She was cooperative and showed personal responsibility in adhering to the 15-minute limitation on sitting and did not need any reminders from the nursing staff. Mrs. Wallis needed assistance in applying the back brace when getting out of bed, and Mr. Wallis became extremely shaky and appeared awkward when trying to align and comfortably position the brace for Mrs. Wallis. Mr. Wallis always called for the nurses to assist Mrs. Wallis with the brace, and he left the room during his wife's dressing period.

Standardized Plan	Individualized Plan
Nursing Diagnosis:	**Nursing Diagnosis:**
Risk for injury related to lack of knowledge of postoperative position restrictions and log-rolling technique	Risk for injury related to lack of knowledge and skill in the use of a back brace
Expected Outcomes:	**Learner Objective:**
1. The client will demonstrate correct positioning and logrolling techniques within 8 hours. 2. The client will verbalize feeling necessary activity precautions by the end of this shift.	1. Client will demonstrate correct application of the back brace. 2. Mr. Wallis will express a feeling of confidence in assisting Mrs. Wallis in donning the back brace. 3. The client will demonstrate proper application and use of the back brace.
Intervention:	**Intervention:**

1. Teach client to use arms and legs to transfer weight properly when getting out of bed.
2. Encourage walking, standing, and sitting for short periods as soon as permitted after surgery.
3. Teach the client precautions to maintain proper body alignment:
  a. Log-rolling techniques
  b. Side-lying position in bed
  c. Positions to avoid
  d. Standing and weight bearing
	1. Demonstrate the proper use of a back brace:
	  a. Explain the mechanism and purpose of the back brace.
	  b. Show Mr. Wallis proper positioning of brace while it is being worn by Mrs. Wallis.
	  c. Demonstrate how to secure the back brace.
	  d. Demonstrate and explain how to minimize skin irritation from wearing the brace.

4. Teach the proper use of a back brace, if indicated.
5. Teach client to avoid:
   a. Prolonged sitting
   b. Twisting the spine
   c. Bending at the waist
   d. Climbing stairs
   e. Automobile trips

e. Show pictures and describe skin breakdown to be assessed each time the brace is applied and removed.
f. Demonstrate skin care and massage after brace removal.
2. Encourage Mr. Wallis to discuss his concerns about responsibilities in helping his wife put on the back brace.
3. Give verbal praise each time Mr. Wallis participates or takes charge in assisting his wife to put on her back brace.

EXPECTED OUTCOMES/LEARNING OBJECTIVES

Learning objectives are similar to the outcome statements used for nursing care plans in general. Learning objectives should be client-centered, measurable statements of what the client will say or do to give evidence of learning. Verbs in learning outcomes should be consistent with the three domains of learning:

- Cognitive learning objectives use verbs describing the results of the thinking process: "The client will state how diet intake affects his blood sugar levels."
- Affective learning objectives use verbs that disclose the client's feelings, attitudes, and values: "The client will express feelings about his colostomy stoma."
- Psychomotor learning objectives use verbs that clarify client actions and skills: "The client will demonstrate aseptic technique when self-administering an insulin injection."

The more specific the desired outcomes are, the easier it will be for the client to pursue learning and for the nurse to evaluate progress. A single general objective, such as "Mr. Martin will become independent in colostomy care," may be accurate but is too global and does not provide enough direction for meeting the client's individual needs. Having several objectives (Display 12.9) can make the teaching plan easier to implement segmentally, gives the nursing team clearer direction, and enables the nurse to evaluate client learning better.

display 12.9 Learning Objectives for Mr. Martin's Individualized Teaching Plan

1. Mr. Martin will empty and change the colostomy bag using the proper technique.
2. Mr. Martin will perform colostomy irrigation independently.
3. Mr. Martin will accurately assess skin area and describe the management of skin irritation if it occurs.
4. Mr. Martin will describe plans for resuming his preoperative lifestyle.
5. Mr. Martin will discuss feelings about the stoma with significant others.

Interventions

When learning objectives have been identified, the nurse chooses teaching strategies appropriate for the type of content, the client's learning style, and the outcomes to be achieved. As discussed, any number of teaching methods and materials may be available, but they will not be effective if misapplied. A demonstration will not facilitate a change in attitude or values if there is no opportunity to express feelings; the best-planned and best-delivered lecture will not achieve psychomotor skills if there is no opportunity to practice. In most client situations, integration of several teaching methods may be required. Nurses must use their own creativity to develop and use teaching interventions to implement their teacher role.

Implementation

When the teaching plan is implemented, the nurse should stay alert and sensitive to the client's needs and responses. If the nurse or client becomes frustrated with the process, the nurse should take a step back and review the objectives and interventions. Were they made with the client? Be prepared to adjust the teaching approach and modify the pace or setting according to the client's progress. The client may have more discomfort or fatigue than expected, so the teaching session may need to be delayed or shortened. Learning a new skill, such as dressing changes, ostomy care, or self-injection, may be more complex for the client than anticipated, so additional practice sessions will need to be provided.

Do not forget that the nurse is part of a team, so some parts of the teaching plan may be delegated to another health care professional. For example, Mr. and Mrs. Willis may be assisted with mobility and brace education by a PT. Drug information for Mr. James can be obtained by the unit pharmacist. In many instances, they can be part of the teaching team. Dr. Lotte may have an advanced nurse practitioner that assists him in the ongoing care of his clients. However, regardless of the support personnel, it is Mary's responsibility to assess, plan, coordinate, and evaluate the teaching.

When possible, include family members and support people in the teaching plan and instructional sessions. Their involvement will help them assist in the client's home care and can reinforce the client's learning.

Evaluation

Evaluation of an individual teaching plan should include the achievement of desired outcomes, adequacy and appropriateness of teaching materials/methods, and effectiveness of the nurse as a teacher. Do not assume that learning has occurred without some type of validation. Such evaluation of learning flows logically from the learning objectives of the teaching plan if the teaching–learning process is developed systematically from the nursing process.

Learning can be evaluated in a variety of ways, including written tests, questionnaires, oral questioning, observation, return demonstration, and home follow-up calls or visits. The method of evaluation should be consistent with the type of learning: Cognitive learning can be evaluated by questioning (written or oral), affective learning through client responses, and psychomotor learning by client return demonstrations. Although questionnaires are sometimes used to evaluate group learning, written tests are not commonly used in clinical settings.

To be effective, evaluation should occur throughout the teaching–learning process and at completion. The nurse should always be alert for staff frustration, client confusion, inaccurate information, or improper return demonstrations by the client. Early correction will ensure that the client does not learn inaccurate information or practice skills incorrectly.

Evaluation of learning should also include an assessment of the adequacy and appropriateness of the materials and methods used. If the assessment shows that the resource library contains adult education materials only in English, it is essential to get a variety of materials (printed and audiovisual) that include pictures or languages appropriate to other client populations.

Just as with other nursing roles, teaching requires practice and experience. The nurse should always complete a self-evaluation to improve his or her approach. Some questions the nurse might ask include the following:

1. Did the client achieve the learning objective?
2. How was I the most (or least) helpful to the client's learning?
3. What factors facilitated (or blocked) the client's success?
4. How could I improve this teaching session next time?
5. Nurses should also seek client feedback about the teaching–learning experience. Much can be learned from the client's perception. An anonymous questionnaire using a standardized form in an objective format (requiring circled or checked responses) should be provided to the client on discharge. Communication of the results should be shared with staff and quality changes made accordingly.

● DOCUMENTATION OF CLIENT TEACHING

Documenting client teaching is an important nursing responsibility required by the following:

- State nurse practice acts
- State home health agency licensure laws
- Medicare and Medicaid program regulations
- The ANA, which established a standard of care that includes teaching as a measure of accountability for quality of nursing care rendered, where the latter must be demonstrated through documentation
- The Joint Commission (formerly known as Joint Commission on Accreditation of Healthcare Organizations), which requires that teaching (involving the client and support system) must be shown by documentation for a facility to receive accreditation

Documentation of teaching and learning is set by agency policy and procedures. Each agency must determine the method of documentation and the types of clinical records that meet the agency's requirements for client teaching. Teaching may be written on a care plan, in nursing notes, or on a separate teaching record, but

display 12.10 **Focus on Charting: Client Teaching**

Problem:	The client requested that the nurse change the newborn son's wet and soiled diaper after circumcision procedure. The client asked many questions about how to care for a circumcised son, including diaper change and bathing instructions.
Intervention:	The nurse taught postcircumcision care with diaper changes and explained and demonstrated cleansing the circumcised penis. The nurse answered questions and will supervise the mother in the next diaper change and reinforce teaching.
Evaluation:	The mother returned a demonstration of diaper and circumcision care as taught. She now requests nursing support for instruction on bottle-feeding the infant.

it must be part of the client's official record. Generally, documentation of client teaching should include the following:

- Learning needs
- Teaching interventions planned
- Teaching interventions implemented
- Client outcomes achieved or not achieved
- Revisions or changes in teaching methods used

Whatever charting format or record is used, the nurse's charting must be clear, concise, accurate, and complete. The charting entries must show what was taught and how well the client or significant other demonstrated learning. An example of documentation of client learning is shown in Display 12.10.

● CLINICAL APPLICATIONS OF THE TEACHING–LEARNING PROCESS

Now that we have reviewed important principles of teaching and learning and applicable teaching strategies for varied clinical settings, we use the teaching–learning process to help Mary complete Mrs. Duncan's preoperative teaching (Display 12.11).

Assessment for Mrs. Duncan. Before using the hospital's guidelines for preoperative teaching (standardized plan), Mary assessed Mrs. Duncan's previous experiences with surgical experiences and hospitalizations, knowledge about the procedure to be performed, and her emotional state regarding surgery. In her assessment, Mary found that Mrs. Duncan had two previous hospital experiences (childbirth at age 26 years and appendectomy at age 14 years), which she found to be satisfying and uneventful, except for postanesthesia nausea and vomiting after her appendectomy. Mrs. Duncan cannot recall what the nurses and physicians expected of her after her previous surgery, but she is apprehensive about postsurgery pain management and nausea and the postoperative length of stay, because she has no sick leave accrued from her new job as a legal secretary and needs to return to work as soon as possible. Mrs. Duncan gives a good description of her surgeon's instructions regarding display **12.11** **Individualized Preoperative Teaching Plan for Mrs. Duncan**

NURSING DIAGNOSIS:

Anxiety related to insufficient knowledge about current anesthesia side effects and pain control management practices

Outcomes:

1. Mrs. Duncan will effectively verbalize specific fears and concerns regarding surgery and anticipated recovery before surgery.
2. Mrs. Duncan will verbalize postoperative pain management routine with the use of patient-controlled analgesia before surgery.

Interventions:

1. Provide an environment with privacy and minimal disruptions to encourage the expression of feelings and concerns.
2. Listen actively, and clarify and reflect feelings as expressed by the client.
3. Return demonstrates preoperative and postoperative activities with emphasis on the use of patient-controlled analgesia.

NURSING DIAGNOSIS:

Deficient knowledge (deep breathing and coughing) related to unfamiliarity with postoperative care activities

Goal:

1. Mrs. Duncan will verbalize knowledge of perioperative care before surgery.
2. Mrs. Duncan will demonstrate correct deep breathing and coughing techniques before surgery.

Interventions:

1. Explain usual preoperative and postoperative activities and expectations for Mrs. Duncan's procedure. Include family members and how the hospital staff will keep them informed of Mrs. Duncan's situation.
2. Demonstrate deep breathing and coughing using an abdominal splinting technique. Have Mrs. Duncan's return practice and demonstrate techniques.
3. Demonstrate incentive spirometry and have her practice and return demonstrations.
4. Show videotape on postoperative respiratory care.
5. Coordinate visit by respiratory therapy for use of mininebulizer treatments.

her procedure and potential complications that may arise with her surgery. She expresses confidence in her physician and trust that the nurses will give her good care. On physical examination, Mary finds that Mrs. Duncan's lungs are clear to auscultation and learns that she was a moderate smoker for 10 years but has not smoked in the last 2 years. Based on her assessment and the efforts of Mary and Mrs. Duncan's family, the nurse and client developed and implemented the individualized teaching plan outlined in Display 12.11.

● CONCLUSION

This chapter focuses on the nurse as a teacher. To institute sound teaching effectiveness, the nurse must first be a good communicator. Through the proper application of the principles of communication, teaching, and learning, the nurse gains the trust and respect of his or her clients in meeting their many self-care needs for the maintenance and promotion of health and recovery from illness or injury. Respect for the client's unique needs is necessary for a successful teaching–learning experience. When possible, the client and the nurse must work as a team toward meeting mutually agreed on objectives, goals, and interventions. The nursing process provides an effective framework for assessing, planning, implementing, and evaluating client learning. The use of varied strategies with direct personal interactions between the nurse and the client is essential to the client's learning. Nurses as health professionals must play a major role in meeting the public's health education needs. The nurse–client interactions provide an excellent opportunity for ongoing client health education.

References

American Nurses Association. (1998). *Standards of clinical practice* (2nd ed.). Washington, DC: Author.

Barclay, L., & Vega, C. (2005). Newest vital sign may be effective quick screen for health literacy. *Annals of Family Medicine, 3,* 514–522. Retrieved July 4, 2007, from http://www.medscape.com/viewarticle/518659_print

Bastable, S. (2008). *Nurse as educator: Principles of teaching and learning for nursing practice* (3rd ed.). Boston, MA: Jones and Barlett.

Berman, A., Snyder, S., McKinney, D. (2011). *Nursing basics for clinical practice.* Upper Saddle River, NJ: Pearson Education Incorporated.

Canobbio, M. (2008). *Mosby's handbook of patient teaching* (3rd ed.). St. Louis, MO: Mosby.

Carpenito-Moyet, L. J. (2008). *Nursing diagnosis: Application to clinical practice* (12th ed.). Philadelphia, PA: Lippincott Williams & Wilkins.

Dip, C., Wilkie, R., McKenzie, K., & Powell, H. (2005). Health promotion: Practice and research. *Learning Disability Practice, 8*(7), 16–19.

Institute of Medicine. (2004). *Health literacy: A prescriptive to decrease confusion.* Washington, DC: National Academics Press.

Lamb, A., Finlayson, M., Mathiowetz, V., & Chen, H. (2005). The outcomes of using self-study modules in energy conservation education for people with multiple sclerosis. *Clinical Rehabilitation, 19,* 475–481.

Lawton, S., & Carrol, D. (2005). Communication skills and district nurses: Examples in palliative care. *British Journal of Community Nursing, 10*(3), 134–136.

Lorenz, J. (2005). Avoiding self-medication: Use education to curb common misuses of medications by patients. *Advance for Nurses, 7*(24), 23–26.

Merriam, S., Caffarella, R., & Baumgartner, L. (2007). Learning in adulthood: A comprehensive guide (3rd ed.). San Francisco, CA: John Wiley Sons.

North American Nursing Diagnosis Association International. (2009). *Nursing diagnoses: Definitions and classifications, 2009–2011.* West Sussex, UK: Wiley-Blackwell.

Rankin, S., Stallings, K., & London, F. (2005). *Patient-education in health and illness* (5th ed.). Philadelphia, PA: Lippincott Williams & Wilkins.

Taylor, C., Lillis, C., LeMone, P., & Lynn, P. (2011). *Fundamentals of nursing* (7th ed.). Philadelphia, PA: Lippincott Williams & Wilkins.

Weiss, B., Mays, M., Martz, W., Castro, K., DeWalt, D., Pignone, M., et al. (2005). Quick assessment of literacy in primary care: The newest vital sign. *Annals of Family Medicine, 3*(6), 514–522.

White, L. (2005). *Foundations of basic nursing* (2nd ed.). Clifton Park, NY: Thomson Delmar Learning.

Wilkinson, J. (2009). *Prentice Hall nursing diagnosis handbook: With NIC interventions and NOC outcomes* (9th ed.). Upper Saddle River, NJ: Prentice-Hall.

Suggested Reading

Craven, R., & Hirnle, C. (2009). *Fundamentals of nursing: Human health and function* (6th ed.). Philadelphia, PA: Lippincott Williams & Wilkins.

Griggs, S. A., & Dunn, R. S. (Eds.). (1998). *Learning styles and the nursing profession.* New York, NY: NLN Press.

Knowles, M., Holton, E., & Swanson, R. (2000). *The adult learner* (5th ed.). Houston, TX: Gulf.

Mayer, G., & Rushton, N. (2002). Writing easy to read teaching aids. *Nursing 2002, 32*(3), 48–49.

Mennies, J. H. (2001). Teaching adult patients with learning disabilities. *Nursing Spectrum, 10*(21), 15–18.

Ruhall, L. (2003). Tips for teaching the elderly. *RN, 66*(5), 48–52.

Springhouse. (1999). *Patient teaching made incredibly easy!* Philadelphia, PA: Lippincott Williams & Wilkins.

Wagner, J. (2001). Patient education: Teaching older adults. *Advance for Nurses, 3*(20), 15–17.

Ward-Collins, D. (1998). 'Noncompliant': Isn't there a better way to say it? *American Journal of Nursing, 98*(5), 27–32.

On the (WEB) *http://www.literacyvolunteers.org/NetCommunity/Page. aspx?pid=191&srcid=-2:* Information on functional illiteracy (Last accessed 3.3.2011)

www.healthAtoZ.com: Consumer health information; maintained by health care professionals (Last accessed 3.3.2011)

http://www.srhs.org/body.cfm?id=128&fr=true: Australian Web site maintained by health care professionals for clients (Last accessed 3.3.2011)

http://www.heart.org/HEARTORG/: Web site of the American Heart Association (Last accessed 3.3.2011)

www.pharmweb.net: Medication information (Last accessed 3.3.2011).

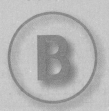

PART

B

Manager of Care

13

Managing Unique Client Care

● LEARNING OUTCOMES

By the end of the chapter, the student will be able to:

1 Discuss the following concepts related to diversity: culture, subculture, customs, beliefs, attitudes, values, and ethnocentrism.

2 Recognize that cultural competency is an ongoing process that requires continuing education.

3 Define the concepts of culture relevant to health and health-seeking behaviors.

4 Discuss how values, beliefs, and attitudes affect the nurse–client relationship.

5 Use communication skills that allow open discussion of similarities and differences with each client.

6 Use a variety of techniques to perform an accurate assessment of the unique variables for each client.

7 Apply concepts of uniqueness in the nursing care planning process.

8 Analyze how diversity impacts the nursing care planning process.

● KEY TERMS

acculturation	ethnocentrism	sexual orientation
assimilation	LGBT (lesbian, gay,	stereotyping
attitudes	bisexual, and	subculture
beliefs	transgendered)	uniqueness
binary opposites	heritage	values
cultural competence	marginalized	
cultural relativism	race	
cultural sensitivity	racism	
enculturation		

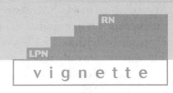

vignette

Sacred Heart Hospital administrators have recruited José Cruz, LPN, from his native Puerto Rico to help staff their community hospital. José has been enjoying his orientation to the telemetry unit and has made a valuable contribution, especially with the large Hispanic population. The nurses within the hospital have welcomed José and other actively recruited Puerto Rican nurses. José has entered the accelerated LPN–RN program at a local community college and is talking to one of his professors.

PROFESSOR: How are you doing, José?

JOSÉ: I'm happy to be in America, although I miss Puerto Rico and my family. The conveniences and the living are much easier here than in Puerto Rico, but the pace is very fast. I am having some problems communicating with the Anglo nurses and physicians. They talk so fast. Sometimes they use words that I know, but I still don't understand what they are trying to say. We don't have as many different meds in Puerto Rico, either. There have been multiple transcription and medication errors. Even though we speak the same language, communication is difficult at times. Everyone here is so strict about time, too. In my country, we are much more relaxed.

PROFESSOR: What do you think would be helpful to you?

JOSÉ: I think if people would just slow down and be more patient. Maybe if they could go to another country and work. Then they would see how difficult it is to think and understand in a different language. Having John Cruz, the Hispanic nurse manager in PACU, mentoring me has meant a lot. We have had many similar experiences.

PROFESSOR: Yes, in the United States, we tend to be pressured about time, and we need to slow down. John was a graduate of our program. It makes me happy that he is helping you out. Would you be willing to share what you are experiencing in class? It would help the other students to see another cultural perspective.

JOSÉ: Sure. I want people to learn how different and similar we are.

Nurses strive to assess, plan, and intervene based on an individual's response to illness. You have spent most of your time learning about the various anatomical and physiological responses to illness. You have undoubtedly worried about the intricacies of hormonal regulation, adverse reactions to medications, and variations in laboratory values and testing procedures. You know what to assess and how to plan and intervene while working with a client. You are aware of the resources available to blend variables such as age and chronic conditions into a plan of care. However, nurses interact with clients and other members of the health care team, like José, from different cultural, social, and religious backgrounds. Being culturally knowledgeable, sensitive, and competent is imperative in the changing environment of nursing.

● UNDERSTANDING UNIQUENESS

According to the U.S. Census Bureau Community Survey of 2006 to 2008 (2010), the breakdown of population per cultural group reveals that around 84.9% were not Hispanic or Latino, 15.1% were Hispanic or Latino, and 65.9% were White alone. These numbers only reflect previously established large cultural groups; they do not in any way reflect the multicultural aspects of many populations. Population statistics have increasingly become more fluid with groups formerly called minorities becoming a majority of the population. Lowe and Archibald (2009) estimate an additional 1/2 million non white nurses will be needed to minister to larger minority populations. Because most nursing care is and has always been provided by white female nurses, the potential for a one-sided view far from the patient's perspective is great.

This challenge has been brought forth by many of the organized health care organizations in the United States. Cultural uniqueness is not just a fad to be fostered; health care education in the client's language is a law and an ethical right of all individuals. The American Nurses Association (ANA, 1998) position on discrimination and racism states that nurses must respect and act taking uniqueness into consideration. Disparity in care among different cultural groups has led to the federal law mandating that any health care be provided in the patient's language. Communication and understanding of how uniqueness impacts the basis of competent and compassionate care is imperative. Nurses are in a unique position to lessen potential conflict and increase understanding in their daily interactions with clients.

Merriam-Webster's On-Line Dictionary (2010) has defined uniqueness as "being without a like or equal." Uniqueness is affected by many factors, including culture, race, gender, sexual orientation, socioeconomic status, spiritual orientation, and education. Each factor is the result of an individual's life journey. Cultural competence is defined as a carrier-long endeavor "to become increasingly self-aware, to value diversity, and to become knowledgeable about cultural strengths" (Maier-Lorentz, 2008, p. 37).

● DEFINITIONS

One of the challenges of learning about human uniqueness is that there is little consensus on what the concepts involved with diversity and culture mean (Storey, 2009). Many of the terms are used interchangeably. Anthropologists and educators define human culture as learned behavior acquired by individuals as members of a social group. The ANA (1998) stated that culture is broadly conceptualized to encompass the belief systems of a variety of groups. Purnell and Paulanka (2008) broadly defined culture as the "totality of socially transmitted behavior patterns, arts, beliefs, values, customs, and lifeways and all other products of human work and through characteristics of a population that guide their world view and decision making" (p. 5). Examples of the cultures to which an individual may belong are family units, nationality, religions, social classes, and professions. Culture is the binding resin of families, neighborhoods, and communities in a relationship of shared meaning. When a nurse renders culturally sensitive care, he or she becomes a part of this shared experience.

Each human society has a body of norms governing behavior and other knowledge to which an individual is socialized or enculturated, beginning at birth or at the time the individual becomes a member of the social group. Culture is learned through socialization with those near to us (Craven & Hirnle, 2009). The socialization process comes from heritage, which is comprises the things that are passed down from generation to generation (Berman, Snyder, Kozier, & Erb, 2007). An individual may or may not incorporate heritage learned into the luggage of life. Therefore, everyone must be considered an individual and be treated as such. To assign characteristics to an individual based on his or her looks or on preconceived ideas is called stereotyping. Because of stereotyping, this individual becomes marginalized with his/her feelings, values, and customs as an individual unrecognized as being different.

The United States is composed of many cultures with social groups (subcultures) coming together to form a larger social group (dominant culture). A subculture is defined as those individuals who have a distinct identity and yet are part of the larger cultural group. For example, although the Asian American population is considered one group statistically, there is a large disparity of language (250 dialects spoken) and many distinctly different subcultures, which include people from Japan, China, Indonesia, India, and Pakistan (James, 2005). Compounding this is a growing number of clients that are bi- and multicultural. They have special needs, because they may identify with the main culture, with the minor culture, none of the cultures, or a blend of them. Therefore, the nurse needs tools to assess the unique elements of culture that the client possesses. Tools for the assessment of diversity are referred to at the end of the chapter. However, elements of uniqueness are defined now. These elements are customs, beliefs, attitudes, and values.

Customs are learned behaviors. These behaviors are shared and practiced by individuals who belong to a particular group. Customs are based on beliefs, attitudes, or values. The importance of a custom is related to the importance of the belief, attitude, or value on which it is based. Many customs that are important to a particular client are easily assessed because they can be observed or elicited by direct questioning. For example, an older custom in the nursing profession is to wear a pin signifying the school from which the nurse graduated. Another example comes to us from the Hopi tribe of Native Americans. The symbol of the thunderbird gives the wearer good luck and spiritual protection.

Beliefs include opinions, knowledge, and faith. A belief is the acceptance of truth or reliability of something with or without proof. Another term for a belief is supposition. A dominant American belief is that the right of the individual is most important. Another belief by Hmong Laotians, who are Buddhists, is that there are 32 spirits *in a person*; injury and illness may be caused by the loss of one of these spirits (Johnson, 2005).

An attitude is way of feeling about or behaving toward a person, object, or idea. Attitudes are comprises many beliefs. If the nursing staff working with José believes that he has made multiple errors in transcription, then they may conclude he is an incompetent nurse and should not be allowed to practice. Judgments of good and bad are called binary opposites and are derived from attitudes.

Values are a set of personal beliefs and attitudes about the truth, beauty, and worth of any thought, object, or behavior. They are action oriented and give direction and meaning to life. Values develop from associations with people, the environment, and self. They are derived from life experiences. Values that are important to many Americans include individualism, accumulating items for self, having a nuclear family, and competition. These values are vastly different from the Native American culture, in which dependence and bonding to the family or group, sharing with others, extended family relationships, and cooperation are more highly valued (Purnell & Paulanka, 2008).

● SELF-ASSESSMENT

People naturally believe that their way of viewing the world is the only right way. This is the way they were socialized into the world as they know it. This narrow one-sided view is called ethnocentrism. Ethnocentrism "is the universal tendency of human beings to think that their ways of thinking, acting, and believing are the only right, proper, and natural ways" (Purnell & Paulanka, 2008, p. 6) Terminology involving ethnicity has many negative connotations and is a barrier to giving individualistic care. Atrocities of one group against another have been widely documented throughout history. The feeding of the Christians to the lions by the Romans, the partial extermination of millions of European Jews by the Nazis, and wars between Bosnian Serbs and Croatians are extreme examples of the hatred and genocide of one subculture by another.

Stepping out of one's comfort zone to learn about another culture is the binary opposite of ethnocentrism called cultural relativism. We have never lived in one-size-fits-all environments; as inquisitive creatures, we have the capacity to learn valuable lessons from each other. Because we live in a multicultural society and because it is impossible to know everything about all cultures, the journey toward cultural relativism is a lifelong process. For a nurse, this process requires that he or she become culturally competent. Individual cultural competence is the "complex integration of knowledge, attitudes, beliefs, skills, and encounters with those from cultures different from one's own that enhances cross-cultural communication and appropriate and effective interactions with others" (Andrews & Boyle, 2008, p. 16). It is the ability to work within a patient's environment. This environment includes the patient, his/her family, the community, cultural values, behaviors, and beliefs. Learning more about your own cultural background is the first step in understanding culturally diverse client populations. Display 13.1 provides suggestions on how a nurse can become more culturally sensitive.

thinking critically

Make a list of the culture/subcultures to which you belong. Write down what you value most about communication, space, social organization, and time. Find another friend, student, or nurse and ask him or her to do the same. What is the same? What is different?

---

display 13.1   **Suggestions to Enhance Cultural Sensitivity**

- Engage in student foreign exchange programs.
- Take a foreign language course.
- Visit other countries on guided tours.
- Talk to nurses from other countries about their experiences.
- Read books and journals.
- View videotapes and movies with cultural themes.
- Enroll in courses with culturally diverse teachers/populations

---

thinking critically

Watch DVDs about different cultures. Some examples might be "Witness," "Iron and Silk," "Dances with Wolves," "Crash," and "Avatar." Write down what the main characters valued most about communication, space, social organization, and time. Now compare these to the values you have written down about yourself and a friend.

One challenge for the RN is the assessment of each client's uniqueness. As discussed in Chapter 10, the nursing care plan must be individualized for each client. Following are some suggestions for data collection strategies for assessing each client's unique characteristics:

Customs: The most easily identifiable unique behaviors are those that can be observed or elicited by questioning.

Beliefs: An individual's beliefs can be ascertained in discussion.

Values: Distinct values, those that form the basis for beliefs and customs, are most difficult to uncover during conversation or observation. The nurse must be sensitive to a client's values, even if they differ from his or her own.

Read the following examples to see how sensitive assessments are performed.

EXAMPLE 1

A 3-year-old Hmong child is hospitalized for dehydration. As the nurse prepares to start an intravenous (IV) line, he notices an embroidered cloth bracelet on the child's wrist. The nurse wants to remove it so that he can start the IV on the child's forearm without interference. The sterile insertion of the IV is extremely important because the child needs to receive fluids to get better. Before snipping the bracelet, the nurse performs an assessment: "Tell me about your bracelet." He learns by direct questioning that placing a bracelet on a child is a Hmong custom. The nurse pursues the discussion and learns that the custom is based on the belief that the bracelet will protect the child from harm. The nurse is sensitive to this belief and allows the bracelet to remain, instead starting the IV in the opposite arm.

EXAMPLE 2

A 6-month-old Mexican infant is brought by her mother to the clinic for immunization. The admitting nurse says, "Your baby is so beautiful!" To which the mother responds, "Oh, this is the ugliest, naughtiest child." The nurse questions, "What makes you say such things about your baby?" By direct questioning, the nurse learns that it is the custom to say negative things about an infant. The mother believes that this will ward off the *mal de ojo*, or evil eye. She explains that admiration of infants by strangers attracts this curse. The nurse uses this information and acts in a way that is sensitive to the beliefs of the mother.

To incorporate uniqueness into the plan of care, the assessment skills used by the nurses in these examples were finely tuned. In both cases, the nurses used wide-angle observational skills (the bracelet, the comments). Their communication was open, accepting, and free from judgment. The nurses did not ask "why" questions or judge the worth of the stated customs.

Remember that your best source of information about the particulars of social, cultural, sexual, and spiritual uniqueness is the client. It is all right to ask the patient to help you understand his or her experience, but then it is also necessary to listen carefully. Seek to understand first and then to be understood.

It is also good to ask another more culturally knowledgeable nurse and/or your unit/organization educator or manager for help. They are in a position to bring needed institutional resources into your environment if they are made aware of the challenges facing nurses in the field. A difficulty recognized now is that there are increasingly fewer culturally diverse nurses; growth in the number of diverse nurses has not kept up with recent changes in population. This increases the homogeneity of the nursing profession, which eliminates a potentially valuable resource—a culturally diverse workforce.

As an LPN, you have undoubtedly recognized the impact of cultural influences. Display 13.2 shows how you fit into the cultural competency staircase model developed by Kersey-Matusiak (2001). This tool increases in level of complexity and

thinking critically

This exercise is designed to stimulate discussion about how the attitudes, beliefs, and values of the nurse may affect the caring, collaborative relationship when the client holds different beliefs and attitudes.

Role play three situations: One person will play the client; another, the nurse; and a third, the observer/recorder. Change roles for each situation.

Situation 1

Client: You are a 30-year-old lesbian hospitalized for a total abdominal hysterectomy. You are crying when the nurse walks into the room.

Nurse: Use therapeutic communication to allow your client to express her feelings.

Observer: Note the nonverbal techniques that are used; note any statements that are judgmental or effectively neutral.

Situation 2

Client: You are a 43-year-old confirmed speed (amphetamine) abuser. You are not interested in giving up your lifestyle. You are hospitalized for a skin staphylococcal infection from IV drug use.

Nurse: Teach the client the causes and preventive measures for infections.
Observer: Note the nonverbal techniques that are used; note any statements that are judgmental or effectively neutral.

Situation 3
Client: You are 56 years old. You are 5 ft, 2 in. tall, weigh 420 lb, and have been hospitalized with low back pain.
Nurse: Discuss the impact of increased weight and the complications associated with low back pain.
Observer: Note the nonverbal techniques that are used; note any statements that are judgmental or effectively neutral.

After completion of this exercise, have each member of the group answer the following questions:

1. How did it feel to play the client character? What was difficult for you?
2. How did the interaction affect you and your responses? Did you feel your character was supported in his or her unique problems?
3. What approach did you take during the interaction as the nurse?
4. What statements or questions were easiest for you to answer? What other information did you gather?
5. What communication techniques were used during the interaction? Which techniques were facilitative and which blocked the interaction?

shows the need for education, communication, and development of self-awareness and sensitivity to similarities and differences among individuals.

The nursing process begins with accurate assessments and continues as the nursing care is carried out, the plan is evaluated, and reassessments are made. The rest of this chapter presents a framework for assessing unique client systems, thereby enriching the level of nursing care provided.

The client is viewed from four different sets of assessment variables. These variables look at the client as a member of smaller social groups or subcultures. The four groups considered are cultural, personal (interpersonal and intrapersonal), sexual, and spiritual. Accurate assessment of these variables in each client provides the basis of information necessary for holistic nursing care planning.

As you become more adept at recognizing the uniqueness of each client, you will develop your own sensitivities. Your personal experiences will give you a list of assessment variables much longer than any chapter or book could contain.

● THE CLIENT AS A MEMBER OF A CULTURAL GROUP

A client may be of a particular cultural group, such as a Japanese man or a Muslim woman. He or she may identify solely with that culture or group or may have adopted or blended values and customs from another group into his or her lifestyle. This blending or adaptation is called acculturation. An example of acculturation would be a Muslim woman coming to the United States and adopting a Western style of dress but continuing to practice Islam by wearing the hijab. The nurse needs to demonstrate cultural competency in this situation; that is, he or she needs to assess this woman based on the client's individual beliefs and values, not on

---

display 13.2   **Cultural Competency Staircase Model**

Step 1: Limited knowledge

Lowest competency level: Nurse fails to recognize the importance of culture. May have graduated before this was incorporated into school curriculum.

Step 2: Growing awareness

Nurse has a growing awareness but limited self-awareness about cultural groups.

Step 3: Acquired knowledge

Nurse has begun to develop cultural awareness about one or two cultures and is attempting to integrate information into the plan of care.

Step 4: Expanding network

Nurse has strong cultural awareness and has a network to draw on to get more information about diverse groups. Consistently includes this knowledge into the plan of care.

Step 5: Applied expertise

Nurse is highly self-aware and not only readily applies knowledge but can also anticipate potential problems.

Step 6: Problem solvers

Nurse has attained a high level of self-awareness, a broad knowledge of other cultures, and can problem solve across cultural groups and mentor other nurses with this knowledge. There is still room for growth.

Adapted from Kersey-Matusiak, G. (2001). An action plan for cultural competency. *Nursing Spectrum,* *10*(7PA), 21–24.

---

preconceived ideas about Muslim women. Assimilation occurs when acculturation is complete. In other words, the individual no longer identifies with his or her culture but has a new cultural identity. Many children who come to the United States have assimilated but have parents living here who have not.

Stereotyping would occur if the nurse assumes that all members of a group are alike. An example of stereotyping would be if you knew that Juanita was Mexican and assumed that Juanita was also Catholic when, in fact, Juanita may be Jewish.

Impact of Physical Characteristics

Physical characteristics are biologic markers that can impart social status, which we call race. Racism is when people use biologic markers to such as skin color to discriminate against a person (Craven & Hirnle, 2009). Each client will display unique physical characteristics (e.g., skin, eye, and hair color; facial shape) attributable all or in part to a definite racial or ethnic group or gender. A sensitive assessment of the accuracy of your assumptions will allow you to uncover the unique aspects of the individual.

A client may resemble a particular group but possess cultural characteristics that resemble a different group. The nurse's initial assumption based on these attributes can be incorrect and incomplete. An example is assuming a dark-skinned client with the last name of Rodriguez speaks Spanish when she really is Portuguese and has married a Hispanic man. A careful interaction with this client would have made her primary language apparent.

Another example is that of an African American woman who, when registering at the emergency room, is asked for her welfare card. The woman, who holds a doctorate in economics and is a faculty member at the local university, must now wonder what other false assumptions will be made during her treatment.

Impact of Language

There are many variations of idiomatic expression. The classic example is "bad" meaning that something is exceptionally good. English-speaking populations have great variation. For example, the term "bloody" has quite a few meanings, depending on where one resides. Consequently, when caring for a client, it is important to clarify meanings.

Slang terms are also difficult for a person speaking English as a second language. The patient may actually be looking for the nail and the hammer if the nurse states, "You've hit the nail on the head." Instead, a simple "That is right" or "Correct" would be best. Never assume English literacy. Because of the enacted federal mandates and HIPAA regulations, institutions can no longer use the patient's friends and family members as translators. If the client requires a language translator, it is important to obtain a translator who can interpret idiomatic phrases. If your client is from Puerto Rico, he or she may have a hard time understanding a Spanish-speaking translator from Spain.

Language also includes nonverbal communication. Head nodding while smiling can be interpreted as signifying an understanding. However, among some groups, these nonverbal messages are a sign of respect only.

Impact of Customs, Beliefs, and Values

This chapter has already discussed how customs, beliefs, and values are assessed. This is an area in which mistakes in assessment data can be made. In the Arab/Muslim culture, it is taboo for a woman to be uncovered for a physical examination or to be examined without the presence of her husband. It is impolite among certain Native American people to look into someone's eyes. Time, personal space, customary healing foods, and rituals for the dead are some of the issues around which poor assessment techniques can have deleterious effects. If the nurse is sensitive and tries to integrate the customs, beliefs, and values of the client whenever possible, he or she will be able to provide sensitive, culturally competent care.

NCLEX–RN *Might Ask*

13.1

The nurse is caring for a Hindu client. The nurse would be culturally sensitive to this client if the nurse

- A. bases interactions on preconceived knowledge about Hindus.
- B. assesses this client for individual preferences.
- C. assigns this client to another nurse.
- D. teaches him to change his diet based on Western ideas.

· See Appendix A for correct answer and rationale.

● THE CLIENT AS A SOCIAL BEING

The social aspects of each person include interpersonal relationships, educational status, and intrapersonal sense.

Impact of Family, Friends, and Community

When we use the word "client," we refer to an individual, a family, or a community. Each person plays a particular role, and each role affects the other client systems. Family is more loosely defined at present and may not be what the nurse defines as family. A family may be composed of two or more persons who are joined by emotional closeness or bonds of sharing and who identify themselves as being part of a family (Andrews & Boyle, 2008). It is important when dealing with families to know that their relationships have developed over a period of time, where the main function of a family is stability through their interpersonal relationships.

The many diverse types of family—single-parent households, homosexual couples, multigenerational families, and biracial families—present challenging situations for the nurse to manage. Although diverse families have been in existence since the early pioneer days, the intermingling has been masked by the way we statistically analyze groups and other social factors. According to Tashiro (2005), the taxonomy we use has not changed much since the early times of Linnaeus' taxonomy of *Homo sapiens*. She challenges us to think about diversity as being a kaleidoscope that may show that diversity within groups is greater than the diversity between groups. Her arguments strongly support that we are so unique that each individual needs to be valued for just that—his or her own unique state of being.

One thing that makes each family distinctive is whether the dominant member is male or female. A man may be the main homemaker and caregiver of the children, which is considered nontraditional in North American society. A nursing care plan developed to allow him to express his concerns about the daily management of household chores in his absence may be appropriate. The client who is ill may not only be taking care of her children but may also be the caregiver of elderly parents. When planning discharge teaching, the nurse needs to know what family, friend, or community support is available. It is also important to assess the beliefs and values that the individual holds about independence versus dependence. Nurses also need to help preserve the family, yet help deal with the intense interpersonal processes. Many feel unprepared to deal with these interactions, especially in the decision-making process. Display 13.3 provides some tips on how to respond with sensitivity when dealing with decisions a family may have to make.

---

display 13.3   Ten Tips for Effectively Dealing With Families

---

1. Be prepared for family chaos. Critical illness can trigger this in the most stable families.
2. Have a fact-finding family conference involving the health care team and all stake holders. Reassure them that no decisions will be made at this time.
3. Assess the family's coping mechanisms.
4. Seek to reestablish a sense of control for family members.

5. Distraction may come in the form of unresolved conflicts. Redirect attention back to the client's needs.
6. Use an organized, simple, straightforward manner to give medical information.
7. Give the family time to ask questions. Provide written booklets and educational tools when needed.
8. Permit emotional expression.
9. Provide a safe haven to allow emotional composure if emotions become difficult to control.
10. Agree to a plan. Remind all family members that they need to step outside themselves and view any decisions in light of what the patient would want.

Impact of Economic Status

Each client has a unique means of financial support. When planning nursing care, we must understand how the client's financial support will be affected by his or her illness. Loss of the ability to earn money is a major concern, especially in today's turbulent economic environment. A prolonged illness may bankrupt even the more financially secure. Many households are managed by single parents, whose incomes pay the rent and buy food. Elderly clients may not be able to pay for the medications or nutritional supplements that are prescribed or suggested. A homeless individual or migrant farm worker may not know how to access available support systems for basic needs and health care.

When assessing economic status, the nurse can learn through direct questioning and by careful listening to the client's concerns. The nurse should not be lulled into false assumptions by material trappings. The client may be well dressed but may have lost his or her job recently. It is appropriate to ask: "How will you purchase medications? What support systems do you have in place? What will you need to attend to your needs?" This will help the nurse plan what institutional or community resources would be appropriate for the client.

Impact of Self-Esteem

The client who feels a lack of control over the situation may not be able to participate in care, and a client who believes that he or she deserves to be ill may be an unwilling participant in his or her recovery. At particular risk are people in violent relationships, people with addictions, and people with chronic diseases that require lifestyle changes to remain healthy. When assessing in this area, the nurse needs to listen for clues. A client may say, "I can't," "I shouldn't," or have excuses for the inability to agree with a plan of care. This is often a sign that the person does not have the ability to make independent healthy decisions. Early psychosocial interventions in the form of counseling or therapy groups may be necessary before the client is willing to take control of his or her own life.

● THE CLIENT AS A SEXUAL BEING

Sexuality is another unique subculture of the client that contributes to the diversity of society. It is value laden for most people. We all have attitudes and opinions about sexuality, based on our own experiences. Sex is a basic human need that all nursing students learn about, following Maslow's hierarchy. It is becoming increasingly important that nurses consider how sexuality affects the client's life—the client's own sexuality and the sexuality of those in his or her support system.

Although most nurses agree that sexuality should be integrated into the plan of care, they often have difficulty doing this (Magnan, Reynolds, & Gavin, 2005; Weber, 2010). The barriers to communicating sexual information to the client include items listed in Display 13.4. Studies show that nurses are more inclined to be passive in introductory remarks leading to a discussion of a sexual nature. The ironic thing found in research is that the patient would prefer the nurse to initiate conversations on this subject. Ultimately, this results in no communication, which leads to untreated and unresolved medical/social problems for the client. Once again, a common threat with diversity is self-discovery; that is, the nurse needs to feel confident in his or her self-awareness. The nurse needs to be accepting and open when assisting the client with sexual issues. For more help on this, see Display 13.5.

Variations in Expression

A person's sexuality is also expressed in the context of his or her own culture. Openly discussing sexual matters may be comfortable to one person and intimidating to another. The nurse needs to be knowledgeable about his or her own attitudes about sex before he or she can be comfortable with a client's ability to express sexual concerns. As with the discussion of sexual problems, possible issues with sexual orientation need to be brought up by the nurse. The first step is often to give permission to the person to discuss sexual concerns in an open way.

---

display 13.4 **Barriers to the Nurse's Discussion of Sexual Issues**

1. Inadequate education and application
2. Perceived embarrassment to the nurse and client(s)
3. Low priority for the client in view of other physiological needs
4. Lack of time and heavy workload
5. Perceived anxiety generated on the part of the nurse and client(s)
6. Inability to intervene or follow through with a client's sexual problem

---

display 13.5 **Tips for Helping the Nurse Discuss Sexual-Related Problems**

Do not expect the client to bring up the subject. Patients expect the nurse to start the conversation.
Ask for educational programs to help with competence and confidence.
Role play difficult situations with a knowledgeable advanced practice nurse, unit manager/educator, social worker, or psychiatrist.

Variations in Orientation

Sexual orientation is a term that refers to the preferred gender of the partner of an individual (Taylor, Lillis, LeMone, & Lynn, 2011). Sexual orientation may be heterosexual, homosexual, or bisexual. "In biomedical literature, these groups are often categorized together under the term sexual minorities or LGBT (lesbian, gay, bisexual, and transgendered)" (Scott, 2010, p. 381). Sexual variations are often not apparent. The nurse may frequently feel unqualified or unable to address these distinct issues (Display 13.6). When interviewing, it is important for the nurse to use questions that are neutral. For example, one common question asked of people in their reproductive years is "What type of birth control do you use?" This question assumes a partner of the opposite gender. This assumption does not allow the homosexual client to discuss health related to sexual practices. A neutral question that would elicit more information would be "What precautions do you take when practicing safe sex?"

NCLEX–RN *Might Ask*   (13.2)

The nurse is caring for the child of a biracial couple. Recognizing that this couple's choice is based on a value system different from the nurse's is known as

   A. prejudice.
   B. enculturation.
   C. ethnocentrism.
   D. cultural relativism.

• *See Appendix A for correct answer and rationale.*

● THE CLIENT AS A SPIRITUAL BEING

We are all spiritual beings. Spirituality is an individual's journey to find the purpose behind his or her life. Religion and spirituality are often thought of as being the same. However, religion is an organized system of beliefs about a higher power (Taylor et al., 2011). Therefore, religion is under the umbrella of spirituality. Religious groups practice worship, prayer, meditation, or healings and may practice in a church, temple, synagogue, or mosque. Usually, there is a religious leader who plays a pivotal role in the development and guidance of religious aspects of life; this may be a priest (Catholicism), pastor (Fundamentalist Christianity), rabbi (Judaism), elder (Anabaptist Christianity [Amish]), or imam (Islam) (Purnell & Paulanka, 2008).

The nurse needs to have a grasp on what kinds of religions are in the health care population that is served. Once again, the openness and accepting nature of the nurse helps foster the bonds needed for care. The best way to become open to others' ideas

---

display 13.6   **Barriers to Discussion of Sexual Orientation (Nurse-Focused)**

1. Fear of awakening change in sexual orientation of the nurse
2. Fear of contagion (especially with homosexuality/multiple sexual partners and AIDS)
3. Fear of unwanted and unwarranted sexual advances
4. Personal, religious, or cultural revulsion to practice or behavior

is to know and be comfortable with your own spirituality. As you become open, the client is allowed to be open. It is this intersection of communication in which each person (the nurse and the client) is touched in some way by the other.

Impact of Religious Beliefs

Each organized religious group has its own values and beliefs. Occasionally, these affect either the client's ability to participate in his or her own care or the nurse's ability to give care. For example, people who practice as Jehovah's Witnesses do not believe in receiving blood. The challenge in this case is to give judicious care without violating the religious beliefs of the client. The nurse must be able to clarify his or her own values and to help the client clarify his or hers. It is not necessary for the nurse to agree with the client, but it is necessary to respect the client's beliefs. One of the ways the nurse can assist with religious beliefs is to incorporate the client's spiritual leader into the plan of care.

Impact of Religious or Spiritual Symbols or Treatments

Many religious or spiritual groups use symbols, talismans, or special treatments as part of their rituals. Many of those treatments are being researched and have been used longer than organized Western medicine. The use of a crystal, candles, folk medicine, or herbal remedy is therapeutic when supporting a client's personal belief system. Practices such as acupuncture and acupressure, meditation, therapeutic touch, tai chi, or Reiki are examples of nontraditional health belief choices that a client might consider therapeutic. Incorporating these choices into the plan of care can promote the health of the client by respecting his or her belief system.

● NURSING CARE PLANNING

Uniqueness affects the nursing process in the following ways.

Assessment

The ability to obtain a full assessment depends on communication skills. Asking questions in an open way will allow the nurse to gain valuable information about the way each individual will achieve a state of health that is personally satisfying.

Which questions are asked and the way in which they are asked are important. Display 13.7 provides some questions to start with in a cultural assessment.

---

thinking critically

Locate the Health Research and Educational Trust (HRET) Web site at www. hretdisparities.org. Find the HRET Disparities Toolkit for collecting race, ethnicity, and primary language information from patients. Then, contact the health care organization that you work for and ask if they use a tool for collecting information. If they do, compare this to the HRET tool. What are the similarities? What are the differences? What is the impact of these various tools on the quality of nursing care for the client? If they are not using a tool find out if they are interested in using one.

display 13.7	Assessment of Cultural Uniqueness

1. What are your views on health and health care?
2. Tell me about your family and community relationships.
3. What is the language spoken at home?
4. Do you have ties to another country or another part of this country?
5. Describe some of the types of foods you usually eat.
6. What religion do you follow? How much of a part of your life is it?
7. Tell me about how you view childbirth and child rearing. Who is the decision maker at home?
8. What are your views about death/death rituals?

Diagnosis

The NANDA-I uses nursing diagnoses to include cultural, spiritual, and social variations (Display 13.8). However, according to Carpenito-Moyet (2008) and Doeges, Moorhourse, and Murr (2009), the work on nursing diagnoses has not yet taken cultural aspects into consideration. More work is needed by nurses from a diverse cultural background. Only then can these diagnostic statements be more clinically and culturally relevant. There is much work needed to support nursing research in this area.

NCLEX–RN *Might Ask* 13.3

The nurse is formulating a nursing diagnosis for a client who speaks only Chinese. Which of the following nursing diagnoses would be *most* appropriate?

A. Knowledge Deficit related to surgical procedure
B. Impaired Communication related to inability to speak and read English
C. Social Impairment caused by inability to hear
D. Spiritual Distress caused by hopelessness

· See Appendix A for correct answer and rationale.

Planning and Goal Setting

True planning and goal setting require collaboration between the client and the nurse. The client's family, if he or she wants, can also be important players. A

display 13.8	Cultural/Social/Spiritual Nursing Diagnoses

Powerless related to inability to make verbal needs known
Risk for spiritual distress related to limited access to spiritual advisor
Impaired communication related to inability to speak and read English
Role strain related to recent divorce and newly declared lesbian status
Altered spiritual function related to absence at spiritual group meetings while hospitalized

spiritual advisor may also be part of the client's decision-making team at the client's request. This collaboration must include sensitivity to the nurse's and the client's values and beliefs. Behavior that one nurse might interpret as noncompliant might actually be behavior that signifies respect.

Interventions

The impact of uniqueness during this phase of the nursing process should be clear. Why include warm foods in your plan of care if your client has the belief that cold foods have healing properties when one has a fever? How can an intervention be written to monitor vaginal bleeding if the female client holds spiritual beliefs that only allow her to show her body to a relative? How can a Muslim prayer rug be incorporated into the busy mix of a medical—surgical unit? How do you deal effectively with a lesbian couple? Display 13.9 gives interventional strategies that can be used by the nurse to be more culturally sensitive.

Evaluations

When uniqueness is considered throughout the nursing care planning process, the evaluation phase may reflect satisfaction. If the evaluation of the plan is unsatisfactory, one should consider that there are unique factors at play. If the client is not able to express the reasons for using insulin, you must assess the impact of education level on understanding health teaching or the client's cultural beliefs about using medications. An important thing for the nurse to remember is that this is a process. Failure, although unintended, may cause the nurse to think more creatively and increase the use of resources that would not have been considered previously. Continuing to try, as well as noting what works and what does not, are key. Evaluation always leads back to the assessment phase of the nursing process. Review the areas of uniqueness that might need to be reassessed when goals are not met.

---

display 13.9   **Interventions for the Culturally Sensitive Nurse**

- Be aware of how your ethnocentric tendencies color your world.
- Analyze your community for major cultural groups using the health care setting.
- Listen with a sensitive ear.
- Ask for help from the patient, family, or other health care worker, if needed.
- Ask for in-services or continuing education regarding diversity.
- Apologize for making mistakes; this is a learning process.
- Use a "wide-angle lens" with observational skills.
- Speak slowly, and try not to raise the voice tone.
- Avoid medical terminology and slang.
- Use gestures, pantomime, or pictures.
- Incorporate practices/ideas from the client's health care beliefs.
- Use the dominant family member/spiritual advisor for support if the patient approves.
- Respect food preferences when possible.
- Use a nonfamily, culturally similar interpreter.

• CONCLUSION

This chapter provides an overview of the management of unique client systems. The nurse can better assess and individualize care planning by viewing the client as a member of a cultural group and as a social, sexual, and spiritual being. Several clinical examples and exercises are provided. The nurse's ongoing clarification of his or her own values fosters a greater sensitivity to those of the client.

References

American Nurses Association. (1998). *ANA position statement: Discrimination and racism in health care* [Online]. Retrieved December 12, 2010, from http://www.nursingworld.org/MainMenuCategories/EthicsStandards/Ethics-Position-Statements/Copy%20of%20prtetdisrac14448.aspx

Andrews, M., & Boyle, J. (2008). *Transcultural concepts in nursing care* (5th ed.). Philadelphia, PA: Lippincott.

Berman, A., Snyder, S., Kozier, B., & Erb, G. (2007). *Fundamentals of nursing: concepts, process and practice* (8th ed.). Upper Saddle River, NJ: Pearson Prentice-Hall.

Carpenito-Moyet, L. (2008). *Nursing diagnosis: Application to clinical practice* (12th ed.). Philadelphia, PA: Lippincott Williams & Wilkins.

Craven, R., & Hirnle, C. (2009). *Fundamentals of nursing: Human health and function* (6th ed.). Philadelphia, PA: Wolters Kluwer.

Doeges, M., Moorhourse, M., & Murr, A. (2009). *Nursing diagnosis manual: Planning, individualizing and documenting client care* (8th ed.). Philadelphia, PA: F. A. Davis.

James, E. (2005). Caring for Asian-Americans. *Advance for Nurses, 7*(10), 12.

Johnson, T. (2005). Intensive spiritual care: A case study. *Critical Care Nurse, 25*(6), 20–26.

Kersey-Matusiak, G. (2001). An action plan for cultural competency. *Nursing Spectrum, 10*(7PA), 21–24.

Lowe, J., & Archibald, C. (2009). Cultural diversity: The intention of nursing. *Nursing Forum, 44*(1), 11–18.

Magnan, M., Reynolds, K., & Gavin, E. (2005). Barriers to addressing patient sexuality in nursing practice. *MEDSURG Nursing, 14*(5), 282–290.

Maier-Lorentz, M. (2008). Transcultural nursing: It's importance in nursing practice. *Journal of Cultural Diversity, 15*(1), 37–43.

Merriam-Webster's On-Line Dictionary. (2010). Retrieved from http://merriam-webster.com/dictionary/unique

Purnell, L. D., & Paulanka, B. J. (2008). *Guide to culturally competent health care* (3rd ed.). Philadelphia, PA: F.A. Davis.

Storey, J. (2009). *Cultural theory and popular culture: An introduction* (5th ed.). Harlow, UK: Pearson Education Limited

Tashiro, C. (2005). Health disparities in the context of mixed races: Challenging the ideology of race. *Advances in Nursing Science, 28*(3), 203–211.

Taylor, C., Lillis, C., LeMone, P., & Lynn, P. (2011). *Fundamentals of Nursing: The art and science of nursing care* (7th ed.). Philadelphia: Wolters Kluwer/Lippincott Williams and Wilkins.

U.S. Census Bureau. (2010). Retrieved December 13, 2010, from http://factfinder.census.gov/home/saff/main.html?_lang=en

Weber, S. (2010). A stigma identification framework for family nurses working with parents who are lesbian, gay, bisexual or transgendered and their families. *Journal of Family Nursing, 16*(4) 378–393.

Suggested Reading

Christensen, M. (2005). Homophobia in nursing: A concept analysis. *Nursing Forum, 40*(2), 60–71.

D'Avanzo, C. (2007). *Mosby's pocket guide to cultural health assessment*. St. Louis, MO: Mosby.

Galanti, G. (2008). *Caring for patients from different culture* (4th ed.). Philadelphia, PA: University of Pennsylvania Press.

Magnan, M., Reynolds, K., & Galvin, E. (2005). Barriers to addressing patient sexuality in nursing practice. *MEDSURG Nursing, 14*(5), 282–289.

Muñoz, C., & Hilgenberg, C. (2005). Ethnopharmacology: Understanding how ethnicity can affect drug response essential to providing culturally competent care. *American Journal of Nursing, 105*(8), 40–49.

Nardi, D., & Siwinski-Hebel, S. (2005). Cultural issues in home care. *Advance for Nurses, 7*(12), 23–28.

On the (WEB) *http:// tcn.sagepub.com:* Transcultural Nursing Web site. (Last accessed 7.24.2011).

www.tcns.org/journal: Journal of Transcultural Nursing. (Last accessed 7.24.2011).

http://www.hret.org: Health Research and Educational Trust. (Last accessed 7.24.2011).

chapter

14

Managing Time, Conflict, and the Nursing Environment

● LEARNING OUTCOMES

By the end of this chapter, the student will be able to:

1 Summarize factors that influence time management.

2 Describe strategies to manage time more effectively.

3 Discuss various contexts in which conflict occurs.

4 Identify the process for conflict resolution.

5 Apply the guidelines for conflict resolution to a hypothetical situation.

6 List the steps in the decision-making process.

7 Compare the role of the RN to that of the LPN/LVN in decision making.

8 Recognize the role of the nurse in cost-containment activities.

9 Analyze the role of the nurse in managing a safe environment.

10 Give examples of the LPN/LVN-to-RN role transition in managing client care.

● KEY TERMS

chunking	effectiveness	Q-tip principle
conflict	efficiency	time management
conflict resolution	mediator	unlicensed assistive
cost containment	multitasking	personnel
decision making	Pareto principle	worksheet
delegation	perfectionism	

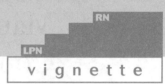

vignette

Nancy is the preceptor to Juanita, a new RN graduate who was formerly an LPN. Juanita has to "pay back" her student loan at New Berry Hospital by staying in their employment, and due to staff turnover, Juanita is orienting on the same unit where she was functioning as an LPN before graduation. Nancy is discussing her orientation with Juanita.

NANCY: You are progressing well. The patients are complementary about your care, and your assessment skills and nursing care planning speak highly of your school preparation. If you could pinpoint an area where you need the most help, what would that be?

JUANITA: I believe conflict management. I seem to be irritating the other aides and LPNs that I have worked with for years. Suddenly, since I have assumed this new role, they don't seem to want to do what I am delegating to them. Every time I turn around, I am "putting out fires" with people I have always gotten along with. I find myself doing things myself just to avoid conflict, which I know isn't a good use of my time. This is much more difficult for me than the actual tasks I have to do. Any words of advice?

NANCY: I can understand what you are saying. Sometimes it is better to either change units or change hospitals, especially if the institution is small and people really know each other. It is especially difficult being on the same unit because people often have difficulty adjusting to you in your newly expanded role. The first step is to always assess the situation. You have already done that in identifying the problem. Now, you need to assess how frequently it occurs and with whom. Keep track of the issues factually and unemotionally if you can. I would try to identify the MOST problematic person and deal with that person in a nonthreatening way, say, after work. Pick a time, and try to approach it in a humanistic manner. Maybe you can meet up with the person at the end of your shift, ask to walk along to his or her car, and engage him or her in what you are seeing. Confrontation is not a bad thing; it often gives both parties time to air the issues. If you can't come to some resolution here, you may need a neutral third party to discuss the issues.

Today's health care system requires that RNs be prepared to assume the management of care for large, diverse groups of clients. This includes completing assigned tasks in a timely manner, delegating work to others, managing conflict, making wise decisions, and maintaining a safe environment for all clients. Juanita is cognizant that she has a time management issue. She has successfully identified that she needs to settle relationships with coworkers in order to be a successful time management steward.

The frustration that Juanita is feeling is not a new one. You can probably remember what it was like transitioning into the role of an LPN/LVN. Unless you were placed in a new unit or had mentors who taught you how to deal with other staff while transitioning into your new role, you probably had similar conflicts with your role change.

Any transition is difficult, and the transition to RN is no exception. Delegation and time management are crucial skills, and they can be tough to learn. Unless you have had some excellent mentors, you may not have developed the tools to deal with different situations and manage your time effectively. A toolbox of varied skills is essential in transitioning from LPN/LVN to RN.

Managing client care requires the nurse to assess the needs of the clients; plan, organize, and direct the implementation of care; and evaluate its effectiveness. The definition of manager of care is centered on the combed roles of care provider, coordinator, and overseer. It also involves the ability to organize time effectively, establish priorities, delegate appropriately, and ensure effective and efficient client care. The concepts of conflict management and decision making are also important components of the manager of care role.

In this chapter, we introduce strategies to manage your time more effectively while providing and managing client care. You also learn about methods to deal with issues of conflict and conflict resolution in the work setting. Other aspects of managing client care involve decision making and managing resources. This chapter is designed to provide you with a better understanding of organizational and management skills as you change roles and expand your responsibilities.

● MANAGING TIME

Time is static and finite, but it cannot be replaced. If everyone were a good manager of time, it would not be studied and written about so frequently in our fast-paced society. Although we cannot add time to a day, we can work toward managing time more effectively. Time management is the use of tools and processes to increase productivity. Time is one of our most valuable resources and one of the most difficult resources to manage amidst the nursing shortage. In managing client care, the task of time management becomes more complex and extremely variable. Time management is similar to the nursing process. It involves assessing current activities, establishing an estimated time for completion, planning and setting goals and priorities, and evaluating the results (Table 14.1). In the next sections, methods for examining time usage are described.

Do You Have a Time Management Problem?

Self-assessment will help determine whether you need to adopt better time management strategies. Take a retrospective look at your past work week and answer the following questions. Have you experienced:

- An increase in the number of hours to complete your daily work?
- Feelings of resentment about the lack of "free time"?

table

14-1 COMPARISON OF TIME MANAGEMENT AND THE NURSING PROCESS

Time Management	Nursing Process
1. Assess daily jobs to be done and who will do them. (Allow time to plan.)	1. Assessment of the client
2. Develop a daily plan.	2. Diagnosis
3. Set priorities. (Pick the highest priority task and finish it.)	3. Planning
4. Complete assignment tasks.	4. Interventions
5. Set new priorities as needed. (Reprioritize based on new data or remaining tasks.)	
6. Evaluate the results of the plan.	5. Evaluation

- An increase in regularity of completing work items at home or on weekends?
- An increase in the feeling of being rushed or "out of control"?

If you are experiencing any of these, do not despair. You can learn to manage time more effectively. In fact, you have taken the first step by realizing that better time management needs increased personal work.

Time Assessment

In your role as a student RN nurse, you recognize that managing your time with respect to client care is dictated by the number of clients to whom you are assigned and the role that you have for that particular clinical day. For example, if you are assigned to two clients, you are able to plan the care based on the needs of those two people. Although your time is somewhat controlled by what else happens with your clients or by having to wait for an instructor to supervise you in a procedure, you are able to complete the requirements of the assignment with appropriate planning. As an LPN/LVN, you are also familiar with caring for a larger number of clients and not having as much flexibility in planning your time. The shift is dictated by predetermined schedules for care and procedures and by multiple interruptions.

Time management strategies can be used for home, work, school, and personal management of time. Time becomes crucial when you try to simultaneously balance these activities; however, the same principles can be applied.

As you move into the RN role, you will have little free time, time that is not dedicated to assessment, implementation, accomplishing interventions, and evaluating the results of those tasks. In your new role, you will have to anticipate that there will be both "good days" when everything goes smoothly and "bad days" when your "best" is not good enough. Highs and lows are the nature of nursing. However, unless your professors show you how to implement planning strategies at the RN level, you might not progress from the "not good enough" mode. This is not an uncommon scenario for nurses, regardless of the level they have attained.

Time management is the process of organizing "and using your time efficiently" (Ellis & Hartley, 2008a, p. 498). One of the principles of time management is called the Pareto principle (2008). This principle states that in order to manage time we need to shift into the planning mode. When we do this, 20% of our effort will result in 80% results. If we fail to plan, 80% of efforts will result only in 20% results. However organized, the plan needs to be flexible in order to provide for sudden interruptions that comprise a nurse's unpredictable days.

When assessing your time as a manager of care, it is helpful to formulate a Time Activity Log that tracks every 30 minutes of your shift. Display 14.1 shows an example of this type of log. You can also revise this log to include half-hour time increments. After you have listed the hours appropriate to your shift, indicate the activity in which you were engaged for that quarter hour; be as specific as possible. It is helpful to do this for at least 3 days to determine what interruptions you experience and what happens when the unexpected occurs. Keeping a log for several days also helps you analyze how you cope with interruptions, what strengths you have in keeping things organized, and when you are the most productive. You will be able

display 14.1   Time Assessment

Day 1		Day 2		Day 1		Day 2	
Time	Activity	Time	Activity	Time	Activity	Time	Activity
7:00	___	7:00	___		___		___
	___		___	12:00	___	12:00	___
7:30	___	7:30	___				
	___		___	12:30	___	12:30	___
8:00	___	8:00	___				___
	___		___	13:00	___	13:00	___
8:30	___	8:30	___				___
	___		___	13:30	___	13:30	___
9:00	___	9:00	___				___
	___		___	14:00	___	14:00	___
9:30	___	9:30	___				___
	___		___	14:30	___	14:30	___
10:00	___	10:00	___				___
	___		___	15:00	___	15:00	___
10:30	___	10:30	___				___
	___		___	15:30	___	15:30	___
11:00	___	11:00	___				___
	___		___	16:00	___*	16:00	___*
11:30	___	11:30	___				

*Continue until you need a break.

to identify how you save time and how you waste it. In the next section, strategies for managing time more effectively and common ways time is wasted are described.

Planning

The notion of planning when working as a manager of care is sometimes viewed as unnecessary or useless because the work is already dictated by time constraints and unit policies. One of Juanita's problems in the vignette was that she failed to anticipate problems with other staff in her new role. Juanita could adjust, but the other staff needed help "seeing" her in a new position. Managing conflict with her coworkers was more time consuming than she had anticipated, but the plan her preceptor has suggested may help her deal with the problems she is facing and regain some of that wasted time.

However, in nursing care, one shift never mirrors another, and careful planning is one of the best ways to maximize efficiency. Start by developing a time schedule, which can be done by using a worksheet (see Display 14.2). It can actually help you get back on track, assisting you in dealing with the unexpected and changing gears as needed. At the beginning of a shift, you should take a few minutes to examine what needs to be done (goal setting) and then develop a plan to accomplish those goals. It is important to estimate the time required to complete assigned tasks. If you fail to plan, you will have no sense of control; time will rule you and not vice versa. As you gain experience in the RN role, being realistic with time requirements for the work to be done will become easier, and you will develop a basic routine. Obviously, this daily plan cannot account for crises, but it should allow for flexibility and reorganization when those unexpected interruptions occur. Also, consult your instructor or other more experienced nurses comparing how they plan the day. See whether they can give you timely tips and advice on organizing the day.

Setting Priorities

When developing a daily plan, the activities that need to be accomplished will obviously emerge. Many nurses find it useful to make a worksheet from the daily plan (Display 14.2). This worksheet simply lists what must be done for each patient.

---

display 14.2   **Sample Worksheet for Medical–Surgical Unit**

Room #	Patient Name MD Diagnosis PMH	Vital Signs/ Input & Output/ Weight (Delegation) IV	Dx. Studies Labs	Abnormal Assessments	Treatments

table
14-2   PLANNING PRIORITIES HIERARCHY*

Care Priorities	Types of Care	Examples
Urgency of care	ABCs of care (airway, breathing, circulation) Life-threatening situations	Blocked airway, hypotension
Safety of care	Change in assessment status Protection from injury	Avoiding medication errors, prevention of falling, seizures
Patient's priority of care	Tasks to be done routinely or at client's request Partner with the client to set priorities; remember that the patient is the champion of his or her own care	Administering medications and treatments, informed consent, patient education
Ongoing care	Not essential; could be put off until a later time	Following up with psychologist on low self-esteem needs; nutritional consult

*This may change with the situation. For example, if a patient's self-esteem needs are so low that she or he is suicidal, then it becomes a safety issue and is a priority.

It also assists you in establishing priorities by determining what is essential and what is important but not critical. Items to perform can also be separated into the "do now," "delegate," "do later," "do whenever," and "don't do" priorities.

Each LPN/LVN comes with a different level of experience. As an experienced practitioner, you probably already have a way that you determine priorities. These might have been learned by trial and error or by modeling another LPN/LVN. Or an experienced RN might have assisted you along the way. However, as the planner of care and as the one at the bedside 24/7, you must coordinate priorities of client care and for most of the members of the health care team. Your "to do list" should be thought of in terms of urgency of care, safety of care, patient's priority of care, and ongoing care (Table 14.2).

It is often beneficial to indicate what must absolutely be done by highlighting or color-coding different priorities. For example, preoperative patients take priority and so you may develop a plan to color-code them in red. Early regular insulin and blood glucose checks are also a priority but can have a bit of flexibility. You might color-code these in blue. Although this seems rather simplistic, if you are in hurry, this can save time by enabling you to identify priorities at a glance.

thinking critically

As an LPN/LVN, you have probably used planning sheets (reports) to weave through a workday. Meet with other students in your class. Compare and contrast the various types of time management sheets. Take the best of each sheet and combine them into one. Use this sheet in clinical. The following week, report back to the group what worked or what did not. Also, discuss how you felt about your clinical time. Were you more or less organized?

Another aspect of developing and maintaining a worksheet is to get in the habit of writing things down. Although some nurses have an ability to remember everything, most nurses find it useful to jot down key facts. The worksheet is an excellent place to do this, either beside the listed items or on the back of the paper. This information can include abnormal assessment findings, laboratory results, and PRN medications given. It is not meant to replace appropriate documentation, but it is a method to assist you in being accurate and continually updating the establishment of priorities for critical tasks.

A final aspect of the worksheet is to determine who needs to be doing what. You may color-code in green what is done by the unlicensed assistive personnel (UAP) (vital signs, glucose checks, and walking a client). You can use this color-coding to help verify that the work was accomplished and the outcomes. This is an essential component of managing client care and an important aspect in your role transition.

One of the extremely rewarding functions of planning or using a worksheet is that you get to check off or cross out tasks that have been completed. This will give you a basis for documenting what still needs to be accomplished by the oncoming shift and a sense that you have accomplished that 80% of the Pareto principle.

Hospital management teams are realizing the importance of planning and "quiet time" for nurses. They realize humans need time to complete complex thinking required in the duties and responsibilities of a nurse. Some hospitals have designated no-interruption zones especially during medications passes. If your facility has not looked at research on this topic, it might be a place where you could start evidence-based changes to allow thinking time.

EVIDENCE-BASED RESEARCH

Waterworth's (2003) qualitative study of 22 senior nurses in the United Kingdom found that nurses use a wide variety of time management strategies but predominately used routinization and prioritization to manage clinical practice. This rather individualistic approach by nurses ignores the importance of team building, organizational, and other influences that could be used during the workday.

Delegation

The process of delegation often proves troublesome for new nurses and for those who are making the transition from LPN/LVN to RN. The reasons for this are as follows:

- Lack of understanding about the process of delegating
- Inability to assess what should be delegated and to whom
- Guilt about not doing as many tasks as the rest of the team members are doing
- Desire to be liked by everyone
- Inability to organize
- Distrust of others' abilities or the need to take care of everything personally
- Being caught in the trap of "we've always done it that way"

Delegation is covered in more depth in Chapter 11. Because delegation is an important feature in today's nursing world, be sure to review this chapter.

NCLEX–RN *Might Ask*

The RN's patient assignment team includes one LPN and two UAPs for 10 clients on night shift. Before assigning tasks to perform, the RN must

    A. free herself or himself to deliver care to only the most acutely ill.
    B. assess the skills of the workers assigned.
    C. check on every task assignment by the nurse.
    D. assume that all standards of care are upheld.

* See Appendix A for correct answer and rationale.

Efficient and Effective Use of Time

Some of the components of managing time assessment, planning, setting priorities, and delegation are essential to being efficient and effective. However, some other factors can assist you in managing your time. Zerwekh and Claborn (2009) distinguished between "efficiency" and "effectiveness" in the following way: *Efficiency* is the process of doing something right; *effectiveness* is doing the right thing right. As simplistic as this may seem, as a nurse, you have to make choices about what needs to be accomplished and then do it right. Table 14.2 may be helpful in planning for efficiency and priorities throughout the day.

One of the best methods for increasing effectiveness is to know yourself. Assess your own energy levels as they relate to the time of day. Are you a night owl or a morning lark? You can probably determine at what time of day you are the most productive, allowing for some variation regarding the time of year and the multiple demands on your time. Although you may not always be able to work according to your time clock, it is useful to pay attention to the high-energy periods and plan to do the things that require more energy at those times. It is also helpful to recognize that your efficiency may not be as great at the low-energy times, even though you need to accomplish some important tasks. During these times, you may work with less speed and focus. Methods to augment your energy needs include providing for basic human needs, such as eating appropriately, sleeping adequately, and planning regular exercise.

A second method for increasing effectiveness is to be careful about assisting others or asking for help. Although this may seem to be in direct conflict with the notion of teamwork, effective time management means that you have to learn to ask for help, just as you need to learn when it is not appropriate to provide assistance. Because job conflict is a real and present cause of stress and tension among coworkers, some units agree that all RNs will not sit down until they ask each other if they need help. As you may recall from Chapter 1, having the ability to say "no" or the recognition that you need help will assist you in coping more efficiently and effectively with time management.

One of the issues that you face as you make the transition from LPN/LVN to RN is related to the need to demonstrate that you can do everything without help. You may have felt overburdened with work as an LPN/LVN and are determined not to impose on other members of the team. What was difficult to appreciate at the time was the need for the RN to manage client care, make judgments, make decisions, and delegate. The RN needs time to reorganize, set priorities, delegate the appropriate tasks to the best people, and generally manage time. You will accomplish this by treating others as you would yourself. You would want help when you need it and so would they. So, ask for help when appropriate and give it accordingly. Also the more experienced nurses can assist you by telling stories about their tips and time savers. Much can be shared by storytelling (Dawes, 1999).

A final method for increasing efficiency and effectiveness is to assess the paperwork dilemma. One way to do this is to reduce the amount of paperwork to which you attend. You cannot avoid the requirements of the agency for which you work, but you can decrease the amount of paper. For instance, if you use a worksheet, limit yourself to one piece of paper so that you are not dealing with multiple pieces and having to shuffle through them. Keep the worksheet easily accessible so that you know where it is and are not spending valuable time looking for it. Create a worksheet that meets your needs and improves the efficiency in managing the care for a group of clients. If you think that paperwork issues could be more streamlined, develop and suggest methods to do that. Changes are often made because someone is able to demonstrate a more streamlined approach. Because paperwork is such an issue, many institutions are going "paperless." They are standardizing forms that can be accessible to all need-to-know professionals. This eliminates the "where did I put it" syndrome and decreases interruptions of nursing time to report retrievable information. Marquis and Huston (2008) have the following suggestions: Gather the supplies that you will need before engaging in an activity or group them in the same area, if possible. In addition, use time estimates to complete tasks and document them as soon as possible. Remember that nursing care is frequently "around the clock." You may not always be able to complete everything in your allotted time. It is important to communicate to the following nurse what remains to be done and its priority.

Handling paperwork more efficiently will make you more effective in managing client care. Display 14.3 will give some help with personal effectiveness, and Display 14.4 gives important tips on preventing paperwork from handling you.

---

display 14.3   Tips for Personal Effectiveness

- Pay attention to basic human needs (sleep, nutrition, exercise).
- Plan frequently (daily, weekly, yearly).
- Take breaks (more frequent for mental work).
- Declutter and organize any work areas.
- Find a quiet place without interruptions when doing paperwork.
- Work as a team when possible.
- Delegate appropriately.
- Handle paper only once.

display 14.4	Handling the Paper Flow

- File
- Forward
- Respond
- Delegate
- Discard

Identifying Time Wasters

The last aspect of managing time is the identification of things that waste time or decrease your ability to be efficient and effective. You are undoubtedly able to identify factors that waste time or generally impede your ability to get a job done. Some of these things are personal time wasters, and others are outside factors. In the following paragraphs, some of these issues are highlighted, with suggestions on how to control or minimize the things that interfere with your efficiency and effectiveness (Display 14.5).

INTERRUPTIONS

An interruption can be defined as being stopped in the middle of one activity to give attention to another. Some of these interruptions are necessary and essential to the well-being of a client or to the general management of a group of clients. Other interruptions are less urgent and should be limited for greater efficiency. The task for the nurse is to determine which interruptions are positive. Many cannot be avoided and are part of the job. For example, if a call bell is on, it is prudent to answer the call, just as it is necessary to answer the telephone to speak with family members or the physician. The use of mobile handheld telephones is common and can allow the nurse to manage telephone calls while performing other tasks and decrease travel time to a stationary phone. However, handheld telephones do interrupt the nurse in the process of completing tasks, and so the nurse needs to reorganize once the call is answered. Personal phone calls (nonemergent) are negative interruptions and should not interfere with your job performance. You must

display 14.5	Common Time Wasters

- Interruptions
- Socialization
- Personal disorganization
- Poor communication (lack of information or feedback)
- Meetings
- Paperwork
- Perfectionism
- Procrastination

determine how to deal with interruptions. You need to stay focused as much as possible on completing what you start and moving on from there. With multiple interruptions, you may start many things but never complete any.

Multitasking is the ability to handle many different tasks simultaneously. A nurse rarely has the chance to finish one task prior to starting another. For example, it is not unusual for a nurse to be balancing teaching a diabetic, handling a preoperative patient, giving medications, and performing colostomy care all in one day. It would be helpful to make a "to do list" and adjust it as needed. A quick glance at this list will allow a nurse to juggle many tasks at one time.

SOCIALIZING

Socializing is possibly the biggest factor in wasting time (Ellis & Hartley, 2008b). All of us participate in various social conversations while at work and enjoy the camaraderie that we have with fellow employees. Although you may not plan to have an extended conversation, it can occur anyplace, anytime, with anyone. An alternative to socializing in the workplace is to plan to socialize during breaks or at lunch. It will take some willpower on your part, and perhaps some planning, to minimize socializing except on planned breaks and outside work.

POOR COMMUNICATION

A nurse may start out with an excellent plan for the day and find out that something that was a low-level priority is now at the top of the list. Chaos can reign when there is poor communication or lack of information that helps in decision making. Before proceeding, the nurse should seek clarification regarding key bits of information. Proactive planning could occur to solve these problems by use of consistent charting forms or report data. Nursing care plans are an excellent medium to communicate what has been done, the success of it, and any further needs of the client. The nurse should also seek feedback, especially if the task or project she or he is assuming is a new one. Feedback would alleviate redoing work if the nurse was going offtrack with the assignment.

PERSONAL DISORGANIZATION

In your nursing programs (both LPN/LVN and RN), planning ahead for procedures implied that you would have the necessary supplies gathered before you begin a procedure. Nothing wastes more time than going back and forth for needed items. Patient units in many hospitals have tried to minimize this issue by having some commonly used supplies in the client's room. However, careful planning will still help alleviate wasted steps. Saving time can also be accomplished by combining several requests from clients into one trip. Personal organization is further reflected in how you organize your work. The use of a worksheet, daily or weekly planners, or calendars will assist you in being more organized.

Personal organization can be enhanced by judicious use of "downtime." Each of us has time that we spend waiting. Instead of wasting this time by doing nothing, productivity can be increased by carrying work, articles, correspondence, and small segments of larger time-consuming projects that will fit those time slots nicely. Bringing paper and pencils to write down ideas at bedtime or during a commute can help you to find some spare minutes in a day that is full to the brim with activities.

PROCRASTINATION

Procrastination ranks high in the list of time wasters (Cherry & Jacob, 2008). Marquis and Huston (2008) described procrastination as delaying a project or item without a cause. It is frequently prevalent "when a person is faced with an unpleasant task, difficult task or difficult decision." For a personal example, no one enjoys doing their income tax, but if this task is spread out from January to April or done by investing a small amount of time each month, then the deadline does not seem so overwhelming. Although there are times when delaying a particular task is advantageous, waiting to complete something will generally have only negative results. A professional example of this is if there is a particular procedure to be done sometime during the shift, it is more beneficial to do it as soon as you have time because the unexpected may occur, preventing you from getting it done at all. In addition, tasks that are delayed often become bigger than they were when they first needed to be done.

There are several things to do to avoid procrastination. First, recognize and admit that you are procrastinating. Next, identify the consequences of the delay (ie, I won't get my promotion, the job won't get done, I will look inefficient, I will feel bad about it). Next think, if this task could be most efficiently delegated to someone else? If not develop an action plan. Start early by breaking a task into small steps that seem more manageable (sometimes called "chunking"). Remember that perfection is not always necessary as long as standards are maintained (Kelly & Marthaler, 2011). Finally, reward yourself for accomplishing the dreaded chore (Display 14.6). Reward becomes important here. If you reward yourself within reason, then there is positive reinforcement for your actions. Over time, the anticipation of this reward will lead to a decreased lag time in task completion.

EVIDENCE-BASED RESEARCH

Brubaker, Ruthman, and Wallock (2009) researched the impact of institutiong personal data assistants (PDAs) into their nursing program. Their small convenience sample found that using PDAs to look up information help their students save time on clinical.

---

display 14.6   **Tips to Prevent Procrastination**

1. Recognize that procrastination is occurring and determine why.
2. Analyze what is being avoided.
3. Start the task with planning.
4. Divide tasks into small pieces over a period of time (chunking).
5. Don't take past failures personally.
6. Don't dwell on the past; move on to the next project.

PERFECTIONISM

Nurses are acculturated in their training to be the perfect nurse. In nursing school, we are educated to do things and practice them until we do them right! However, all tasks do not have to be 100% correct unless they involve nursing care standards. A nurse striving for the perfect teaching tool or the perfect paper may not complete it or meet class deadlines. You may have to settle for "good enough" over perfect in order to meet time constraints. Try not to set such high standards unless it is extremely important that the task be perfect. If your expected outcomes are too high, you may never complete the task. Also, things do not have to be original. As the saying goes, "Why reinvent the wheel?" If you know something works, stick to it, modify it, and continuously evaluate it.

Learning to Say "No"

Nurses often try to be all things to all people. In doing so, they often tackle the impossible by trying to accomplish too much. Once you have written your "to do list" and have prioritized it, think of what can be delegated on this list (see Chapter 11). The nurse should not be assuming tasks that can be delegated to a more appropriate team member. If someone to whom you have delegated asks for help, further assessment is needed into the nature of that help and what is going on with the client. Perhaps the nurse is working with a UAP who needs further help with his or her own priority setting abilities. Steps must then be taken to communicate this to the proper leader, and appropriate remediation or disciplinary action must be taken. One of Juanita's frustrations is that she knows how to delegate, but the staff members do not want to do what she says, and this leads to contention, conflict, and wasted time.

Although you cannot say "no" to a client in pain or a UAP who has abnormal findings, you can opt out of committee work if it is too much on top of your personal responsibilities. But it takes real assertiveness techniques and good communication skills to let the proper management people know that the time is not right for you. It should be clearly communicated, though, when you can resume your extra activities so that you are not seen as disinterested or lazy. Most managers are empathetic and will take steps to "lighten" a student's load if they know the situation.

Time management is crucial as you make the transition from LPN/LVN to RN. Although you may naturally be good at keeping everything organized, you may have to acquire or improve your skills. Managing care for a group of clients requires that you be knowledgeable, flexible, thorough, responsible, and accountable. Take the time to assess your time management abilities and identify methods that will help you be more skilled in this area. This activity will prove invaluable in your role transition.

In the following sections, we introduce other components of managing client care. The RN role requires that you have the ability to handle conflict, make decisions, and manage resources. The Thinking Critically activities give you an opportunity to consider issues you may encounter as you move into the RN role.

NCLEX–RN *Might Ask*

14.2

The RN should be efficient and effective in delivering client care. A common time waster a nurse should avoid is

   A. socialization.
   B. handling a paper once.
   C. organizing supplies ahead of time.
   D. calling physicians to report changes in clients' assessed condition.

* *See Appendix A for correct answer and rationale.*

MANAGING CONFLICT

Conflict occurs when there is tension or disharmony between individuals or groups about ideas, values, or beliefs. Because no one thinks identically to another, conflict is an inevitable part of life. Conflict can occur between people and within organizations is not necessarily a negative phenomenon, although it may be viewed as damaging to the relationships in a work environment. Some believe that conflict is needed to build stronger bonds and promote organizational change. Examples of positive outcomes of conflict include innovative change, exchange of ideas, and a greater understanding of another person's feelings. However, conflict is uncomfortable to most people, producing tension, which can cause people to engage in uncharacteristic behaviors.

When managing client care, you will be faced with various conflicts related to care of the client and to other health care workers. This conflict may lead to antagonism and incompatibility between individuals or groups and can be disruptive. Unfortunately, conflict is common within health care agencies. It may be that the business of taking care of clients produces a certain amount of tension at all times. Whatever the reason, nurses are often in the midst of conflict-producing situations.

Types and Causes of Conflict

Types and causes of conflict within nursing are numerous. Zerwekh and Claborn (2009) identified some common factors that contribute to conflict in nursing. The types of conflict that a nurse may experience are role, communication, goal, personality, and ethical or value conflict.

ROLE CONFLICT

Conflict can occur when people share similar responsibilities but the boundaries are not well delineated. For example, shift-to-shift conflict about who is responsible for particular procedures during certain hours is common. Role conflict may also occur when a community nurse enters a home for a visit. Decisions need to be made with the patient and family about who will do what in the care of the client. This conflict may be ongoing or related to a specific treatment.

COMMUNICATION CONFLICT

This type of conflict has several levels. One is that communication is not understood or is misinterpreted. Another is that differences are recognized but not discussed between the individuals or groups. The final one is that information is not communicated because it was forgotten or overlooked. Whatever the reason, because communication involves two or more parties, a break in the process may lead to conflict. The conflict becomes greater when it is not discussed with the appropriate person but with everyone else instead.

GOAL CONFLICT

In some situations, individuals may prioritize differently. For example, one individual may place a higher priority on achieving personal goals than on working for the goals and objectives of the patient, group, or organization. A patient's goals need to be taken into consideration in formulating nursing goals, or goals will not be achieved. As a nurse working for an organization, you need to be keenly aware of your organization's mission, goals, and values, both the written and understood culture (Catalano, 2009). Choosing a conflict that is in direct violation of those values can result in negative consequences.

PERSONALITY CONFLICT

This factor is unfortunately common. No one has a perfect personality, and there are instances when we may not deal with a situation appropriately. Health care restructuring has had a major effect on the expression of distress in the workplace. Families are often angered about the care of their loved ones. When too few nurses are spread too thin, this anger is often directed at the nursing staff. In addition, some individuals seem to lack a sense of humor, rarely display common courtesy, or have other social interaction shortcomings. Because conflict is defined as disagreements about something important to each individual, there will always be conflict and difficult people in the work setting.

ETHICAL OR VALUE CONFLICT

This type of conflict can pose a real dilemma. For example, disagreement about the code status of a client or the type of treatment to be used for a terminally ill client can be a source of conflict. In Chapter 17, we examine ethics as they relate to nursing practice. You will have more opportunity to discuss the potential for conflict in relation to ethics and values.

The factors described in the preceding paragraphs contribute to conflict within nursing. In the next paragraphs, guidelines for resolving and dealing with conflict are examined.

Conflict Resolution

Resolving conflict within a health care setting is not easy and is a situation in which you may not want to participate. However, it can be learned and as you move into

NCLEX–RN *Might Ask*   14.3

An RN has delegated the obtaining of vital signs on a six-client assignment to a UAP. When the RN checks the vital sign sheet, only four have been recorded. When the RN draws the UAP's attention to this, the UAP states, "I thought I only had these four to do." This type of potential conflict is known as a(n) _____ conflict.

    A. role
    B. communication
    C. goal
    D. personality

· *See Appendix A for correct answer and rationale.*

---

the RN role, it will become more imperative that you deal with conflict. Some individuals are selective about the conflicts in which they engage, and others seem to enjoy conflict for the challenge it represents. Methods for dealing with conflict include accommodation, avoidance, competition, compromise, and collaboration. Choosing or participating in any of these methods will be determined by the situation, your comfort level, and your reaction to the conflict. Nurturing workplace environments has become so critical to nursing that the American Association of Critical-Care Nurses (AACN, 2005) developed six standards for health care work environments. Display 14.7 shows these six standards. Because collaboration is one of these, greater emphasis will be placed on describing this strategy. An examination of the various methods of conflict resolution follows.

ACCOMMODATION

Accommodation is also called "smoothing over" or "bowing to the wishes of another." Juanita has tried to adjust to the conflict with the staff by doing the work herself that she would normally delegate. However, this leads to Juanita being behind in her work and being less efficient.

One advantage to this strategy is a short-term lessening of the potential for disruption that the conflict has caused. Another advantage to this is that the nurse may believe that the issue is not high on his or her priority list; other issues are more of a concern. Politically, the nurse may also do this if there is a large power differential between her or him and another individual (eg, a cardiothoracic surgeon).

---

display 14.7   **AACN Six Standards for Establishing and Nurturing Healthy Work Environments**

1. Skilled communication
2. True collaboration
3. Effective decision making
4. Appropriate staffing
5. Meaningful recognition
6. Authentic leadership

The underlying concept is "a little sugar goes a long way." The fourth reason why this is used is that the individual wants time to plan a solution to the conflict. The disadvantage of this strategy is that if it is used frequently, resentment and hostility can fester. Anger may also be displaced to people who have no stake in the issue, such as a client.

AVOIDANCE

This method also is referred to as "denying or ignoring" conflict. Generally, nurses who are uncomfortable with conflict avoid addressing conflict situations or try to remain neutral. There are times when avoiding conflict is preferable, such as when insufficient information is available or when the particular problem represents a minute portion of the overall difficulty. The main idea here is to "leave it alone, and it will go away." However, in most instances, avoiding conflict is not a positive way to deal with issues. Many of the same negative results encountered with accommodating can also rear their ugly heads when avoiding conflict. In some instances, nurses have gone so far as to quit their jobs rather than deal with interpersonal work conflicts. This can lead to regret and guilt about avoidance behaviors with a work record that shows it.

COMPETITION

Resolving conflict in a competitive manner usually means that a person wants to force the issue or achieve personal goals. In this situation, the person or group has a strong need to win the conflict and asserts this desire by outtalking, outshouting, and possibly threatening the opponents. This is a winner–loser situation. The advantage of this strategy is that it might be the best solution if one of the parties is more knowledgeable than the other. A competitive approach may be beneficial if the conflict warrants moving beyond a deadlock, but it rarely does much to resolve a problem. The obvious disadvantage to this approach is that someone always loses. The negative feelings, as with any of these strategies, may last longer than the original conflict. Despite all the education on conflict management, health care providers are concerned that this mode of dealing with conflict is too often the one of choice.

COMPROMISE

The method of compromise or negotiation implies that a conflict will be resolved by considering all aspects of the conflict and creating solutions that are agreeable to all participants. It also ensures that the issues are handled in a more direct way because all parties are aware of what is transpiring. In compromise, each side makes concessions and demands. Compromise is seen at the bargaining table in union or collective bargaining negotiations. The advantage to this is that it is participative. Parties have a voice in the negotiations. Focusing on the outcomes and not on the individual will help decrease feelings of tension that occur when handling compromising conflict tactics. The disadvantage is that both parties settle for a less than desired outcome. It is also time consuming for face-to-face interaction and dialogue. Another problem is that a third party may be needed if negotiations are bogged down. In a union situation, a neutral third party is called a mediator. Due to

Conflict Resolution Strategies

Accommodating: "A little bit of sugar goes a long way"; schmoozing.
Avoidance: "Leave it alone … it will go away."
Competition: "I win… You lose."
Compromise: "One for you, one for me. Two for you, two for me."
Collaboration: "The more heads, the better!" "None of us is as smart as all of us."

the uncomfortable feelings that many people have with conflict, many nurses would rather avoid or accommodate rather than compromise.

COLLABORATION

This is the preferred method of conflict resolution. This method builds on the method of compromise yet is more committed to creating a solution to the conflict that all participants feel good about and can support. This requires more effort but has long-reaching benefits. Collaboration is strongly advantageous as it builds teamwork and harmony. Blanchard, Bowles, Carew, and Parisi-Carew (2001) called this the "none of us is as smart as all of us" technique or "synergistic harmony." The AACN (2005) stated that "true collaboration is a process, not an event." Respect of each contributor's knowledge and abilities is inherent in collaboration.

Ellis and Hartley (2008a,b) remind us that "this approach requires a commitment on the part of all persons to be supportive and considerate of one another, to listen to one another and to try to understand the other person's point of view." This is necessary to sustain and nurture patient and family needs in today's complex heath care arena.

You may recall from Chapter 1 that a method of win/win was used to reach agreements with significant others. When considering the conflict resolution methods discussed, collaboration has the most potential to produce a win/win agreement (Display 14.8).

In the following Thinking Critically activity, you build on the conflict that you presented or created with your classmates and determine the benefits of the various methods used to resolve the conflict.

thinking critically

Recall a conflict that you or your classmates have had recently. Develop possible methods of resolving this conflict using accommodation, avoidance, competition, compromise, and collaboration. Contrast the advantages and disadvantages of each method for resolving the conflict.

Guidelines for Dealing with Conflict

Whenever more than one person interacts with another, conflict has the potential to occur. Resolving daily conflict when managing client care may seem to be unrealistic; however, you will encounter many situations that require using conflict resolution methods. As an LPN/LVN, you have seen conflict and have used some of the strategies discussed to deal with it. Although each confrontational situation is unique, there are some basic guidelines you can use to help defuse tempers and emotions when someone's "hot buttons" have been pushed (see Chapter 11).

ASSESSMENT

Using the nursing process approach, assess the problem first. Identify the issue, and ask questions to clarify the scope of the problem. When you ask questions, your concern is apparent and true involvement develops. Identify the key stakeholders and the strength of their issues. What is the source of the problem? If it is something simple, take steps to fix it. If calmly and quickly addressed, conflict can help team building and cementing relationships with renewed energies unleashed with all benefiting.

Now more than ever, it is an important time to review those therapeutic communications skills in Chapter 11. One of the first skills was active listening. But in situations with conflict overtones, you need to listen "aggressively." When Captain S. Michael Abrashoff took command of the USS Benfold in 1996, he knew he had many conflicts within his ranks and within the US Navy itself. One of the reasons he was so successful in his leadership was using a technique he calls "aggressive listening." He not only listened but also actively sought out what his crew had to say about problems and issues. "I decided that my job was to listen aggressively and to pick up every good idea the crew had for improving the ship's operation" (Abrashoff, 2002, p. 44). As a result, Captain Abrashoff developed a team aboard that ship that was effective, efficient, and happy. Taking the time to listen to patients, families, staff, physicians, and administrators will assist you in looking at issues from multiple perspectives. They can give you a more overall, comprehensive picture than that of your own vision. This will help you take responsibility for yourself in the issues.

PLANNING

Once the problem or issue is clearly identified, some quick planning for a successful outcome is important. The emphasis is on creating a win/win situation, or a collaborative one. Captain Abrashoff made the decisions in a participative manner. Everyone was involved from the cooks to the officers. Whenever possible,

- Seek a quiet environment without interruptions
- Find a place that is neutral to put people at ease
- Enhance the privacy of all involved

As a nurse, you want to create a positive environment conducive to clear, private, and calm interaction.

INTERVENTIONS

Now comes the real work of conflict management. Focus on the problem or the issue. Avoid getting caught up in the emotions or the moment. Goleman (1998) display **14.9**   **Conflict Management Strategies**

1. Focus on the issues, not on the personalities.
2. Take responsibility for your part in the conflict.
3. Communicate openly.
4. Listen aggressively.
5. Seek to understand first, and then to be understood.
6. Move to a neutral, private area.
7. If aggressive behaviors occur, use assertiveness strategies.
8. Let intelligence and not emotion rule.
9. Seek possible solutions.
10. Stress consequences of unresolved behaviors on the team.

called this working with "emotional intelligence ... Emotional intelligence refers to the capacity for recognizing our own feelings and those of others, for motivating ourselves and for managing emotions well within ourselves and our relationships." It might be helpful to state how you feel by stating and emphasizing the "I" word. "I feel frustrated when...," "I feel angry due to...," "It upsets me when...." Take responsibility for your actions. There is an old saying, "It takes two to tango." If there is a personality conflict, it would not occur without both parties (Display 14.9).

Look for situations that both parties can live with—the win/win solutions. While you are doing this, look for nonverbal communications that convey lack of understanding or continuing disagreement. If a person or family becomes emotional and aggressive, make them aware of their behaviors and how you feel about them. For example, if a physician is angry at you, you might want to say, "Dr. Brown, you may not realize this but you are shouting at me. This makes me feel uncomfortable and prevents us from problem solving." Do not lose your composure. Remain calm and in control.

Lastly, stress the team element focusing on consequences. What will happen to the group if conflict continues? Suggest possible solutions. Test to see if these are acceptable in striving for consensus (Schuster & Nykolyn, 2010).

You may not always come out of a session with agreement. In some instances, such as with union settlements, an impartial third party such as a nurse manager, legal counsel, or ethics committee may be needed to mobilize all resources and help in complex situations.

Try to keep an open mind. The Q-tip principle might be something to keep handy Quit Taking It Personally. By altering your reaction to a situation, you might avert escalating an unpleasant situation. Try not to back anyone into a corner. People tend to increase aggressiveness and defensiveness if put on the spot.

When a decision has been made, stop and review or summarize the key issues and steps toward resolution. Once again, observe for any behaviors that tell you the opposite of what you have both agreed to do. In some instances, a written statement or summary can be helpful.

If people were naturally skilled at conflict management, humanity would never be at war. Conflict management is not easy. You are not born knowing how to do it, but practice will help. There is a reason why there is so much written in self-help books about it. If you are unhappy about always using avoidance or accommodating strategies, and know true teamwork will improve outcomes, ask for programs or in-services on assertive behaviors in a periodic manner. Invite a psychologist to your unit or workplace and help role play interactive situations. Keep working at it and periodically attend workshops, read books, and reflect on what has worked and what has failed.

Managing client care involves a greater responsibility for the RN to deal effectively with conflict. The method that you select will depend on what meaning the conflict has for you and how it affects the nature of the care being provided to the client or group of clients. Successful resolution of conflict requires that the nurse be committed to resolution and that communication and trust are maintained. In the rest of this chapter, other issues related to managing client care are presented. These issues build on the use of conflict resolution methods.

• MAKING DECISIONS

As you make the transition from LPN/LVN to RN, an important element in your role is the ability to make decisions for client care based on the information that has been reported to you or that you have observed. "Decision making is the process of choosing among alternatives" (Lipe & Beasley, 2004, p. 37). Decision making involves judgments that can affect client care negatively or positively. Along with problem solving, it is part of the critical thinking process (see Chapter 8). Although the words are used interchangeably, decision making is different from problem solving. Problem solving involves selecting various alternatives that will solve an issue. Making a decision does not necessarily solve a problem, and it is not necessarily the result of a problem. Nurses are good decision makers but often fail at solving the long-term problems that occur. Factors influencing decision making are values, life experiences, perceptions of the issue, possible risks involved, and personal approaches to making decisions. Decision making incorporates personal ability with learned skills. As the health care system becomes more concerned with cost containment and client outcomes, the need to be an effective decision maker will become more important.

The process of making a decision consists of five steps, as shown in Table 14.3. The first step is to *identify the problem or concern*. This identification will be based on the nurse's perception of the issue. Another nurse may view the same situation differently. Once the problem has been identified, the nurse will obtain more information to become more knowledgeable. This process is similar to the assessment step in the nursing process. After the data have been gathered, it is important to *analyze the information*. The third step is to *establish goals*. In developing goals, the nurse determines what is realistic and whether the measure would produce an improvement or positive change. Seeking alternative solutions or strategies ensures that the issue is being considered from all sides. Analysis of each strategy will help you determine whether it is beneficial and cost effective and whether the resources needed are available. The selection of a strategy will be based on the methods of implementation available, time involved, and resources.

The next step is to *implement*. Nurses are good at short-term interventions to support immediate decisions. Using muscle power of staff to lift patients might have

table 14-3	DECISION MAKING AND THE NURSING PROCESS

Decision-Making Steps	Nursing Process
1. Identify the problem and gather data.	Assessment
2. Analyze the data.	Diagnosis
3. Establish goals, outcomes, and plans of action.	Planning
4. Implement the plan.	Implementation
5. Evaluate the results.	Evaluation

been an acceptable way to move patients in the past, but newer equipment is safer for the staff and patient. Speaking up for organizational change so that the short-term patch does not become the norm is important. Short-term decisions, although giving the illusion of efficiency, foster long-term inefficiency and might endanger quality.

Implementation may be done by the nurse or be delegated. That is part of the decision-making process. However, the nurse will be accountable for overseeing the implementation. The final step of the process is *evaluation*. As with any evaluation, the nurse compares the results of the implementation with the goals.

For many of the decisions that they must make, nurses do not have the luxury of time to conduct such a formal process. Many decisions must be made within seconds. However, when learning to make more effective decisions, it is useful to use the decision-making process as much as possible. This process will enable you to be more efficient and effective, particularly as you gain more experience with it.

Managing client care involves being effective in making decisions. The quality of client care is affected by the quality of decisions made. Other aspects of decision making and managing client care include managing resources.

thinking critically

As a new nurse in a long-term care facility, the oncoming charge nurse tells you that you spend too much time giving report. Although your feelings are hurt, you also face the dilemma of needing to shorten report and passing along what you feel to be essential information. Using the six steps of the decision-making process, make a decision that will solve this dilemma.

● MANAGING RESOURCES

Resources, by definition, are things that are necessary to do a job. Resources include work space, supplies, equipment, budgeted funds, and services. In today's health care world, the attention to resource management has greatly increased. The expectation is that high-quality care will be delivered to a large number of clients by fewer people (particularly professional people) with a cost-conscious use of resources. In addition, the environment will be conducive to maintaining high standards and a safe environment. This is an enormous responsibility for nurses and other health care workers and one with which you will be more acquainted as you gain experience in the RN role. This section gives you a brief overview of managing resources.

One of the first steps in managing resources is to develop cost awareness. This involves having an understanding of budgetary constraints related to salaries and resources. Many health care agencies have developed strategies to deliver client care services in a different way so that fewer professional services are needed. There is also more emphasis on conserving supplies and equipment. Knowledge of the standards for client care is important as you learn to balance client safety, environmental safety, and cost awareness. It will be helpful for you to gain a greater understanding of what is involved in cost-saving measures in the agency where you will be employed.

A second step in managing resources is related to cost containment. This term applies to any efforts that are made to reduce rising health care costs. It may include decreasing ineffective use of resources and time, finding more efficient and cost-effective methods to deliver care, and developing more businesslike approaches to managing the care of clients. Ellis and Hartley (2008) stated:

Staff nurses cannot control all the elements that impact on health care costs; however, they do have control over certain resources in the clinical setting, and to keep costs down they must use these resources responsibly. (p. 69)

The future of health care will continue to be linked to financial concerns. Your role as an RN will combine the need to continue to provide high-quality, safe, and responsible care to clients, with the necessity of being cost conscious and efficient. Standards of care and safety will need to be followed and not compromised. This is the continuing challenge, which also may prove to be ethically challenging. Theoretically, if safety and standards are maintained, client care will be cost effective.

● CONCLUSION

The role of the RN as manager of client care is crucial in health care today. The changes occurring in health care are geared to cost containment with the use of less-skilled and less-trained personnel. RNs will be required to manage the care of larger groups of clients and will be less supported by professional staff. As LPN/LVNs moving into the RN role, you will discover that this transition will mean that your skills as managers and your ability to provide expert clinical care will be highly valued.

Your role as an RN is that of a decision maker, deciding who is qualified to provide a particular aspect of care, what will best preserve a client's dignity in the face of increased technology, and how to restore hope when fear and suffering threaten to overcome clients. Your role will be one of managing time in a cost-effective and efficient manner, resolving conflict so that clients receive optimal care, problem solving, and ensuring that the client environment is safe in all respects.

The role of the RN will continue to expand. It will be your job to maintain the caring components of nursing practice so that the client is not forgotten in the quest to contain costs and to provide support in a cost-effective way. Your role as manager of client care will be complex and challenging. Acquisition of management skills is as important as the skills that you have acquired to provide client care.

student exercises

1. Consider the following scenario:

   Diane, a new ADN graduate, is working on a 30-bed adult surgical unit, where she had previously been employed as an LPN. After she completed her orientation, she began working three evenings a week. When Diane arrives at work one evening, she is assigned to team lead for half of the unit, which currently has 12 clients. Her team consists of one LPN and two patient care technicians. During report, she learns that there are five new postoperative clients, all of whom are having problems with nausea. Two clients are scheduled for surgery in 1 hour. The postoperative client from yesterday who had a colon tumor removed just tore off his colostomy bag and is screaming that the nurses are trying to kill him. Four of the clients are elderly and require assistance with activities of daily living. The client in Room 4 has just fallen out of bed. The unit secretary for the floor has called in sick, and the float unit secretary cannot be in for 1 hour. Diane tells the charge nurse that she is concerned she will not be able to attend to everything. The charge nurse is orienting a new team leader and tells Diane that she will be there but cannot be too available. The charge nurse thinks that Diane's experience on the unit as an LPN will help her get through and that she will not need any more help.

   a. What does Diane need to do to get organized?

   b. What should the work plan or worksheet include?

   c. What should a client care assignment look like in this situation?

   d. What does Diane need to know about the people assigned to her team?

   e. Does Diane need additional personnel? If yes, what skill level does she require?

   f. What is Diane's role in this situation? What should her assignment include?

   g. What advice would you give to Diane?

   h. What might you discuss with the charge nurse if you were in this situation?

2. Consider the scenario with Juanita and Nancy in the vignette. Imagine you are in the same situation.

   a. How can Juanita enhance her relationship with coworkers who are no longer her peers?

   b. How does a situation like this lead to inefficient utilization of resources?

   c. Using what strategies for conflict resolution offers some solutions to this situation?

   d. When would management need to intervene, and what could they do to help Juanita's transition?

References

Abrashoff, D. (2002). *It's your ship: Management techniques from the best damn ship in the Navy*. New York, NY: Warner Books.

American Association of Critical-Care Nurses. (2005). AACN standards for establishing and sustaining health work environments: A journey to excellence. *American Journal of Critical Care, 14*(3), 187–197.

Blanchard, K., Bowles, S., Carew, D., & Parisi-Carew, E. (2001). *High five: The magic of working together*. New York, NY: HarperCollins.

Brubaker, C., Ruthman, J., & Walloch, J. (2009). The usefulness of personal digital assistants (PDAs) to nursing students in the clinical setting. A pilot study. *Nursing Education Perspectives, 30*(6), 390–392.

Catalano, J. (2009). *Nursing now: Today's issues tomorrows trends*. Philadelphia, PA: F. A. Davis.

Cherry, B., & Jacob, S. R. (2008). *Contemporary nursing: Issues, trends, and management* (4th ed.). St. Louis, MO: CV Mosby.

Dawes, B. (1999). Perspectives on priorities of time management, and patient care. *Association of Operating Room Nurses Journal, 70*(3), 374–377.

Ellis, J., & Hartley, C. (2008a). *Nursing in today's world: Trends, issues and management* (9th ed.). Philadelphia, PA: Wolters Kluwer Health.

Ellis, J. R., & Hartley, C. L. (2008b). *Managing and coordinating nursing care* (5th ed.). Philadelphia, PA: Lippincott Williams & Wilkins.

Goleman, D. (1998). *Working with emotional intelligence*. New York, NY: Bantam Books.

Kelly, P., & Marthaler, M. (2011). *Nursing delegation, setting priorities, and making patient assignments* (2nd ed.). Clifton Park, NY: Delmar Cengage Learning.

Lipe, S., & Beasley, S. (2004). *Critical thinking in nursing: A cognitive skills workbook*. Philadelphia, PA: Lippincott Williams & Wilkins.

Marquis, B., & Huston, C. (2008). *Management decision making for nurse* (6th ed.). Philadelphia, PA: Lippincott Williams & Wilkins.

Pareto Principle. (2008). *The 80–20 Rule*. Complete information Retrieved at www.mintools.com/tmintrohtml

Schuster, P., & Nykolyn, L. (2010). *Communication for nurses: How to prevent harmful events and promote patient safely*. Philadelphia, PA: F. A. Davis.

Waterworth, S. (2003). Time management strategies in nursing practice. *Journal of Advanced Nursing, 43*(5), 432–440.

Zerwekh, J., & Claborn, J. C. (2009). *Nursing today: Transitions and trends* (4th ed.). Philadelphia, PA: WB Saunders.

Suggested Reading

Covey, S. (1989). *The seven habits of highly effective people*. New York, NY: Simon & Schuster.

Fisher, M. (2000). Do you have delegation savvy? *Nursing 2000, 9*, 58–59.

Forman, H. (2001). Difficult people? What's the problem? *Nursing Spectrum, 10*(12), 10.

Gladwell, M. (2005). *The power of thinking without thinking*. New York, NY: Little, Brown and Company.

Habel, M. (2005). Emotional intelligence helps RN's work smart. *Nursing Spectrum, 14*(16), 17–19.

Harvard Business School. (2005). *The results-driven manager. Taking control of your time*. Boston, MA: Author.

Klein, R. (2005). *Time management secrets for working women: Getting organized to get the most out of each day*. Naperville, IL: Sourcebooks, Inc.

Libel, d., & Watson, N. (2005). Consolidating medication passes. It can lead to more time with patients. *American Journal of Nursing, 105*(12), 63–64.

Lyon, B. (2001). Positive situation focusing: Pollyanna or a powerful stress prevention strategy? *Reflections on Nursing Leadership, 27*(2), 38–39.

Minar-Baugh, V. (1998). Survival strategies: Improving time management skills. *Ostomy/Wound Management, 44*(5), 79.

National Council State Boards of Nursing. (1995). *Delegation: Concepts and decision-making process*. Chicago, IL: Author.

Pagana, K. (1994). Teaching students time management strategies. *Journal of Nursing Education, 33*, 381.

Parsons, L. (1997). Delegation decision-making: Evaluation of a teaching strategy. *Journal of Nursing Administration, 27*(2), 47–52.

Ventworth, S. (2003). Time management strategies in nursing practice. *Journal of Advanced Nursing, 43*(5), 432–440.

On the (WEB) *www.dayrunner.com:* The Day Runner. (Last accessed 7.24.2011).

http://daytimer.com: The Day-Timer. (Last accessed 7.24.2011).

www.eiconsortium.org: The Consortium for Research on Emotional Intelligence in Organizations. (Last accessed 7.24.2011).

www.ncsbn.org/index.htm: The NCBSN. (Last accessed 7.24.2011).

www.nurseadvocate.org: The Nurse Advocate. (Last accessed 7.24.2011).

http://nursingworld.org: The ANA. (Last accessed 7.24.2011).

http://familytime.com/default.aspx: The Family Time. (Last accessed 7.24.2011).

http://supercalendar.com: The Super Calendar. (Last accessed 7.24.2011).

Member of the Discipline of Nursing

15

Professional
Responsibilities

● LEARNING OUTCOMES

By the end of the chapter, the student will be able to:

1 Recall the four qualities of the professional discussed in Chapter 1.

2 Discuss the commonalities of, and differences between, the LPN/LVN and the RN in the role of member of the discipline of nursing as outlined by the NLN.

3 Describe areas of responsibility of the RN in the role of member of the discipline of nursing.

4 Critique your verbal statements and behaviors and those of others for their portrayal of how nursing is valued and their subsequent impact on nursing's image.

5 Describe areas of professional growth to which the RN is committed as a member of the profession.

6 Develop a professional plan for your growth needs to respond to societal changes.

7 Describe ways in which the RN promotes and maintains standards of nursing practice.

8 Describe the role of the RN in clinical practice regarding generating questions for research and applying research findings to practice.

9 Describe the RN's role in professional stewardship and the advancement of nursing.

10 Compare and contrast the roles of the LPN/LVN and the RN as client advocate.

accountability	learning management	professionalism
advocacy	system (LMS)	referrals
bilingual	image	responsibility
blog	integrity	role modeling
client advocacy	magnet hospitals	really simple
clinical research	mentor	syndication (RSS)
evidence-based	modeling	self-regulation
practice	multiculturalism	stewardship
global community	peer review	valuing
healthy work	proactive	wiki
environments	profession	

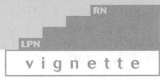

v i g n e t t e

Jennifer and Courtney have been friends since LPN school 5 years ago. They have maintained their friendship via e-mail and texting despite distance and time factors. Jennifer is in her second semester of RN school as an advanced placement student, and Courtney is considering returning to school. This is an e-mail transmission of their conversation.

COURTNEY: Sometimes I get so discouraged. It seems like we are going nowhere in nursing. The work is hard, the hours are difficult, some new graduates are making more money than the experienced staff, and you hit a ceiling where you can't advance if you stay at the bedside. Is it a waste of time, effort, and money for me to go back to school?

JENNIFER: You sound pretty overwhelmed and discouraged right now but are raising some serious and important questions. I think it might be helpful to focus on nursing as a young profession that is still experiencing growing pains. Despite the very real challenges you bring up, it has never been a better time to become an RN. The professional responsibilities are really awesome. I never imagined the responsibility to the public we have. RNs continue to be respected in the public eye, and we want to keep it that way. We are also moving toward more professional unity, collaboration, autonomy, and evidence-based practice. These are all hallmarks of a profession.

What the two of us have been doing for years is networking. Now, thanks to school and computers, I have other RNs—mentors, colleagues, teachers, and professors—who are networking with me. School is also teaching me more about power and how to intervene effectively in speaking for the client and to the public. I feel a renewed sense of spirit in my nursing endeavors. Yes, it is time-consuming, hard work, and expensive, but school has truly been an eye-opening, positive experience.

COURTNEY: You sound so excited and full of energy. I hope this will rub off on me. I need a shot of something! I don't really see the need to get more education when I see little difference in what an RN does and what I do now!

JENNIFER: Well, one thing we need to do is keep in touch. I can also help you by sending you some other online resources to help you get excited, engaged, and energized. These documents talk about the differences in roles from an LPN to RN. I am attaching them now. I will e-mail you later this weekend and see what you think about them.

COURTNEY: Thanks, Jen. You've really made my day and restored my confidence in nursing and its future role. I'm going to also work on that application to nursing school now and send it in. I'll text you later about how I make out.

The conversation Jennifer and Courtney are having is not a new one. In fact, it is probably one you had several times with many fellow nurses before you applied to nursing school. What is the difference in practice between the LPN and the RN? Is it worth my while to further my education? This chapter provides you with the opportunity to reflect on what you have learned in previous chapters and to answer such questions as: What are my professional responsibilities as an RN? In what ways, and how, will I assume a more expanded role with greater accountability within the profession? What role will I play in research and stewardship of the profession as an RN?

It may be helpful to look at *Educational Competencies for Graduates of Associate Degree Nursing Programs* (Display 15.1) by the National League for Nursing (NLN, 2000). Both LPN and RN graduates practice within their respective scopes and adhere to legal and ethical standards. Both are client advocates and engage in continuous learning and professional growth. However, the associate degree nurse has more formalized education in communication skills, assessment, and teaching–learning. Much more time is spent in knowing not only how but also *why* a nurse performs certain skills. The RN also organizes, collaborates, and manages care using the nursing process as a model. She or he is a role model to other members of the nursing team and assumes a proactive role in governance, self-regulation, and advancement of the profession. Some of the documents Jennifer sent Courtney involved role differentiation. Until the LPN/LVN "steps into the RN's shoes," he or she may not be aware of the RN's level of functioning.

This chapter presents RN responsibilities in the role of member of the discipline of nursing (Display 15.2). Responsibilities are presented in seven major areas:

1. Modeling and valuing nursing
2. Professional growth
3. Standards of nursing practice
4. Nursing research
5. Professional stewardship and the advancement of nursing
6. Client advocacy
7. Legal and ethical practice

Legal and ethical issues are presented in more depth in Chapters 16 and 17.

---

display 15.1   RN Core Competencies

Professional behaviors	Managing care
Communication	Teaching–Learning
Assessment	
Clinical decision making	
Collaboration	

Adapted from National League for Nursing. (2000). *Educational competencies for graduates of associate degree nursing programs*. Boston, MA: Jones and Bartlett.

• MODELING AND VALUING NURSING

Perhaps the most important responsibility you will have in the role of member of the discipline of nursing as you transition to the RN level is that of modeling and valuing nursing. But what exactly is modeling and valuing nursing? Modeling is defined as "to plan or form after a pattern" (*Merriam-Webster Online Dictionary,* 2010). Nurses need to set professional examples in all that they do. They also need to be more vocal about their decision-making and critical thinking abilities so the general public will view them as having a pivotal impact on their health care journey (Salvage, 2006; Kalisch, Kalisch, & Benner, 2005). Nurses need to know their role models and consult them frequently regarding issues.

"Nurses have to believe in who nurses are and in what nurses do. This requires valuing the name of nursing and reclaiming the name and practice" (Cherry & Jacob, 2008, p. 40). In its *Code of Ethics for Nurses with Interpretive Statements,* the American Nurses Association (ANA, 2004a) stated that nurses are client advocates who work to protect the health, rights, and safety of the clients they serve. One of the ways that nursing has survived despite the sweeping changes in the health care system has been to remain focused on the deeply rooted values (high-quality, individualized care) and beliefs that have been its strength.

According to Gordon (1997), nurses receive little reward for what they do and can be devalued daily in discussions with patients, families, and physicians, even though it is a nurse who often finds problems. She called this creating the invisible nurse.

> … when a nurse makes a contribution into patient care—one that could illuminate what she really knows and really does—the system often gives credit for her actions and contribution to the physician. This means that the nurse is stuck in the most pernicious Catch 22 of all: Whatever the nurse does confers credit on the physician. (Gordon, 2005, p. 48)

One of the things nurses can do to decrease their invisibility is to increase their sense of value and power. Working within their institution, nurses can create an environment that empowers nurses. The magnet hospital concept capitalizes on the strength of nursing. The ANCC (2011) described the magnet hospital program as such: "The Magnet Recognition Program® was developed by the American Nurses Credentialing Center (ANCC) to recognize health care organizations that provide

---

display 15.2   **RN Responsibilities in the Role of Member of the Discipline of Nursing**

Responsibilities of the RN in the role of member of the discipline of nursing include the following:

1. Modeling and valuing nursing
2. Making a commitment to ongoing professional growth
3. Ensuring that high standards of nursing are practiced
4. Contributing to and using nursing research in practice
5. Practicing professional stewardship to support the advancement of nursing
6. Serving as a client advocate
7. Practicing within the legal boundaries and ethical framework of nursing

---

display 15.3   **Daily Ways to Display Modeling and Valuing Nursing**

1. Refer to yourself as Mr./Ms. _____ and state that you are the RN in client interactions.
2. Encourage the use of business cards for yourself and other nurses.
3. Volunteer to be on committees at your institution that promote the professionalism of nursing. This includes trying to achieve magnet status.
4. Emphasize the positive impact you make on reduction of costs, complications, and death.
5. Get involved with community service activities.
6. Inspire interest in nursing early; appear as a guest speaker for Brownies or Cub Scouts or at the local schools, community centers, or places of worship.
7. Capitalize on the fact that you are a college-educated scientist and critical thinker, not just involved with menial tasks.
8. Use nursing research to add power to your image.
9. Refer to the nursing shortage as an opportunity.
10. Join and participate in local, regional, and national nursing organizations that are promoting nursing politically.
11. Be positive about the impact of nursing, and lessen the emotionalism regarding your life and career.
12. Donate money, supplies, or support to a nursing student in another country.

---

nursing excellence. The program also provides a vehicle for disseminating successful nursing practices and strategies." Requirements for designation as a magnet hospital are stringent; more than 65 standards must be met. These workplaces identify that nurses need to be supported and valued. They have a low nurse turnover and a high rate of nursing satisfaction because they know that nurse satisfaction and patient safety are intertwined and important (Donley, 2005). Display 15.3 gives the RN student ideas for daily presentation to increase the sense of modeling and valuing nursing.

Nursing's Image

The image of nursing within the health care industry and in the eyes of the public affects policy development, decision making, funding, recruitment of new nurses, autonomy and development of the profession, and nursing's role in the structure and governance of health care systems. The nursing profession has struggled to accurately portray who a nurse is and what a nurse does. Kalisch and Kalisch (1982, 1987, 1995), Kalisch, Kalisch, and Scobey (1981), Gordon (1997, 2005), and Strasen (1992) have done extensive work on the image of nursing. As they reported, the public forms its view of nursing from the media, particularly through television, films, newspapers, books, and research.

In the 1950s and 1960s, the nurse, nearly always a woman, was portrayed as a handmaiden to the physician. The nurse as an independent care provider, decision maker, patient teacher, manager, and member of a profession was noticeably absent from the media. In addition, the nurse was not represented in such advanced roles as clinical specialist, educator, researcher, and administrator.

Nursing's image was further compromised in the 1970s, when in addition to being underrepresented in the media, the profession was grossly misrepresented, with nurses portrayed as overbearing and sadistic (Bridges, 1990; Duncan, 1992).

Muff (1982), in examining the portrayal of nurses in the media and novels, identified several categories into which the nurse fell: ministering angels, handmaidens, battle-axes, fools, and whores. These portrayals have also been seen in children's books, comic strips, greeting cards, and other media, all contributing to the denigration of nursing. This low point in nursing's image during the 1970s heightened the need for nurses, acting as members of the discipline of nursing, to take a proactive role in strengthening nursing's image. Nurses learned from influences in the women's movement that they had the power to play a pivotal role in political decision making and health policy (Kagan, 2009).

In 1982, the NLN formed the Task Force on Nursing's Public Image to provide leadership for nurses to take a proactive role in changing nursing's image. During the rest of the 1980s and into the 1990s, several media campaigns were launched and recruitment videos produced that had a positive impact on the profession.

Nursing's image had improved by the late 1990s and 2000s. In June 1999, Sigma Theta Tau International consulted with the Louis Harris Association to conduct a US public opinion poll on 1,006 individuals considered to represent average Americans. This poll indicated that 92% of those polled trusted nurses as much as their physician with regard to information presented to them; 85% said they would be honored if their offspring chose nursing as a profession (http://findarticles.com/p/articles/mi-qa4022/13_200401/ai_n9378872). The Gallup polls of 2000, 2002, and 2003 indicated that the public ranks nursing as the most ethical of all professions.

In the new millennium, changes in the mix of nursing staff, dissolution of the primary nursing model, and the continued spiraling health care costs helped dismantle many one-time meccas of nursing power (Wineberg, 2003). The image of RNs as an unnecessary, costly commodity contributing to skyrocketing costs of health care is now being disputed as new research emerges. Studies such as the one by Needleman, Buerhaus, Stewart, Zelevinsky, and Mattke (2006) appealed to the "dollars and cents" or business end of nursing. Although RNs may increase costs, they postulate that greater use of RNs results in fewer deaths, decreased lengths of stay, and lower hospital-linked complications. Nurses need to understand and capitalize on research to support that they prevent complications, save lives, alleviate suffering, and reduce costs (Buresh & Gordon, 2006; Stainton, 2005).

Nurses need more recruits into nursing to help decrease the nursing shortage and improve the profession. Yet, many potential candidates perceive a negative image of nursing (Erickson, Holm, Chelminiak, & Ditomassi, 2005; Fletcher, 2007). Nurses need to be vocal regarding the critical linchpin they are in the health care arena. They need be active in political policy making and recognize their influence and power with the general public.

The Nurse as Role Model

Each RN has a role to play as a member of the discipline to strengthen the image of nursing through modeling. As an LPN/LVN transitioning to the RN level, you will be assuming more of a leadership role in promoting the image of nursing. Role modeling will become even more important. When referring to the vignette, which nurse has a more future-oriented outlook on nursing? Which represents the attributes of the professional? Each comment you make about nursing and your action or inaction in matters dealing with nursing's image will have a positive or negative impact on the profession.

thinking critically

What is your response when someone asks you what a nurse does and how you like being a nurse? How do you reply to the person (male or female) who is considering nursing as a career choice and asks you for your advice? How do your answers and the answers of thousands of other nurses affect the image and progress of the profession? Your words, actions, conduct, and fulfillment of your nursing responsibilities demonstrate the degree to which you value nursing. Image changes start with you. How you think, act, and talk about nursing and its future is important!

This can seem like a daunting task; however, never underestimate the power of one person. To show how the power of one can be extremely important, several sources may inspire you. Greg Mortenson, an emergency nurse from California, had a vision of promoting education among the poor of Pakistan's Karakoram Himalaya (Mortenson & Hosseini, 2010; Mortenson & Relin, 2006). He has built 55 schools and, in the process, helped change America's image in a terrorist-breeding hotbed. *The Tipping Point: How Little Things Can Make a Big Difference* by Malcolm Caldwell (2002) is also a good reference to read about planned and unplanned change, how it can occur, and the role of the individual in making things happen.

● PROFESSIONAL GROWTH

As a member of the discipline of nursing, the RN makes a commitment to ongoing professional growth. The NLN's (2000) *Educational Competencies for Graduates of Associate Degree Nursing Programs* stated that an ADN graduate must participate in lifelong learning and develop and implement a plan to meet self-learning needs.

You may be saying, "I already attend in-services and subscribe to nursing journals as an LPN." But do you have a plan for continued growth and goals that lead in that direction? As you transition to the RN role, you will assume a leadership role in the profession, including a broader scope of responsibility and accountability (as discussed in Units I and II). By making a commitment to professional growth at the RN level (Display 15.4), the nurse continually strives to maintain an updated knowledge base, remain technologically current, apply the latest research to practice, and respond to societal trends, such as those described in Chapter 4.

display 15.4   Areas for Professional Growth at the RN Level

The RN continually strives:

- To maintain a current knowledge base
- To remain technologically current
- To apply current research to practice
- To respond to societal changes

Maintaining a Current Knowledge Base

Maintaining a current knowledge base in nursing is an ongoing challenge for any RN, yet it is a critical responsibility as a member within the discipline of nursing. Longevity, seniority, and the passage of time do not necessarily equal expertise. Nurses are frequently heard saying, "I've been a nurse for 20 years, I think I know what I'm doing." But has this nurse made plans for new learning, or has she or he had the same experiences repeatedly in that period of time? On what areas should the nurse focus when seeking to update her or his knowledge base? Chapter 8 discusses RN competencies as a member of a professional discipline. As new information becomes available in the biological, physical, behavioral, social, and nursing sciences, each nurse must seek ways of gaining this new knowledge and applying it in each of the three nursing roles.

Maintaining a current knowledge base can be accomplished in several ways. In-service programs are available in most health care agencies, but the nurse should never wait for them to occur. That is, if health care agencies cannot provide the necessary updating, the RN should take the initiative. Local, state, regional, national, and international conferences are held regularly in nursing and in disciplines that support and inform nursing. Schools of nursing often offer courses, clinical updates, refresher programs, and some independent study options with an advisor, mentor, or preceptor. In addition, numerous nursing periodicals (journals) feature articles and case studies to maximize dissemination of new knowledge in nursing, and most journals offer online continuing education that can be accessed within the work or home setting. Nurses can also subscribe to online services providing the latest journal articles, as well as bulletins on new advances in procedures, drugs, or other practices. Nurses committed to lifelong learning have positive attitudes toward—and even embrace—change. They realize that change can positively charge them and increase their growth experiences if actively sought.

thinking critically

A plan for designing learning lies squarely on the shoulders of each nurse. You obviously had a plan when you chose to further your nursing education. But do you have a yearly, 5-, 10-, or 20-year plan? Have you ever thought of what you want to accomplish prior to retirement? What educational needs would you need to meet to complete these plans? Share your projections with the members of your class either during a discussion or in an online chat room or student café. A wise person once said that "Planning is everything, but the plan itself is nothing."

Remaining Technologically Current

Equally important for professional growth is the nurse's need to be technologically current to practice competently in the care provider and manager roles. New technology continues to emerge, including cardiorespiratory diagnostic and supportive devices, pharmacotherapeutics, and computer-based treatment devices and client documentation systems. In-services are often provided as new technology is introduced in health care agencies, and schools of nursing may provide workshops or courses for technology upgrade.

According to Roux and Halstead (2009), nursing informatics "is a specialty that integrates nursing science, computer science, and information science to manage and communicate data, information, knowledge, and wisdom in nursing practice." This is a growing field in nursing with a need for nurses with advanced training in use of informatics within nursing. In their effort to provide safe, timely, and current nursing care, nurses will need to know how to access and enter databases, use e-mail to receive and communicate with others, use learning management systems (LMS) such as WebCt or Blackboard for continuing education, use clinical simulators to spruce up on critical thinking and interventional skills, and use the Internet to help with evidence-based research and patient education (Display 15.5). The ANA has developed the scope and standards of practice for nursing informatics in 2008, and its 10 measurement criteria about nursing informatics can be ordered online at http:// nursingworld.org.

Applying Evidence-Based Research

Sweeney, Saarmann, Flagg, and Seidman (2008) conducted a study in Southern California with 473 nurses enrolling in asynchronous online free tutorials. Only 52% of enrollees completed the tutorials. They suggest that nurses who have had previous computer classes and have technical and enrollment support have a better chance of completing online tutorials.

Applying Current Research

A third area of professional growth for the RN as a member of the discipline of nursing is the application of research to clinical practice. To meet the needs of clients and promote health, nurses must continue to incorporate nursing research into their practice. The link between nursing informatics and evidence-based practice needs to be valued and strengthened. Nurses need to request that time is provided to do this, as well as privately using resources. Nursing research expands the nurse's ability to use the nursing process for assessment and diagnosis, thereby providing comprehensive care planning. The usefulness of nursing research is presented later in this chapter.

---

display 15.5	Computer Competencies for the Technologically Current Nurse

1. Personal digital assistants (PDAs)
2. iPad; iPod; podcasting
3. Medication administration via bar coding/automated systems
4. Use of point of care technology
5. Telecommunications
6. Internet with use of blogs, wikis, and really simple syndication (RSS)
7. Genetic engineering
8. Use of electronic health and clinical information systems

Since the mid-1990s, evidence-based practice has been driving our profession to change what nurses have done by tradition:

> Evidence-based care is an approach to health care that realizes that pathophysiologic reasoning and personal experience are necessary but not sufficient for making decisions. This technique emphasizes decision-making based on the best available evidence and the use of outcome studies to guide decisions. (Craven & Hirnle, 2009, p. 112)

In addition, the North American Nursing Diagnosis Association-International (NANDA-I) continues to update its list of nursing diagnoses based on research findings from clinical practice. This assists in providing a common language for the discipline of nursing, communicating nursing's domain to other health care professionals and the public, and establishing a framework for designing care standards.

In applying Web-based technology, the use of Web 2.0 Technologies is becoming important as the wealth of information now available can be completely overwhelming in its volume. Examples of Web 2.0 Resources are available in Display 15.6.

---

display 15.6   **WEB 2.0 Resources**

Resources	Definition	Example
Blogs*	Web log: usually a diary, journal bulletin board. Updated frequently with general comments that can be added by the public	http://mediblogopathy. blogspot.com
Wiki*	Online site that allows compilation of posting and editing	www.wikipedia.com
Social Web sites*	These allow photographs, commentary, and access to Web sites by others	www.facebook.com
Collaborative editing Web sites	Texts, documents, and spreadsheets may be shared between two or more participants	www.docs.google.com
Survey data complication	Participants of a study or group like students can be surveyed about their opinions	www.surveymonkey.com
RSS	Sends summaries of research documents to users that sign up for results	https://www.mdlinx.com http://smartbrief.com/ana http://medscape.com http://allnurses.com

*Information obtained may not be reputable. Authors of sites must be interrogated before application of resource information.

Responding to Societal Changes

When making a commitment to professional growth, the RN strives to respond to societal changes to meet the needs of clients. A number of societal trends, as discussed in Chapter 4, influence nursing and have professional growth implications for nurses in clinical practice. Four important societal trends to note are changing demographics, health care reform, the emerging global community, and advances that are increasing the amount, cost, and complexity of technology, especially in the health care industry (Donley, 2005; Heller, Oros, & Durney-Crowley, 2002).

CHANGING DEMOGRAPHICS

American society is aging, and the ethnic population is growing. Within the next few decades, the population older than 85 years will dramatically increase. In some areas of the United States, two thirds of clients are of minority populations, calling for nurses to think and act from a multicultural perspective. Such societal changes require RNs to seek professional growth to meet the needs of their changing client population. Many in-service programs, courses, conferences, and publications are available to assist the nurse with professional development in these areas. Following are just a few of the many considerations to keep in mind as our client population ages:

- When caring for the elderly, the nurse must gain additional knowledge on the differing care needs of well, frail, and ill elders.
- What new evidence-based research is available in geriatric nursing and the field of gerontology?
- What nursing intervention is needed for a client who is nearing 100 years of age?
- What safety and preventive measures are required to maintain health in this frail individual?
- What new information is available in the behavioral sciences to support nursing of elders?

The nurse will need many new skills to address the US multicultural population.

Multiculturalism must be considered in every aspect of the care provider role. To meet the increased self-care demands of our clients as the length of stay in health care facilities continues to shorten, our communication skills and client-teaching strategies must be crafted with ethnic differences in mind. At the RN level, these skills are also essential in the manager of care role as the RN finds greater ethnic representation among her or his nursing team. Many RNs are learning a second language, finding that the nurse who is bilingual—or speaks two languages—enriches her or his own life and is better able to fulfill nursing care responsibilities (see Chapter 13).

HEALTH CARE REFORM

One of the more hotly debated concerns as we move into the second decade of the millenium is the health care reform legislation. How this reform will affect nursing is a largely unknown. However, nurses are positive and optimistic about how this will affect public health and nurses specifically. Nurses are in a great position to speak out and be in the forefront confronting issues, and many have been galvanized to speak about quality reforms. Beverly Malone, chief nursing officers of the NLN states that "nurses need to be prepared to deal with the complex, comprehensive patient in the home and in the community. That is a huge issue we will be dealing with. The nation is gearing up for that and nurses need to be leaders in that" (Wood, 2010, Health Care Reform Revamped, para. 4). One of the issues is having enough primary care providers for all the millions medically uninsured. To meet these needs, the nurse's role will need to be expanded. Input from nurses can be sent to Congress via Twitter, Facebook, and e-mails, which are much more convenient messages to those in governmental power. Social networks like Twitter and Facebook are a powerful lobby tool to make voices heard and progressive steps taken for social reform.

GLOBAL COMMUNITY

As technology advances in the information and communication fields, nursing has become a discipline within a global community.

It is now possible for more people than ever to collaborate and compete in real time with more other people on more different kinds of work from more different corners of the planet and on a more equal footing than at any previous time in the history of the world—using computers, e-mail, fiber-optic networks, teleconferencing, and dynamic new software (Friedman, 2006).

The worldwide access to collaboration by a technology has lead to a drawing closer of the global community, or globalization. This has lead to new changes in how business, governments, communities, and individuals interact. Friedman (2006) refers to this in his landmark book as a flattening of the world.

Advances in distance education are creating the opportunity for nurses to participate in professional development activities with colleagues across the United States and internationally. This creates an exciting professional growth opportunity for RNs around the world. In addition, this challenges the RN to commit to professional growth to be a participating partner in confronting global issues such as hunger, AIDS, emerging diseases such as the H5N1 virus (avian flu), overpopulation, bioterrorism and disaster preparedness, and preservation of the environment.

ADVANCES IN TECHNOLOGY

Technological advances can be seen in every field, but the rapidly increasing amount, cost, and complexity of technology in the health care industry can be overwhelming to both nurse and patient. As discussed, it is imperative that the nurse remains technologically current. The use of handheld technology, in the form of PDAs and cell phones, can help nurses and patients access data almost immediately. Computer-assisted drug administration in the form of bar coding and automatic delivery systems and access to electronic databases require that the nurse adjust to advances needed for client safety. Although there is evidence to support that nurses do not feel proficient in basic computer skills, nurses need to voice their concerns and demand proper training to assist with client care (Display 15.5) (Starren et al., 2005; Wilbright et al., 2006).

The nurse must also be an astute observer and conserver of costly client resources. At the RN level in the manager of care role, this means ensuring that nursing team members are afforded opportunities to become comfortable and competent with new technology. It also means that every effort is coordinated to reduce costs.

In addition, the RN plays a leadership role in balancing "high tech" with "high touch." Nursing team members must believe that the RN cares about them, is available, and listens to their needs. This is also true of clients. Numerous surveys to determine the satisfaction of clients at discharge from health care settings continue to rank personal, caring activities and listening as essential characteristics of the nursing staff. As flowers and personal belongings are set aside to make room for machines, and as supportive others have difficulty getting close enough to their loved one to touch, hug, or otherwise provide emotional support, the nurse must learn new ways to create the balance between high tech and high touch.

NCLEX–RN *Might Ask*   15.1

Two nurses are developing a nursing plan of care for a community experiencing an outbreak of *Escherichia coli*. These nurses are using evidence-based outcomes to update the community on the latest preventative and treatment methods for this bacterium. The nurses are using which of the following qualities of professional behaviors?

    A. Tradition, shared personal values, and autonomy
    B. Intellectual activities, service to society, and autonomy
    C. Licensure, tradition, and accountability
    D. Coalition building, professional dependency, and tradition

• See Appendix A for correct answer and rationale.

● STANDARDS OF NURSING PRACTICE

A third major area of responsibility for the RN as a member of the discipline of nursing is ensuring that high standards of nursing are practiced. The ANA (2004b) described the nurse's role in safeguarding the client and public, using judgment in her or his own practice, and managing care provided by others.

Promoting High Standards

Contributing to the establishment of high nursing standards and ensuring adherence to them is every nurse's responsibility. Chapter 8 describes standards of practice, differentiating them from regulations and policies, whereas Chapter 4 discusses the role professional nursing organizations play in generating nursing standards. Participation in such organizations by individual practicing RNs generates standards that are comprehensive and based on daily nurse–client interactions in the clinical area. The health care settings in which nurses work have become more diverse, with a greater portion of clinical practice occurring in ambulatory and home care settings. Client care has shifted from a focus of providing hands-on care to one of assisting the client to assume the captainship of his or her self-care. Standards for nursing practice must reflect such changes in the profession.

Nurses also participate in promoting high standards by contributing to the ongoing development of nursing diagnoses and desired nursing outcomes through activities sponsored by NANDA-I and evidence-based practice. This includes the generation and identification of emerging diagnoses with advances in nursing research assessment. It also means critiquing existing and recommended new diagnoses to ensure their applicability to clients of both genders, all ages, and with a diversity of socioeconomic, religious, cultural, and ethnic backgrounds.

Promoting high standards also means that RNs use as part of their autonomous practice such standards in writing appropriate outcomes, revising nursing interventions, and evaluating outcomes. Nursing diagnoses, long- and short-term outcomes, and delineated nursing intervention activities must be clear, concise, and individualized to the client's condition and state of health. In addition, maintaining high standards means that nurses are current in their knowledge base and technical skills and incorporate current clinical research on preventive, therapeutic, and rehabilitative intervention strategies into nursing care plans.

Finally, RNs are mentors and teachers to other nursing staff to foster their knowledge and application of those standards. One of the most severe shortages in nursing today is in the nurse educator field. One of the reasons nursing schools are turning away qualified applicants is the lack of qualified nurse educators. In addition, in the 2010s, most current educators will be retiring (Benner, Sutphen, Leonard, & Day, 2010). According to the NLN, there are ten reasons to become a nurse educator. These are listed in Display 15.7. According to Benner et al. (2010), the following strategies for teaching salience will be imperative for nurse educators to master for the new nursing professional (Display 15.8). These will be important for mentors to continue in their process of orienting new nurses.

---

display 15.7 — **Top 10 Reasons to Become a Nurse Educator**

1. You teach what you love.
2. You change lives.
3. You shape the future of health care.
4. You encourage and educate eager minds and rejoice when your students surpass you.
5. You can teach from the beach or the slopes using technology.
6. You can teach anywhere in the world.
7. Your work has value to society.
8. Your research creates knowledge and advances the field; your publications bring you prestige.
9. You have autonomy and flexibility.
10. You work in an intellectually stimulating environment.

Adapted from Steefel, L. (2006). Educators wanted. *Nursing Spectrum, 15*(8), 12–13.

---

display 15.8 — **Benner's Strategies for Teaching for a Sense of Salience**

1. Create continuity and coherence in learning
2. Use questioning techniques
3. Rehearse for practice
4. Reflect on learning

Accountability

As a member of the discipline of nursing at the RN level, the nurse maintains accountability for the standards of practice. The nurse is also accountable to self, colleagues, and those to whom client care is delegated. Accountability extends beyond the responsibility of incorporating high standards into nursing care plans and assignments of delegated work. Accountability also involves evaluating the actual care implemented to ensure it is consistent with written standards and seeking consultation with health care provider colleagues and others as needed. (Accountability is discussed in more depth in Chapter 16.) Accountability and professionalism are ways in which nursing can increase a power base. In accepting responsibility, nurses have more control over their future and are less likely to be governed by nonnursing groups. As nurses move into the community, autonomy and accountability will be increasingly essential. Without direct access to a more experienced colleague, the nurse will have to decide when they need to consult or seek advice to ensure client safety.

Peer Review and Self-Regulation

In *Nursing's Social Policy Statement*, the ANA (2004b) noted that nursing as a profession gains its authority from the social contract it holds with society. Under its terms, society grants the profession authority over functions vital to itself and permits them considerable autonomy in the conduct of their own affairs. In return, the profession is expected to act responsibly, always mindful of the public trust. Self-regulation to ensure quality in performance is at the heart of this relationship.

The major vehicle for the profession's self-regulation is by way of its professional organizations. Through activities and forums of these organizations, nurses are able to establish and maintain standards for nursing practice. This is discussed later in this chapter.

On the local level, RNs have a number of opportunities and responsibilities to engage in peer review to support standards of nursing practice. Some examples of these include shared governance, peer nurse employee evaluation processes, nursing peer review panels, record audits, quality councils, quality assurance procedures, staffing ratio committees, and ethics committees. In addition, it is every nurse's responsibility to take the initiative to report behaviors or actions taken by nurse colleagues that are inconsistent with standards of nursing practice.

• NURSING RESEARCH

A fourth major responsibility for the RN is in the area of research. It is important that all levels of nursing be involved in research not just at the previously thought of educational level. The practicing RN plays three key roles in the area of nursing research. First, the nurse in clinical practice is in the position to generate questions for research. Second, the nurse can participate in clinical research studies that strengthen client care and health promotion. The practicing nurse notes possible relations between nursing intervention activities and client progress toward health. Third, the nurse in clinical practice fulfills the role of applying research findings to assist clients in regaining, maintaining, and promoting health. The name for this is evidence-based practice. Earlier in this chapter, information is provided on RN responsibilities related to professional growth, including a discussion on applying current research. Take a moment to review that section now.

---

thinking critically

Use an RSS to look at the abstracts of recent nursing journals. Synthesize one or two significant research findings presented. How can you apply these findings in your clinical practice to improve client care or strengthen client health?

● PROFESSIONAL STEWARDSHIP AND THE ADVANCEMENT OF NURSING

A fifth major area of responsibility for the RN as a member of the discipline of nursing is professional stewardship and supporting the advancement of nursing. Chapter 4 provides an in-depth discussion on the transitions that have occurred in nursing.

Through the efforts of individuals, groups of nurse leaders, and friends of nursing, nursing as a profession continues to grow in its knowledge and practice base. As you transition to the RN level of practice, your involvement as a member of the profession will be essential in the areas of governance and decision making, participation in professional organizations, and recruiting/mentoring new nurses entering the profession.

Governance and Decision Making

Nurses have had a recent impact in governmental changes in the health care system. Increasing opportunities exist for the RN in decision making in the health care industry. Many agencies have recognized the importance of healthy work environments for both the client and the nurse. A deepening concern regarding the importance of not only enlisting but also *retaining* nurses has lead to inquiry into what constitutes an environment that fosters a joyful workplace. According to the American Association of Critical-Care Nurses (AACN, 2005),

> The model of a healthy work environment includes six components: skilled communication, authentic leadership, meaningful recognition, appropriate staffing, true collaboration and effective decision-making ... healthy effective work environments exhibit a strong sense of trust between management and employees. These organizations engage and empower employees in decision making, risk taking and personal and professional growth. (Shirey, 2006, p. 258)

Many agencies have established shared governance councils among nursing, medicine, and health care administrators. Staff nurses are assuming a greater role in hiring practices, peer review processes, committees for policy making, creating healthy work environments for nurses, and the development of standards of practice. In addition, at the unit level, staff nurses have increased their involvement in shared governance (scheduling, staffing, and other decision-making processes) traditionally done by the nurse manager.

On the state and national levels, nurses participate in decision making by joining and being active in professional organizations. Technological advances have created new opportunities for nurses that enhance involvement in professional organizations. Newer technologies enable nurses to communicate more easily and enhance nurses' ability to speak with one voice.

Providing Leadership Through Professional Organizations

Another responsibility you will have as an RN is to provide leadership for the discipline of nursing through membership and active participation in professional organizations at the state or national level. Such RN involvement generates rich dialogue and discussions about issues important to nurses. Professional organizations provide a forum for expressing viewpoints from a variety of perspectives, establishing position papers and standards to guide the profession and assist it to speak with one voice, and engaging in cooperative efforts to identify and achieve common goals.

Nurses have not used their professional organizations to their fullest extent. According to the ANA, only 6% of the 2.7 million RNs in the United States are ANA members. Some blame the number and competition among nursing organizations for decreasing its power potential. However, more than 60 nursing organizations have formed a coalition known as the Nursing Organizations Alliance. Its mission is to help increase nursing's visibility and impact on health through communication, collaboration, and advocacy. This is an effort to unite the nurse as a profession into one powerful voice instead of many fragmented ones.

As an RN student, your nursing faculty will encourage you to join and participate in activities via the National Student Nurses Association (NSNA) or the Canadian Nursing Students Association (CNSA). Students established the NSNA in 1953 as an organization for students, managed, financed, and run by students. The goals of the NSNA involve promoting high-quality care and providing educational programs to promote development of the whole person. Involvement in local, regional, and national workshops can help a student grow for the same reasons previously mentioned for the RN. The Web sites of both the NSNA and the CNSA are included at the end of the chapter.

---

thinking critically

Review the content on critical thinking presented in Chapter 9. Visit any of the student nurse organization Web sites provided at the chapter's end. How can you put your critical thinking skills to work through active participation in one of these organizations to provide leadership for the nursing profession?

Chapter 4 provides an in-depth review of the ANA and the NLN. Both the ANA and the NLN are organized at the state level; for example, in California, nurses can join the California Nurses Association or the California League for Nursing and the national organization.

Participating in professional organizations provides the nurse with valuable information on advancements in nursing and the profession's interdependent and collaborative efforts with medicine and other professions. The ANA (2004b) clarified the definition of nursing as a discipline, identifying it as an entity discrete from medicine with its own unique purpose and autonomous practice (see Chapter 8, Display 8.3). Nursing's professional organizations play a key role in further defining the discipline, identifying entry-level competencies, and establishing professional standards of practice. Chapter 8 also discusses the difference between LPN/LVN and RN scopes of practice in their respective nurse practice acts. Professional organizations provide guidance and practice standards for RNs, who practice autonomously and in collaboration with other professionals. Such activity is critical for professional stewardship and the advancement of nursing.

Recruiting and Mentoring New Nurses

As you transition to the RN level, you become an important contributor to the advancement of nursing through your efforts in recruiting and mentoring new nurses. In the vignette, Jennifer is both recruiting Courtney into school and trying to be a mentor to her.

RECRUITMENT

It is estimated that by the year 2020, there will be a shortage of 400,000 RNs. Recent data from the U.S. Bureau of Labor Statistics (2010) show that by 2018 registered nurses will experience a 22.2% job expected growth with the need of 581,500 jobs to fill that need. Nursing is striving to portray itself as a viable profession to young people. With work on a more positive image and working conditions, it is hoped that young men and women will not be "turned off" and instead seek nursing as an attractive profession that provides a happy, fulfilling life.

As mentioned previously, the "graying" of nurse educators is reaching critical mass. Much work needs to be done to provide incentives for prospective nurse educators to further their education to the master's and doctorate levels.

Nursing continues to strive for diversity in an effort to meet the needs of clients. In particular, more men and underrepresented (minority) members are needed in the profession. In addition, as nursing competes with professions such as business, medicine, and law for the best and brightest, the challenge for each RN as a member of the profession is to seek methods to attract these individuals.

MENTORING

Nurses also play a role in mentoring new nurses entering the profession. A mentor takes a special interest in a student or colleague. It is an essential aspect of a profession that the "torch," or previous knowledge, is bestowed on the younger fellows of the profession. They inspire and encourage mentees in their career development. As you begin your practice at the RN level, you will find it essential to confer with more experienced RNs. But the bond between mentor and mentee is much stronger in that it improves satisfaction for both and strengthens the profession (Display 15.9). This is especially true in expanded scope of practice areas, such as the manager of care role and aspects of the care provider role (eg, client education, referrals, responsibilities related to nursing process). Chapter 8 compares and contrasts LPN/LVN and RN knowledge, roles, and competencies. Chapter 9 discusses the

display 15.9	Positive Effects of a Mentor on Professionalism

1. Career success and advancement
2. Personal and professional satisfaction
3. Increased self-confidence and self-esteem
4. Preparation for leadership positions
5. Strengthening the profession

independent (autonomous) and collaborative practice components at the RN level and provides more information in the area of nursing process, describing the use of clinical judgment to formulate nursing diagnoses. A review of these chapters will assist you in identifying areas in which you may need a mentor.

Carpenito-Moyet (2008) and others have worked extensively in the area of nursing diagnosis, its application, and the formulation of collaborative problems. As you transition to the RN level, this new practice expectation may cause you some difficulty. Benner (2001) noted that the ability to cluster data intuitively, identify patterns, and thereby exercise clinical judgment in formulating nursing diagnostic statements increases with experience. By conferring with other more experienced nurses who serve as your mentors, you will develop this intuitive experiential knowledge to move from novice to expert.

thinking critically

Reflect on your own practice in nursing and the competencies you anticipate acquiring as you transition to the RN level. In what areas are you experienced and can offer to mentor others? In what areas might you seek a mentor to assist you? What qualities would you look for in a mentor that are consistent with your philosophy of education?

As nurses gain expertise in assessment, clinical judgment, nursing diagnosis, client education, and management of care, they have a responsibility as members of the profession in a leadership role to model these competencies and serve as mentors (and preceptors) to student and novice nurses entering the profession.

● CLIENT ADVOCACY

A sixth area of responsibility for the RN is that of client advocacy. Advocacy in general can be defined as pleading on one's behalf or acting in support of another. Client advocacy means speaking for the client or representing the client's point of view. This may involve speaking for the client because he or she is unable to do so alone. Or it may involve translating or articulating the client's intent when, in the nurse's view, it is not being heard, perceived, or understood accurately or consistently with the client's original thinking. As an LPN/LVN, you played a role in client advocacy. However, at the RN level, you will have ultimate accountability in advocating for the client and ensuring that the client's desires are understood and his or her rights (and freedom of choice) protected.

Speaking for the Client

At times, the client needs help communicating his or her desires. Respiratory devices, lowered states of consciousness, or other physical impairments may impede or limit the client's ability to express herself or himself. Language or cultural barriers may be present. The client may be illiterate; mentally or learning disabled; or unable to read, comprehend, or communicate adequately. The client may simply not grasp the concept of what is being explained. The RN's educational preparation in communication skills and his or her assessment skills will assist the nurse in ascertaining the client's needs and serving as a spokesperson and client advocate.

NCLEX–RN *Might Ask* (15.2)

The nurse is interceding for a client who has refused radiation treatment for a slow-growing malignant tumor. In this role, the nurse is acting as

- A. teacher.
- B. benefactor.
- C. advocate.
- D. proxy.

• *See Appendix A for correct answer and rationale.*

Informed Decision Making

It is the RN's responsibility to ensure that clients are well informed to make choices and decisions about their care. Information should be provided verbally and in writing and should not be rushed. The nurse uses her or his knowledge and application of effective communication skills to ensure that the client has not only been provided with the information but has also comprehended it. The client should be able to describe to the nurse what procedure or treatment is to be done or his or her understanding of the information given and the consequences of such (both positive and negative). When more than one alternative exists, the nurse ensures that all alternatives are understood. The nurse communicates in a nonjudgmental manner; when uncertainty is apparent, the nurse helps the client acquire more information or obtain a second medical opinion, or otherwise works to remove the client's uncertainty. Informed consent and the nurse's role related to advance directions (eg, living wills) are discussed in Chapter 16. The nurse can teach the client to use the same decision-making techniques discussed in Chapter 14.

Referral

In addition to assisting the client in gaining more information and second medical opinions, the RN is also the client's advocate in making referrals. In transitioning from the LPN/LVN to the RN role, your scope of practice will include the need to make referrals. Referrals are indicated when information or intervention needed by the client is outside the scope of RN practice or when that intervention will occur under another nurse's care (eg, in the transfer from acute to ambulatory care).

Referrals are generally within the health care provider environment but are occasionally to other entities such as behavioral scientists. Advanced technology via the Internet should be used in the age of the informed consumer. Nurses need to play a role to inform the consumer about accurate Web sites but also make them aware that there is no one in control of a Web site's accuracy.

Referrals are written to convey the client's needs and desires and to speak for the client as an advocate. Sometimes referrals by RNs are made in-house to other RNs with specialized expertise, such as enterostomal therapy nurses, lactation nurse specialists, special procedures nurses, oncology nurses, or diabetes education nurses.

Protection of Rights

Finally, in the area of client advocacy, the RN ensures that each client's rights are protected. Chapter 13 discusses the nurse's role in managing diverse and sensitive human situations and systems. The client is viewed as a member of a cultural group, a social being, a sexual being, and a spiritual being. The importance of respecting and protecting each client's individual preferences and confidential nature of needs is emphasized. Client advocacy means supporting the client in exercising individual preferences and exploring intervention strategies that will promote health within the client's belief system. At times, this means serving as an advocate for the client's right to refuse intervention, even if it means a decline in health. More on confidentiality of patient information can be found in Chapter 16.

● LEGAL AND ETHICAL PRACTICE

The seventh and final area of responsibility for the RN as a member of the discipline of nursing is legal and ethical practice. Both the ANA (2004a) in *Code of Ethics for Nurses With Interpretive Statements* and the NLN (2000) in its delineation of competencies for the ADN graduate emphasize the importance of practicing within the legal boundaries and ethical framework of nursing. Through these mechanisms, nursing maintains its accountability to society. Legal and ethical issues are explored in Chapters 16 and 17, as is the role of the RN in regard to these issues.

● CONCLUSION

This chapter examines the professional responsibilities of the RN, including those related to nursing research and stewardship of the profession. Roles of the LPN/LVN and RN as members of the discipline of nursing are compared and contrasted, highlighting competencies identified by the NLN.

Seven major areas of responsibility for the RN are examined. As you complete this chapter and prepare for Chapters 16 and 17 and their focus on legal and ethical issues, respectively, you may find it helpful to reflect on these seven areas of responsibility and their relation to the ANA's (2004a) *A Code for Nurses*. This relationship is provided for you in Table 15.1.

table

15-1   ANA CODE FOR NURSES STATEMENTS RELATED TO AREAS OF RESPONSIBILITY
FOR RNS AS MEMBERS OF THE DISCIPLINE OF NURSING

RN as Member of Discipline Seven Areas of Responsibility	ANA Code for Nurses Statements
1. Modeling and valuing nursing	The nurse participates in the profession's efforts to protect the public from misinformation and misrepresentation and to maintain the integrity of nursing.
2. Making a commitment to ongoing professional growth	The nurse maintains competence in nursing.
3. Ensuring that high standards of nursing are practiced	The nurse acts to safeguard the client and the public when health care and safety are affected by the incompetent, unethical, or illegal practice of any person. The nurse assumes responsibility and accountability for individual nursing judgments and actions. The nurse exercises informed judgment and uses individual competence and qualifications as criteria when seeking consultation, accepting responsibilities, and delegating nursing activities to others.
4. Contributing to and using nursing research in practice	The nurse participates in the profession's efforts to establish and maintain conditions of employment conducive to high-quality nursing care.
5. Practicing professional stewardship to support the advancement of nursing	The nurse participates in activities that contribute to the ongoing development of the profession's body of knowledge.
6. Serving as a client advocate	The nurse provides services with respect for human dignity and the uniqueness of the client unrestricted by considerations of social or economic status, personal attributes, or the nature of health problems. The nurse collaborates with members of health professions and other citizens in promoting community and national efforts to meet the health needs of the public.
7. Practicing within the legal boundaries and ethical framework of nursing	The nurse safeguards the client's right to privacy by judiciously protecting information of a confidential nature.

student exercises

1. Observe a practicing RN in the clinical setting for several hours.

   a. Cite statements made by the nurse or behaviors displayed by the nurse that tell you the degree to which she or he values (or does not value) nursing as a profession.

   b. Who was present at the time of these statements (eg, patients, visitors, students, other health care workers)? How might these observers' perceptions of nursing be influenced (positively or negatively) by what they observed?

   c. How might these perceptions contribute to the evolving image of nursing and progress of the profession?

2. Imagine you have just completed the ADN program and are beginning your career as an RN. Design a professional growth plan for yourself by completing the following outline, identifying your strategies for maintaining competence during your first few years of nursing practice.

   a. Maintaining a current knowledge base

   b. Remaining technologically current

   c. Applying current research to practice

   d. Participating in professional organizations

   e. Responding to societal changes and needs

3. Reflect on who might be your mentor as you transition to the RN role. List individuals, and describe why you have selected them. How do they operationalize the strategies for professional growth using the previous five strategies?

References

American Nurses Accrediting Organization. (2011). American Nurses Accrediting Association Magnet Recognition Program available at http://nursecredentialing.org/Magnet.aspx

American Association of Critical-Care Nurses. (2005). Creating a healthy work environment. Retrieved July 5, 2007, from http://www.aacn.org/_882565100000a416.nsf/0/886943d6d40b0b2b88256 ebb0070e6d?Open Document

American Nurses Association. (2004a). *Code of ethics for nurses with interpretive statements*. Washington, DC: American Nurses Publishing.

American Nurses Association. (2004b). *Nursing's social policy statement*. Kansas City, MO: Author.

Benner, P. (2001). *From novice to expert: Excellence and power in clinical nursing practice* (Commemorative ed.). Upper Saddle River, NJ: Prentice-Hall Health.

Benner, P., Sutphen, M., Leonard, V., & Day, L. (2010). *Educating nurses: A call for radical transformation*. San Francisco, CA: Jossey-Bass.

Bridges, J. (1990). Literature review on images of the nurse and nursing in the media. *Journal of Advanced Nursing, 15*(7), 850–854.

Buresh, B., & Gordon, S. (2006). *From silence to voice: What nurses know and must communicate to the public* (2nd ed.). Ithaca, NY: ILR Press.

Caldwell, M. (2002). *The tipping point: How little things can make a big difference*. New York, NY: Little, Brown and Company.

Carpenito-Moyet, L. (2008). *Nursing diagnosis: Application to clinical practice* (12th ed.). Philadelphia, PA: Lippincott Williams & Wilkins.

Cherry, B., & Jacob, S. R. (2008). *Contemporary nursing: Issues, trends, and management* (4th ed.). St. Louis, MO: CV Mosby.

Craven, R., & Hirnle, C. (2009). *Fundamentals of nursing: Human health and function* (6th ed.). Philadelphia, PA: Lippincott Williams & Wilkins.

Donley, G. (2005). Challenges for nursing in the 21st century. *Nursing Economics, 23*(6), 312–314.

Duncan, P. (1992). Media portrayals of nurses versus the actual work of nurses. Unpublished doctoral dissertation. Syracuse, NY: Syracuse University.

Erickson, J., Holm, L., Chelminiak, L., & Ditomassi, M. (2005). Why not nursing? *Nursing, 35*(7), 46–49.

Fletcher, K. (2007). Image: Changing how female nurses think about themselves. A literature review. *Journal of Advanced Nursing, 58*(3), 207–215.

Friedman, T. (2006). *The world is flat: A brief history of the twenty-first century*. New York, NY: Farrar, Straus and Giroux.

Gordon, S. (1997). *Life support: Three nurses on the front lines*. Boston, MA: Little, Brown and Company.

Gordon, S. (2005). *Nursing against the odds: How health care cost cutting, media stereotypes, and medical hubris undermine nurses and patient care*. Ithaca, NY: Cornell University Press.

Heller, B. R., Oros, M. T., & Durney-Crowley, J. (2002). *The future of nursing education: Ten trends to watch*. Retrieved July 5, 2007, from www.nln.org/nlnjournal/infotrends.htm#1

Kagan, P. (2009). Historical voices of resistance: Crossing the boundaries to praxis through documentary filmmaking for the public. *Advances in Nursing Science, 32*(1), 19–32.

Kalisch, P. A., & Kalisch, B. J. (1982). Nurses on prime-time television. *American Journal of Nursing, 82*(2), 264.

Kalisch, P., & Kalisch, B. (1987). *The changing image of the nurse.* Menlo Park, CA: Addison Wesley.

Kalisch, P. A., & Kalisch, B. J. (1995). *The advance of American nursing* (3rd ed.). Philadelphia, PA: JB Lippincott.

Kalisch, P., Kalisch, B., & Benner, P. (2005). Perspectives on improving nursing's public image. *Nursing Education Perspectives, 26*(1), 11–17.

Kalisch, P. A., Kalisch, B. J., & Scobey, M. (1981). Reflections on a TV image. *Nursing and Health Care, 5*(5), 248–255.

Merriam-Webster Online Dictionary. (2010). Modeling. Retrieved from http://www.merriam-webster.com/model

Mortenson, G., & Hosseini, K. (2010). *Stones for schools: Promoting peace by education in Afghanistan and Pakistan.* New York, NY: Viking.

Mortenson, G., & Relin, D. (2006). *Three cups of tea: One man's mission to fight terrorism and build nations... one school at a time.* New York, NY: Viking.

Muff, J. (1982). *Socialization, sexism, and stereotyping.* St. Louis, MO: CV Mosby.

National League for Nursing. (2000). *Educational competencies for graduates of associate degree nursing programs.* Boston, MA: Jones and Bartlett.

Needleman, J., Buerhaus, P., Stewart, M., Zelevinsky, K., & Mattke, S. (2006). Nurse staffing in hospitals: Is there a business case for quality? *Health Affairs, 25*(1), 204–211.

Roux, G., & Halstead, J. (2009). *Issues and trends in nursing: Essential knowledge for today and tomorrow.* Sudbury, MA: Jones and Barlett.

Salvage, J. (2006). More than a makeover is needed to improve nursing's image. *Journal of Advanced Nursing, 54*(3), 259–260.

Shirey, M. (2006). Authentic leaders creating healthy work environments for nursing practice. *American Journal of Critical Care, 15*(3), 256–267.

Stainton, M. (2005). The power of nursing. *Reflections on Nursing Leadership, 31*(2), 16–22.

Starren, J., Tsai, C., Bakken, S., Aidala, A., Morin, P., Hillman, C., et al. (2005). The role of nurses in installing telehealth technology in the home. *Computer Informatics Nursing, 23*(4), 181–189.

Steefel, L. (2006). Educators wanted. *Nursing Spectrum, 15*(8), 12–13.

Strasen, L. (1992). *The image of professional nursing: Strategies for action.* Philadelphia, PA: JB Lippincott.

Sweeney, M., Saarmann, L., Flagg, J., & Seidman, R. (2008). The keys to successful online continuing education programs for nurses. *The Journal of Continuing Education in Nursing, 39*(1), 34–40.

Wilbright, W., Haun, D., Romano, R., Krutzfeldt, R., Fontenot, C., & Nolan, T. (2006). Computer use in an urban university hospital: Technology ahead of literacy. *Computer Informatics Nursing, 24*(1), 37–43.

Wineberg, S. (2003). *Code green: Money-driven hospitals and the dismantling of nursing.* Ithaca, NY: Cornell University Press.

Wood, D. (2010). *Nursing leaders reveal top trends impacting nurses in 2010.* Retrieved from http://www.nursezone.com/Nursing-News-Events/more-news/Nursing-Leaders-Reveal-Top-Trends-Impacting-Nurses-in-2010_33230.aspx

U.S. Bureau of Labor Statistics (2010). *Occupational Employment and Wages, May 2009.* Retrieved from http://www.nursezone.com/Nursing-News-Events/more-news/Nursing-Leaders-Reveal-Top-Trends-Impacting-Nurses-in-2010_33230.aspx

Suggested Reading

Alfaro-LeFevre, R. (2006). *Applying nursing process: A step-by-step guide* (6th ed.). Philadelphia, PA: Lippincott Williams & Wilkins.

Ellis, J. R., & Hartley, C. L. (2004). *Nursing in today's world: Challenges, issues, and trends* (8th ed.). Philadelphia, PA: Lippincott Williams & Wilkins.

Hannah, K., Ball, M., & Edwards, M. (2006). *Introduction to Nursing Informatics* (3rd ed.). New York, NY: Springer.

Koticki, C. (2006). Translating research into practice. *Nursing Spectrum, 15*(3), 8–9.

Kover, C., Brewer, C., Wu, Y-W., Cheng, Y., & Suzuki, M. (2006). Factors associated with work satisfaction of registered nurses. *Journal of Nursing Scholarship, 38*(1), 71–79.

Malka, S. (2007). *Daring to care: American nursing and second-wave feminism.* Chicago, IL: University of Illinois Press.

National League for Nursing. (1999). *Entry-level competencies of graduates of educational programs in practical nursing.* New York, NY: Author.

Polit, D., & Beck, C. (2007). *Nursing research: Principles and methods* (8th ed.). Philadelphia, PA: Lippincott Williams & Wilkins.

Reverby, S. (1987). *Ordered to Care: The Dilemma of American Nursing, 1850–1945.* New York, NY: Cambridge University Press.

On the (WEB) *www.cnsa/ca/:* The Canadian Nursing Students' Association. (Last accessed 7.26.2011).

http://ebri.bmj.com: Evidence-Based Nursing. (Last accessed 7.26.2011).

http://www.informaticsnurse.com: On line resource for employment opportunities, workshops and much more involving nursing informatics. (Last accessed 7.26.2011).

www.nursingadvocacy.org: Center for Nursing Advocacy. For anyone interested in learning about the media images of nursing. (Last accessed 7.26.2011).

www.nsna.org: National Student Nurses' Organization. (Last accessed 7.26.2011).

www.nursing-alliance.org: The Web site of the Nursing Organizations Alliance, an alliance created for nursing organizations to create "a strong voice for nurses. (Last accessed 7.26.2011)."

chapter

16

Legal Accountability

● LEARNING OUTCOMES

By the end of the chapter, the student will be able to:

1 Describe the origins of US law.

2 List the differences among public, private, and nursing law.

3 Identify the components of accountability and its impact on nursing.

4 Identify the nurse's role in delegation.

5 Define liability, negligence, and malpractice.

6 Discuss methods to avoid litigation.

7 Identify legal issues that affect nursing practice.

8 Differentiate between the role of the LPN/LVN and RN in relation to legal responsibilities.

advance directive
Against Medical
  Advice form (AMA)
civil law
common law
contract law
criminal negligence
defendant
deposition
documentation
durable power of
  attorney

expert witness
health care proxy
HIPAA
incident report
informed consent
invasion of privacy
legal precedents
liability
living will
malpractice
negligence
occurrence report

plaintiff
professional
  boundaries
reckless
  endangerment
risk management
sentinel event
standards of care/
  practice
statutory law
tort

RN

LPN

v i g n e t t e

Cal Thomas is in his second rotation as an RN student at City Community College. He also works per diem as an LPN at busy Willow Glen Medical Center. Cal is talking to his nurse manager, Joann Francheski. Joann has been a practicing nurse for more than 20 years; she, too, started out as an LPN.

CAL: I never really gave much thought to the responsibilities RNs have until recently. There is a big difference as I am living that experience in my school clinicals, but I must remember that I'm an LPN on my job here. It is tempting to practice those advanced skills and delegation while on the job, but I would be stepping out of my bounds of practice as an LPN.

JOANN: Yes, it sounds as if you are feeling a bit of role conflict now; in the future, you will be functioning on a level that is much different from how you have practiced in the past. I found the role transition from LPN to RN to be tough. It was also a challenge for the staff to adjust to my new role as delegator and manager of care. However challenging, it is a rewarding step in your growth as a professional. Come, let's talk about the role conflict you are experiencing. I have lots of success stories to help you understand what you are experiencing now.

The health care delivery system is extremely complex. Health maintenance and health care provision are the primary functions of the health care delivery system. Laws and standards have been developed to protect society and maintain and promote accountability for safe practice in the health care system. In the vignette, Cal is grappling with the change in this role function as an LPN/LVN, as well as the increased responsibility and accountability he has in fulfilling his new role. In this role, Cal will be even more immersed in legal and ethical decisions that affect his clients and his practice. Today's society is very litigious. It is often the nurse as the patient advocate who is the last line of defense in preventing irreparable damage to a client or family (Griffin, 2012). The best defense a nurse has in preventing harm is to follow the standards of care acting wisely and in a prudent manner in client care. This chapter concentrates on how laws affect nursing and how to help protect your license in the event of a malpractice suit.

Laws are defined as rules for conduct and actions within a society. They are binding for all citizens. Laws are developed by the people of that society and are enforced by a particular authority. US and most Canadian laws are based on English common law. Within the United States, laws are created by local, state, and national governments. They are enforced by officers and agencies of the government and courts.

The law influences many decisions made by nurses. As nursing has evolved to a more independent level, they are more responsible for their actions and decisions. Many situations faced by nurses today involve concerns about protecting client rights, carrying out accepted modes of treatment, and maintaining practice standards. Issues related to confidentiality, competence, safety, and optimal care can pose difficult dilemmas for nurses, especially in a fiscally strapped economy. The legal aspects of health care are closely aligned with ethical concerns. Because societal values and views change before law, law enforcement is the carrying out of ethical "shoulds" (Craven & Hirnle, 2009). Frequently, conflicts in the law can arise from an ethical problem (see Chapter 17).

In this chapter, we introduce the general concepts of law. There are opportunities for you to consider legal implications for your own practice. Although you will not emerge as an expert in legal issues, you will have a greater understanding of the concepts and a better appreciation of these principles for your own practice. You will also have an increased appreciation for the role transition that you are making in terms of legal responsibilities.

● LEGAL CONSIDERATIONS

This portion of the chapter provides brief explanations of legal terminology and introduces you to legal concepts that are important in your nursing practice. The expanded work role of the nurse necessitates that each nurse remain informed of current laws and regulations that affect the health care system. Origins and classifications of law in the United States are discussed. In addition, issues related to accountability, contracts, negligence, malpractice, and liability are introduced. An important part of this section is a brief examination of legal issues and public policies that affect nursing practice. You have an opportunity to consider several legal issues and their impact on your work world. Critical thinking activities provide an opportunity to apply legal concepts to the practice world.

● SOURCES OF LAW

The health care system is affected by several sources of law. In the United States, there are four sources: constitutional, statutory, common, and administrative laws.

Constitutional Law

The US Constitution guarantees particular fundamental freedoms to all people in the United States. Constitutional law affects nurses by protecting their basic rights. For example, freedom of speech and the right to privacy are rights that patients and nurses have as US citizens. There are controversies in constitutional laws that can affect health care workers. For example, the right to bear arms in an increasingly violent world and the rights of all citizens to have health insurance affect nurses and nursing care.

Statutory Law

Legislative bodies at the local, state, and federal levels enact laws that are formalized, written, and voted on by the appropriate legislators. Every time a legislative body passes a law, the law expands. The expansion of these and other laws makes their compliance a challenge for health care practitioners, individuals they affect, and health care agencies. For example, the changes in Medicare reimbursement for elder citizens have a profound effect on nursing and health care.

Although the administration of the nurse practice act was passed under administrative law, it is interpreted and enacted on by state statutory law. To change statutory law, amendments or repeals must be agreed on by the assigned legislators. Other federal statutes that fall under statutory law are included in Display 16.1. The Good Samaritan laws enacted in most states and the Oregon Death With Dignity Act of 1994 (which legalizes physician-assisted suicide with some restrictions) are other types of state statutory laws.

Common Law

"Common law derives from common usage, custom, and judicial law" (Ellis & Hartley, 2008, p. 290). This type of law is based on court judgments, decisions, and decrees. The interpretation of the earlier law is called a legal precedent. The principle of *stare decisis* ("let the decision stand") evolved when courts began to present written decisions based on earlier court cases; the same rules and principles are applied. In other words, if one court has previously made a decision for a particular case and another court has a similar case, the same decision will be made, citing the

---

display 16.1   **Examples of Federal Statutes of Statutory Law**

EMERGENCY MEDICAL TREATMENT AND ACTIVE LABOR LAW (EMTALA)

This law prevents hospitals from transferring those who are unable to pay to other hospitals. Also called the "antidumping law."

HEALTH INSURANCE PORTABILITY AND ACCOUNTABILITY ACT OF 1996 (HIPPA)

This federal law was enacted to prevent the release of health information without the patient's authorization.

PATIENT SELF-DETERMINATION ACT OF 1990 AND OMNIBUS BUDGET RECONCILIATION ACT OF 1990

This law was enacted to allow clients to make decisions regarding their end-of-life care and to require medical personnel to inquire if patients have a living will or health care proxy. It is in effect for all federally funded hospitals.

precedent of the earlier case. New rules will be made if the precedent is no longer applicable or is outdated. Although the decisions are considered binding within the court's jurisdiction, they are guidelines for other jurisdictions. These laws were developed so that all would be tried fairly under the law and no one group would be favored over another. Examples of violations of common law include patient abandonment, failure to obtain informed consent, and failure to accept a client's right to refuse treatment.

Administrative Law

Administrative law is sometimes called regulatory law. These laws are created by administrative agencies directed by the executive portion of the government to take the pressure off the courts and the government to try special cases. For example, the nurse practice acts are formed by state statutory law, but the authority to regulate these acts is given to an administrative agency overseen by the state's governor. Regulations developed and approved by that agency are considered to be administrative laws. The National Labor Relations Board is another regulatory agency that can affect nursing, especially in the area of contract law and collective bargaining. Some examples of violations of regulatory laws include practicing nursing with an expired license, failure to report unethical nursing conduct, and writing false information on a nursing license application. These can lead to suspension and possible revocation of a nursing license and sometimes lead to criminal convictions. The vast majority of violations of the nurse practice act involve drugs and alcohol (Cherry & Jacob, 2008).

● CLASSIFICATIONS OF LAW

There are various ways to classify laws. The following types of law presented are those that have direct implications for nursing practice. Three types of laws are presented: civil, criminal, and contract.

Civil Law

Civil law is the protection of individual rights and the governance of conduct between individuals and private organizations (Roux & Halstead, 2009). A violation of civil law is called a tort. Nurses and other health care workers are affected by civil law because malpractice and negligence cases fall within civil law. Torts fall under the category of civil law. "Tort law establishes rules for socially reasonable conduct and imposes liability on a party, a 'wrong-doer', for unreasonable conduction" (Roux & Halsread, p. 364). An intentional tort is one in which there was a conscious intent of harm (eg, assault or false imprisonment). Unintentional torts are occurrences where there was no intent to cause harm. Display 16.2 provides examples of intentional and unintentional torts that could be levied against the professional nurse. By far, the most frequent lawsuits against nurses involve civil law and unintentional torts (Craven & Hirnle, 2009). The result of a guilty verdict in a civil law case means that the defendant (accused) must pay damages to the plaintiff (person suing). In a civil court, the plaintiff has the burden of proof, whereas in a criminal court, the state must prove the defendant guilty beyond a reasonable doubt.

display 16.2	Intentional and Unintentional Torts Leading to Potential Liability

INTENTIONAL TORT

Fraud
Assault and battery
Defamation of character
Invasion of privacy

UNINTENTIONAL TORT

Omitting important assessment data
Failure to establish priorities of care
Teaching not documented
Client falls out of bed or is burned from intervention
Wrong medication given to wrong client

Criminal Law

Criminal law involves crimes an individual commits against society or the public's general welfare. They usually involve a willful intentional act of disregard for the safety, well-being, or life of another. Although the most common criminal violation by nurses is practicing with an expired license (Catalano, 2009), some acts are so serious and reckless that nurses can be brought up on criminal charges (Cherry & Jacob, 2008). Therefore, an unintentional act on the part of a nurse could be tried in criminal court if the nurse's action had dire consequences. This is called criminal negligence or reckless endangerment and is tried as a felony.

There are two types of criminal charges that can be levied against a nurse. The most minor is a misdemeanor. Types of misdemeanors include traffic violations, writing bad checks, or misuse of a controlled substance. The latter is one of the more frequent violations for nurses and can result in action by the local government and the state board of nursing. A misdemeanor usually results in fines, community service, and or a prison term of no more than 1 year.

A felony is a major type of criminal law violation. Conviction of a felony results in a nurse going to jail, heavier fines, and possibly a death sentence. The most recent notorious conviction of a nurse for a multiple murder felonies is the intentional deaths by overdosing caused by Charles Cullen in New Jersey and Pennsylvania.

NCLEX–RN *Might Ask*

16.1

A nurse accidentally administers an incorrect dose of morphine sulfate to a client. Which source of law best addresses this situation?

A. Civil law
B. Criminal law
C. Common law
D. Administrative law

· *See Appendix A for correct answer and rationale.*

Contract Law

Contract law is about the agreements that are formed between two parties in which there is a duty or an obligation involved. Contracts are written or oral, and particular duties may be clearly stated or less definitively implied. Nurses generally become involved with contract law with employee and employer agreements. In the past 20 years, amendments to the original Labor Relations Act have allowed nurses to form collective bargaining units. In the bargaining process, the employer and employees agree on a contract that is legally binding for both parties. The collective bargaining process is complex. If you are employed in a setting that has a union contract, it is essential that you seek the information needed for you to make informed decisions from your collective bargaining representatives.

● ACCOUNTABILITY

The term accountability has become a primary focus for nurses as they have moved toward greater professionalization and independence. Accountability means that the nurse accepts responsibility for her or his own actions or behaviors. According to the American Nurses Association (ANA) standards and the state nurse practice acts, nurses are responsible for demonstrating competence, sound judgment, and critical thinking in their roles as caregivers. As a supervisor of LPN/LVNs and unlicensed assitive personnels (UAPs), the nurse must ensure safe care by delegating only routine care and evaluating the results of the delegated care (Display 16.3). A nurse can delegate tasks, but she or he cannot delegate any aspect of professional judgment or decision making about a client's needs. If the nurse delegates a task that a UAP is not competent to perform, the nurse may be liable if harm befalls the client. However, if the UAP does a task on his or her own without consulting the nurse and the task is beyond his or her scope of training, the UAP, and not the nurse, would be liable for negligence. "Negligence is defined as failure to act in a reasonable and prudent manner" (Cherry & Jacob, 2008, p. 154). The difference between negligence and malpractice is that malpractice usually refers to professional behaviors that are held to a higher professionally agreed upon standards.

As a student nurse, you are also accountable. You should perform only skills you are competent to perform, and you should never attempt anything invasive without

---

display **16.3** **Guidelines for Delegating to Other Healthcare Personnel**

- Is the task delegated "routine care?"
- Do agency policies cover the task delegated?
- Is the person delegated to competent to perform the care?
- Will the delegated individual be able to perform the task in a timely manner?
- Are you available to provide assistance to the person if needed?
- Does the task require assessment, planning, and evaluation? If so, the nurse should assume the task.

the direction/presence of your instructor. The standard of care you are held to is that of a professional nurse, not a student and not an LPN/LVN. Before you perform any skill, ask your clinical supervisor if you are unclear about what to do. Client safety is the most important issue and supersedes your learning experiences.

Evidence-Based Practice and Delegation

Research studies support the lack of education and practice of nurse delegation skills in basic nursing programs (Conger, 1994; Parsons, 2004). Since all models predict the shortage of nurses to perform basic care, this is a role of the nurse that will be enhanced in coming years. "Studies have shown an increase in confidence and job satisfaction in nurses who participate in delegation education and practice" (McInnis & Parsons, 2009, p. 468) using delegation decision-making models like the ANA model. To look up the ANA delegation model, visit this Web site: http://nursingworld.org/MainMenuCategories/ ThePracticeofProfessionalNursing/NursingStandards/ANAPrinciples/Principles-for-Delegation/PrinciplesforDelegationhtml.aspx (Last accessed 2.25.11).

Documentation

A major factor in determining accountability and liability is complete and competent documentation. Nurses are increasingly held responsible or liable for information that is either included or not included in reports and documentation. The work setting does not change the need for accurate and complete documentation. Generally, the nurse remains responsible for a major portion of the client record. Accurate, descriptive, and impeccable documentation provides and ensures that the nurse has met the standard of care. It is also a critical component in preventing lawsuits. If compliance with internal and external standards is met, the case will usually not go to court and may be settled without a trial. The old axiom, "If it's not documented, it wasn't done" holds truth with legal issues. Documentation is the nurses' best defense against legal action brought against him/her. Documentation is one of the first items to be subpoenaed by a plaintiff's lawyer and is usually in his or her hands prior to a nurse's summons.

To reduce omissions and cut down on the time required to chart, many agencies are adopting flow sheets and computerized charting that covers the normal standards of care. Coupled with charting by exception, where only abnormal results and ongoing problems need be addressed, such flow sheets maintain the legal requirements and standards, but the time required to complete them is more in tune with the nurse's busy day. Documentation of falls and of skin and wound disruptions in long-term care is extremely important because these are the first and second leading cases of litigation (Chizek, 2006). Regardless of the setting in which the nurse works, clear, objective, and timely documentation protects everyone. For tips on how to avoid legal problems with your documentation, see Display 16.4.

Standards of Practice

Another aspect of accountability is the need for a profession to determine the aspects for which its members are accountable. The ANA has developed standards

---

display 16.4   **Tips for Preventing Legal Problems With Documentation**

1. Be thorough.
2. Stick to objective data and occurrences.
3. Be honest.
4. Do not blame others.
5. Note correct times.
6. Complete all forms accurately.

Adapted from Springhouse (2005). *Documentation in action.* Philadelphia, PA: Lippincott Williams & Wilkins.

---

of nursing practice, service, and education. These standards provide the means to assess the competency of the nurse members. In general, standards of practice have a common reasonable person rule. This rule assumes that the expected action of a nurse would be held to that of another nurse with similar education and experience (Catalano, 2009). Therefore, during a trial, a nurse expert witness would be called on to verify that standard of practice. The expert witness would be used for the judge and jury.

• LIABILITY, NEGLIGENCE, AND MALPRACTICE

The expanded roles of nurses and the growing knowledge base have increased the responsibility of the nurse. With increased responsibility, nurses are also more likely to encounter issues of liability. In this section, definitions for the terms liability, negligence, malpractice, and risk management are provided. In addition, issues related to risk management and avoiding litigation are presented. You also have the opportunity to differentiate the role of the LPN/LVN and the RN in situations related to liability.

Liability

Liability and legal responsibility are essentially synonymous terms. As a nurse, you are responsible for maintaining standards of care. If an action or lack of an action fails to maintain a standard and results in harm to the client, the nurse is liable or legally responsible. For example, the nurse is expected to administer medications safely and on time. If a client receives the wrong medication and is harmed as a result, that nurse is liable.

Negligence

Negligence is defined as "conduct that fall below a standard of care" (Potter & Perry, 2009, p. 332). It results in harm of another. To be negligent, the actions of an individual, believed to have made a mistake, would be compared with those of a person with similar training to determine if the actions taken were reasonable and prudent or below the acceptable level. Negligence could be levied against a parent if they failed to exercise safe care of their child by leaving a child unattended in a hot car; this is not wise or prudent care of another person by any adult. UAPs can be tried for negligence, but they cannot be tried for malpractice because they are not considered professionals.

Malpractice

Malpractice is also called professional negligence/malpractice. Professionals are expected to maintain a reasonable standard of action that has been defined by the specific profession. A professional is held liable for malpractice when he or she does not practice as his or her professional colleagues with similar knowledge and education would have in a similar circumstance. A negligent act is considered malpractice only if it is done by a professional who is conducting professional responsibilities. An example of professional malpractice might include failure to follow building codes and stresses for a high-rise building by an architect. That architect could be subject to malpractice if that building collapsed. The evolution of nursing to a more professional model has not been without the burden of accountability that comes with it. Due to this and other causes, nurses have been increasingly involved in malpractice suits in the past decades. To differentiate negligence from malpractice, an example is in order. If a nurse caused a car accident, she or he would be held only to a negligence standard, not to a higher malpractice standard because she or he is not exercising professional judgment while driving a car. However, if a nurse infuses intravenous solution into an infant at the rate used for an adult and the action causes brain damage in the infant, the nurse is held to the malpractice standard. Display 16.5 provides definitions of the terms liability, negligence, and malpractice.

For a plaintiff (party with the complaint) to be awarded damages, the lawyer must prove that the actions of the defendant (the nurse) had three essential characteristics: the nurse had a duty to the plaintiff, violated a standard of care (breach of duty occurred), and harm was directly related to the nurse's (direct causation) actions. Finally, the result of these characteristics is that the pain and suffering caused would be (damages) awarded monetarily. Display 16.6 gives a brief explanation of these terms.

Often, the terms described in the preceding paragraphs strike a chord of fear in nurses. Although the following information may not remove the fear, it will make you aware and assist you in prevention of litigation proceedings (lawsuits). As an

---

d i s p l a y 16.5   **Definitions of Liability, Negligence, and Malpractice**

Liability: Legal responsibility for actions that do not reflect the standard of care and cause harm, or a failure to act to prevent harm

Negligence: An unreasonable or careless act or the failure to act in a reasonable and prudent manner that results in harm to an individual or group

Malpractice: Professional negligence; an act or failure to act by a professional in a reasonable and prudent manner in conducting professional duties as defined by members of the profession

---

display 16.6   **The Four Ds of a Successful Lawsuit**

Duty: The nurse has a duty to the client (usually found on assignment sheet or chart)
Dereliction of Duty: A standard of care was violated
Direct Cause: The nurse's actions caused harm (usually hardest to prove by the defense)
Damages: A money amount to be awarded to the client because of pain/suffering.
In order for the plaintiff (person charging the complaint) to be awarded damages, the plaintiff must prove duty, dereliction of duty, and direct cause

---

LPN/LVN moving into the RN role, it is important to differentiate your newer responsibilities.

NCLEX–RN *Might Ask*   16.2

The scope of nursing practice is legally defined by

  A. state nurse practice acts.
  B. professional nursing organizations.
  C. hospital policy and procedure manuals.
  D. physicians in the employing institutions.

• See Appendix A for correct answer and rationale.

● RISK MANAGEMENT

Risk management is a system designed to promote safe practices in the institutional environment (Griffin, 2012). Applied to nursing, it refers to the process of identifying risks, preventing, and reducing the occurrence of potential hazards (Potter & Perry, 2009). Health care institutions employ a person identified as the risk management officer or some similar title. This person has the responsibility of reviewing all the problems that occur at the place of employment, identifying common elements of the problems, and developing methods to reduce the risk of their recurrence. Although this person is an excellent resource, it is the nurses, their managers, and staff who are at the front line 24/7 identifying problems and taking steps to resolve them.

One of the primary tools to review problems is the incident or occurrence report. When an error is made or discovered, or something extraordinary occurs that results in harm or potential harm, an incident report is completed. Near misses or situations where an event almost occurred are also included in incident/occurrence reporting. This report identifies the nature of the incident, who was involved, and what steps were taken to remedy the situation. The incident/occurrence report was not designed to be a punitive tool against employees but is a means to study a problem or series of problems and take steps to prevent recurrence. Information should be as factual and complete as possible. Excuses for behaviors or actions should not be included. In addition, facts about the incident and health care workers responses should be documented in the medical record if a client was involved. However, it is important that no mention of the incident report be included in written form (most authorities recommend that the incident report should not be mentioned). If an event results in death or a serious physical or psychological injury, immediate action in the form of a sentinel event is required by the Joint Commission of Accreditation of Healthcare Organizations.

Risk management can also be applied to the individual employee. Although nurses do not generally call themselves risk managers, many of the procedures and steps that nurses use are methods to reduce harm to clients or employees and reduce the possibility of litigation. As an LPN/LVN, you are aware of the importance of following procedures, documenting your observations, and reporting to the appropriate people. These methods not only ensure quality care of your clients but also reduce the risk of injury to your clients and others, including yourself. As an RN, this will not change, but the responsibility for care that clients receive will be greater and broader scope. You are a care provider and a manager of care (see Chapter 15). This role necessitates that you are managing care for a group of clients but are not necessarily in direct supervision of that care. That also means that it is up to you to ensure that procedures and policies are followed and that client needs are being met.

As you move into the RN role, part of being a risk manager will involve identifying common problems and developing solutions to eliminate or reduce the incidence of particular situations. This should sound familiar on two levels. First, the nursing process uses the method of assessment, diagnosis, planning, implementation, and evaluation. In essence, when a nurse is looking for solutions to common problems, she or he is using a problem-solving method. Second, you may be familiar or involved with some form of quality assurance or quality improvement in your place of employment. This system is used by health care agencies to monitor and identify methods to improve services to the consumer. In that many of the consumer services are care related, RNs are heavily involved in quality assurance or improvement programs. As you progress through your ADN program, you will become more aware of the need to be a consumer advocate and to be involved in the assurance of quality care to clients. You may be asked to identify and implement an in-service or a procedure for a group of employees. For example, you may have observed that certified nursing assistants (CNAs) are unfamiliar with the potential risk in transferring clients without a walker after they have undergone total hip replacement. To provide a constructive remedy, you could develop a procedure/policy or conduct an in-service. As an RN, it will be essential for you to be involved in risk management methods for yourself and your colleagues. Display 16.7 provides some tips on using risk management techniques to avoid legal ramifications.

---

display 16.7   **Risk Management Tips to Avoid Legal Ramifications**

1. Listen to patients and families; they usually sue because they are angry.
2. Stay within the scope of your nursing practice acts and your professional competency level.
3. Act with the client's safety foremost in mind.
4. Know your agency's policies/standards/procedures.
5. Seek continuing education opportunities to increase cognitive, psychomotor, and affective skills.
6. Maintain and understand your professional liability insurance.
7. Promote nursing input by volunteering to be on committees that review incidents.

thinking critically

You have been assigned by your nurse manager to do an in-service for LPNs and UAPs regarding the legal implications of documentation. In your role as an RN, what would you include in this in-service? What is essential to include? What might you use to assist you in illustrating the key points?

● LEGALLY SENSITIVE AREAS THAT AFFECT NURSING PRACTICE

A variety of issues within health care today can have an effect on nursing. The technical advances in medicine and the increased knowledge of consumers have undoubtedly increased the legal implications for nursing. This section addresses a few of these issues. It is not meant to be a complete list.

Advance Directives

Advance directives are documents that competent people execute to have control over their future health care. Examples of these documents are living wills and durable power of attorney. A living will, signed by an individual, indicates that her or his life is not to be sustained by extraordinary measures. Although this document is not always considered legally binding, it does provide information about the desires of the individual. Individuals also use durable power of attorney for future health care decisions. With this type of agreement, a person can assign another individual as a substitute decision maker, or health care proxy, as surrogate decision maker. Generally, if the document is signed and notarized, it is considered binding. A lawyer's advice is not necessary to complete an advance directive. Hospitals and support groups such as Compassion in Dying and Partners in Caring offer websites with examples of advance directives for interested individuals and families. Where problems occur in implementing advance directives are when the family members are not aware of or in agreement with the patient's desires. Issues can also result when individuals have life partners outside of a marriage relationship that is legally binding. In these cases, the partner needs to have a durable power of attorney in order to help make decisions, especially in life-threatening or critical emergent situations (Ellis & Hartley, 2008). Nurses can encourage patients to make their family members aware of the above. The individual initiating the advance directive can change it at any time.

Advance directives can affect nursing in several ways. The first is that the RN must be aware of federal and agency policies regarding advance directives, especially the Patient Self-Determination Act of 1990. For example, agencies that receive federal reimbursement require that nurses ask clients or families about advance directives as part of the admission assessment. It is also the nurse's responsibility to inform physicians about client wishes regarding a living will or if the family is experiencing conflict about the wishes expressed in the document of durable power of attorney. Another responsibility is to provide support for decisions that the client and family have made. Making end-of-life decisions is painful at best. Although advance directives have not solved all issues related to these decisions, they are at least a legal method to ease the decision-making process. Whatever the outcome, it is essential that the nurse document all events that occur in relationship to advance directives.

Informed Consent

Another issue that has many legal ramifications is informed consent. "Under the doctrine of informed consent, the physician or advanced practice nurse has a duty to disclose information so that the patient can make intelligent decisions" (Cherry & Jacob, 2008). By definition, this means that a client must be provided with information about a procedure or treatment that informs the client of the benefits, risks, and alternatives as well as the problems with not having the procedure/treatment. In this way, the client is able to make a voluntary, informed decision about the procedure or treatment. Consent must be given without coercion and may be withdrawn at any time the client changes his or her mind. Clients may also refuse a particular treatment, although there have been incidents in which courts overruled the wishes of a parent or legal guardian. If a client does not believe procedures for obtaining informed consent were followed, he or she may sue for assault and battery (see Display 16.8 for definitions of these terms) or for negligence in failing to obtain informed consent.

The nurse's responsibility in informed consent may be to witness the signature of a client when signing the consent form. The nurse's signature identifies that the client has signed the form. The responsibility for providing risks, benefits, and alternatives to the client rests with the medical provider (physician, nurse practitioner, etc.). Before a nurse witnesses a client's signature, she or he should ask the client if the medical provider has provided an explanation of the procedure. At this time, the nurse may reinforce information given by the physician or inform the physician if the client has any questions or concerns. The nurse can also document the client's understanding of the procedure as related by the client. The RN is responsible for notifying the physician if the client does not understand or is having difficulty accepting what is occurring. The nurse can protect herself by careful, judicious documentation regarding acceptance and refusal and what steps the nurse took to rectify each situation. It is also important for RNs to be familiar with their particular state's laws regarding informed consent and each agency's policies so that RNs can be in compliance with all regulations.

If the patient decides against the procedure and wants to leave the facility against medical advice, the nurse is responsible for notifying the health care provider. She or he is also responsible for explaining the harm that may come to the client if she or he continues with this course of action. Most institutions and facilities have a document known as the Against Medical Advice (AMA) form. An exception to the informed consent doctrine includes emergency situations. In this instance that includes the patient who is unconscious and unable to give consent or incompetent, the institution would do what a reasonably prudent person would do, which is treat the patient (Catalano, 2009).

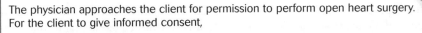

| display 16.8 | Definitions of Assault and Battery |

Assault: An intentional act of one person that causes another person to fear that she or he will be injured or touched in an offensive way; touching does not actually need to occur

Battery: If the act of touching or injuring actually takes place, the act is called battery. Medical treatments and procedures done without prior consent may be considered assault and battery, with exceptions made for emergency treatment

NCLEX–RN *Might Ask* (16.3)

The physician approaches the client for permission to perform open heart surgery. For the client to give informed consent,

   A. the nurse must leave the room.
   B. the client must realize that any information gained from the procedure may be used for research.
   C. the client must be informed about the benefits and risks of the procedure, as well as alternatives to the procedure.
   D. the patient may not withdraw consent once it is given.

· *See Appendix A for correct answer and rationale.*

● CONFIDENTIALITY AND THE RIGHT TO PRIVACY

All patients have the right to have information regarding them honored, respected, and protected. Confidentiality of information is now federally protected under HIPAA. This law states that information regarding the patient may only be given with written authorization of the client, or it could be considered invasion of privacy. Those who are not involved with the care of the client should not have access to the client's information. Although HIPAA is a law, it is only an articulation of what has been a time-honored nursing value: shared trust. As an LPN/LVN, you see, hear, and have become comfortable with confidential information as an everyday occurrence. As an RN student going into a variety of agencies, you have to renew your commitment to patient privacy. This means that as a student nurse who is caring for the client, you must not take identifiable information from the clinical setting. If you do, you can be liable and fines may be levied against the agency involved for any harm that results in the sharing of this information. How could this occur? If you lose patient assignment sheets, nursing care plans, medication information, and charting references with the client's name on them and they can be identified, an innocent breach of confidentiality has occurred. If you include the name, room number, institution, and medical/nursing needs of a client in a school nursing course paper, a breach has occurred. The RN student nurse is held to the same standard as an RN, and the nurse has both a legal and an ethical duty to protect the confidentiality rights of patients in his or her care. Your course professors are valuable resources when it comes to client confidentiality, so you should ask them any questions and concerns regarding client privacy issues.

Patient privacy must be maintained within agencies and for all electronic information. Faxed and computer transmissions of client information are especially vulnerable to interception by those for whom it was not intended. This does not mean that information regarding patients cannot be faxed or sent electronically. It means that the sender must take all reasonable and prudent actions so that it gets to the right place and have the client's authorization to send this information. As a student nurse who is probably using e-mail and the Internet to communicate with your instructor and other students, you should not "talk" online or send any information electronically that can be traced back to a client.

• DEFAMATION

Another legal issue that is related to confidentiality is defamation. An individual may be held liable for sharing information that is considered damaging to that person's reputation. Libel refers to written defamation, and slander is the term for oral defamation. Nurses traditionally have difficulties with defamation issues in relation to client confidentiality. For example, a client is admitted with a medical diagnosis of pneumonia. The medical record reveals the client has multidrug-resistant tuberculosis. Nurses with access to that record tell various people the client has active tuberculosis. The client later claims her business, a beauty salon, endured economic losses as a result of the disclosures by the nursing staff, and sues for slander.

Defamation of character may also be charged by a health care provider who believes that statements made by another professional are false, malicious, and have caused harm. There are accepted mechanisms for confidentially reporting inappropriate care or errors, and these should be used rather than making statements to uninvolved third parties (Ellis & Hartley, 2008).

Defamation issues are often considered by participants to be innocent and harmless but may be injurious to a person's reputation. As an RN, it is essential that you recognize potentially harmful defamation and be alert to issues in which other employees are engaged. You may find it necessary to plan appropriate in-services or to speak with employees you are supervising.

Professional Boundaries

The issue of professional boundaries has stimulated the development of guidelines established for proper nurse–patient relationships in the US state boards of nursing (SBN) and Canadian provinces and territories:

> If someone were to file a complaint with your SBN alleging that you failed to establish and maintain professional boundaries according to your state's practice act or board of nursing regulations, a disciplinary investigation could be brought against you, risking your license (Wright, 2006, p. 52).

What exactly are professional boundaries? The nurse's role is to develop therapeutic relationships with the client or family. There is a breach in the professional boundary when a nurse uses his or her position of power to meet the nurse's needs. The nature of a nurse's work places him or her in close physical and psychological

display 16.9   Examples of Professional Boundary Violations

Physical abuse
Verbal abuse
Emotional abuse
Sexual abuse
Financial abuse
Neglect

contact with another. But with that comes the responsibility to stay in what the National Council of State Boards of Nursing calls the "zone of helpfulness." This means that the nurse must not be either under- or overinvolved with the client. Some kinds of breaches in professional boundaries are intentional and egregious, such as rape or extortion of money. Others are much more innocent in nature, for example, spending more time with one client over another or dating a client. Questions a nurse should ask himself or herself when evaluating professional boundaries might include the following:

- Am I following the constituents of the nurse practice act?
- Is my behavior within the ANA *Code of Ethics*?
- Are my actions in the best interest of this client/family?
- Would another nurse find my actions acceptable?

Some examples of the more infamous violations of professional boundaries can be seen in Display 16.9.

thinking critically

Research a current legal–medical issue that has relevance for nursing practice. For example, examine recent articles about assisted suicide, right to life, medical guardianship, or nurse negligence. Analyze these articles in class with attention to RN role and responsibility.

● CONCLUSION

This chapter emphasizes that nurses have legal responsibilities. Many issues that nurses face require legal knowledge. Legal responsibilities are pertinent to everything a nurse does. Standards of care, licensure laws, negligence and malpractice, and other issues related to liability determine the nurse's responsibilities. Methods such as accuracy in documentation or the performance of a procedure, as well as professional accountability and responsibility ensure legal accountability.

When making the transition from LPN/LVN to RN, students begin to recognize that there are legal consequences for the work nurses do. If a nurse does not practice as defined by legal standards and the client is harmed, the nurse is liable. The most important concern for nurses is the rights of clients, followed by the rights and responsibilities of the nurses' colleagues.

The nursing profession will continue to be challenged by changes in legal issues. Society will be faced with dilemmas that have no answers. The role of government in determining legal answers for ethical questions will bring forth other issues for nurses. Awareness of your personal and professional values will assist you in clarifying legal issues. Continuing self-growth and development will enhance your ability to deal with legal dilemmas. Although you may hope you are never placed in a situation of conflict, it is likely to occur. Be informed. Be prepared. Be knowledgeable.

student exercises

As an RN, you have been hired to be the evening supervisor in a 50-bed, long-term care facility. After an orientation to the role and responsibilities, you are officially the evening charge nurse. There are two units in this agency; one unit is designated for clients with Alzheimer disease. Each unit has one LPN/LVN who acts as the charge person, one CNA with advanced training to administer oral medications, and three CNAs to provide basic care to the clients.

1. As the RN supervisor, what do you need to know from a legal perspective to do your job? Think in terms of delegating, competencies of other personnel, and your responsibility for the care that clients receive.

2. From a legal perspective, what is your responsibility if an employee practices unsafely?

References

Catalano, J. (2009). *Nursing now! Today's issues, tomorrow's trends* (5th ed.). Philadelphia, PA: F.A. Davis.

Cherry, B., & Jacob, S. R. (2008). *Contemporary nursing: Issues, trends, and management* (4th ed.). St. Louis, MO: CV Mosby.

Chizek, M. (2006). Litigation in long-term care. *Advance for Nurses*, 8(1), 32, 41.

Conger, M. (1994). Delegation decision-making. *Journal of Nursing Staff Development*, 9(3), 131–133.

Craven, R., & Hirnle, C. (2009). *Fundamentals of nursing: Human health and foundation* (6th ed.). Philadelphia, PA: Lippincott Williams & Wilkins.

Ellis, J., & Hartley, C. (2008). *Nursing in today's world: Challenges, issues and trends* (9th ed.). Philadelphia, PA: Lippincott Williams & Wilkins.

Griffin, D. (2012). *Hospitals: What they are and how they work* (4th ed.). Sudbury, MA: Jones and Bartlett Learning.

McInnis, L., & Parsons, L. (2009). Thoughtful nursing practice: Reflections on nurse delegation decision-making. *Nursing Clinics of North America*, 44(4), 461–470.

Parsons, L. (2004). Delegation decision-making by registered nurses who provide direct care for patients with spinal cord impairment. *SCI Nurse*, 2(1), 20–28.

Potter, P., & Perry, A. (2009). *Fundamentals of nursing* (7th ed.). Philadelphia, PA: Elsevier Mosby.

Roux, G., & Halstead, J. (2009). *Issues and trends in nursing: Essential knowledge for today and tomorrow*. Sudbury, MA: Jones and Barlett Publishers.

Springhouse. (2005). *Documentation in action*. Philadelphia, PA: Lippincott Williams & Wilkins.

Wright, L. (2006). Violating professional boundaries. *Nursing*, 26(3), 52–54.

Suggested Reading

Ashley, R. (2004). The fifth element of negligence. *Critical Care Nurse*, 24(5), 80–82.

Ashley, R. (2005). Is malpractice insurance important? *Critical Care Nurse*, 25(6), 54.

Brent, J. (2001). *Nurses and the law: A guide to principles and application* (2nd ed.). Philadelphia, PA: W.B. Saunders.

Brooke, N. (2003). How good a Samaritan should you be? *Nursing 2003*, 33(6), 46–47.

Chitty, K. (2007). *Professional nursing: Concepts & challenges* (5th ed.). Philadelphia, PA: Elsevier Saunders.

Frank-Stromborg, M., & Ganschow, J. (2002). How HIPPA will change your practice. *Nursing 2002*, 32(9), 54–57.

Giordano, K. (2003). Examining nursing malpractice: A defense attorney's perspective. *Critical Care Nurse*, 23(2), 104–107.

Grace, P., & McLaughlin, M. (2005). When consent isn't informed enough. *American Journal of Nursing*, *103*(6), 4, 90–104.

Khoury, M. (2003). False statements. *Advance for Nurses, 5*(20), 25–26.

Laboy, A. (2001). How to survive a lawsuit. *Nursing Spectrum, 10*(18), 19.

Manno, M. (2006). Preventing adverse drug events. *Nursing, 36*(3), 56–61.

Martin, R. (2003). HIPPA: Myths and misconceptions. *Advance for Nurses, 5*(26), 29–30.

National Council of State Boards of Nursing. (1995). *Delegation: Concepts and decision-making process.* Chicago, IL: Author.

Polston, M. (1999). Whistleblowing: Does the law protect you? *American Journal of Nursing, 99*(1), 26–31.

Sheehan, J. (2001). Delegating to UAPs: A practical guide. *RN, 64*(11), 65–66.

Springhouse (2004). *Nurse's legal handbook* (5th ed.). Springhouse, PA: Author.

 On the WEB

http://www.safestaffingsaveslives.org/WhatisSafeStaffing/ SafeStaffingPrinciples/PrinciplesforDelegationhtml.aspx: American Nurses Association. Principles for delegation. (Last accessed 7.24.2011)

http://www.aalnc.org: American Association of Legal Nurse Consultants. (Last accessed 7.24.2011)

http://findarticles.com/p/articles/mi_qa3932/is_200301/ai_ n9231380: Information on HIPPA. (Last accessed 7.24.2011)

http://www.nursingworld.org/MainMenuCategories/ANA Marketplace/ANAPeriodicals/OJIN/TableofContents/ Volume102005/No2May05/tpc27ntr16015.aspx: Article on how HIPPA has changed the nursing world. (Last accessed 7.24.2011)

https://www.ncsbn.org/Working_with_Others.pdf: Position paper on delegation from the NCSBN. (Last accessed 7.24.2011)

http://nursingworld.org/MainMenuCategories/The- PracticeofProfessionalNursing/NursingStandards/ ANAPrinciples/Principles-for-Delegation/ PrinciplesforDelegationhtml.aspx: ANA Delegation Model (Last accessed 7.24.2011).

17

Ethical Issues

advocate
autonomy
beneficence
bioethics
code of ethics
· deontology
ethical dilemma
ethics

feminist ethics
fidelity
justice
moral distress
moral outrage
morals
nonmaleficence
nursing ethics

paternalism
standards of nursing
teleology
utilitarianism
values
veracity

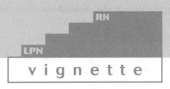

v i g n e t t e

Janet Bieber, LPN, calls you. You are the acting charge RN on a busy rehabilitation unit of a long-term care facility. She tells you Dr. Brown has made rounds. He has ordered a placebo for Mr. Peters, a client who was admitted to your unit several weeks ago after an open reduction and internal fixation of the left hip. Janet says she cannot give the placebo; it is against her beliefs and values. You know that Mr. Peters is frail and elderly with many physiological bases for his pain. You also know that various pharmacological methods have been tried and nothing so far has been able to stop Mr. Peters' pain.

What is the ethical dilemma present in the vignette? What principles of nursing ethics does this involve? Would you, in your new role as charge nurse, have the moral courage to advocate for Mr. Peters? What arguments would you present to Dr. Brown to help sway her away from the placebo and toward more judicious pain management? What kind of a plan would you develop to solve this ethical dilemma?

● ETHICS AND HISTORY

"Ethics is a branch of philosophy dealing with standards of conduct and moral judgments" (Craven & Hirnle, 2009, p. 76). It can also be described as what an individual does to live in relative harmony with his or her fellow man. Ethics are concerned with determining a right act from a wrong act. Often, ethical decisions have to determine the lesser of two evils. Ethical decisions are not based on emotion; instead, they are based on knowledge rather than opinion. Ethics is defined by Marquis and Huston (2009) as

> the systematic study of what a person's conduct and actions ought to be with regard to self, other human beings, and the environment; it is the justification of what is right or good and the study of what a person's life and relationships ought to be, not necessarily what they are. (p. 69)

In the aspect that they define personal choices of good and rightness, ethical decisions transcend those of law. The law is the minimal accepted standard of behavior.

Laws vary from country to country and from society to society. Laws usually change only after the behaviors become acceptable, so laws are slow to change. Where did the discipline of ethics come from, and how did it evolve to the present theories that aid nurses in ethical decision making?

Ethics developed from philosophy (Table 17.1). Grecian thinkers such as Socrates and Plato debated a logical approach to defining what was good or right in human conduct. The Greek, Hippocrates, wrote the Hippocratic Oath, which was the first written code of ethics for physicians. Physicians and philosophers are still debating the tenets of the Hippocratic Oath. Work on theories of ethics continued and included the works of English thinkers such as Jeremy Bentham and John Stuart Mill. They developed and refined the theory of utilitarianism and Immanuel Kant's work on deontology. Nursing ethics developed from these previous theorists and Florence Nightingale's writings. Nightingale supported fundamental nursing concepts such as clean air, good hygiene, improved nutrition, and hospital cleanliness. These were not ideas that were generally supported by the medical community at that time.

Feminists in the 1960s added a woman's perspective to ethical theories. They emphasized that decisions should not be devoid of emotions. "Feminist theories have suggested that another way of being moved to moral action is through the emotions" (Bosek & Savage, 2007, p. 11). Caring and emotional support of patients during experiences are a tie that binds many nurses to those in their care. Many of these concepts were espoused by Florence Nightingale (Display 17.1).

A code of ethics is a document agreed on by practitioners in a discipline that serves as a guide to decision making. It is a professional's moral code and is a public statement about the role of that profession. It is not a static document. Like laws, it evolves to keep pace with a changing profession. Nursing's first code of ethics was born from the Florence Nightingale Pledge. However, it devalued the status of the nurse to that of the "handmaiden" of the physician, and loyalty to the physician was one of its principles. The code of ethics has changed with the changing role of the nurse and has been revised nine times (Bosek & Savage, 2007).

table
17-1   SUMMARY OF NURSING ETHICS HISTORY

Time	Person	Achievement
400–300 BC	Plato, Aristotle Early Christians	Virtue Ethics
400–300 BC	Hippocrates	Hippocratic Oath Father of Modern Medicine
1724–1804	Immanuel Kant	Theory of Deontology
1738–1782	Jeremy Bentham	Principle of Utilitarianism
1806–1873	John Stuart Mill	Refined Utilitarianism
1800–1900	Florence Nightingale	Florence Nightingale Pledge
1960s	Feminists	Emotional, intuitive and relationship aspects of caring

---

display 17.1 **Fundamental Values of Nursing**

Accountability
▸Advocacy
Collaboration
Innovation
Integrity
Leadership
Lifelong learning
Passion and commitment
Quality/excellence commitment
Stewardship

Some of those changes include having the accountability to question a physician's orders, promoting collegiality and collaboration in physician–nurse relationships, and supporting patient self-determination.

● ETHICAL DILEMMAS

An ethical dilemma occurs when a nurse's personal/professional values and morals differ from those of a patient, family, physician, other health care worker; the institution where the nurse works; and the country's laws. In the vignette, Janet Bieber, LPN, does not believe that Mr. Peters' pain will be controlled with the placebo that Dr. Brown has ordered. Janet is acting as an advocate for Mr. Peters and knows that this will not meet his pain control needs. This places Janet and Dr. Brown in conflict. Others variables can add to the dilemma: Perhaps the other staff have pressured Dr. Brown into ordering the placebo. Perhaps the family is not happy with Mr. Peters' pain and is pushing for a solution beyond medication. Display 17.2 lists common nursing ethical dilemmas.

Moral Distress

Because of their close and unique relationship with the patient, nurses make ethical decisions almost every day. At times, a nurse may run the gamut of emotions from a generalized feeling of anxiety to uncertainty to outright moral suffering resulting from this close patient interaction. Moral distress—the feeling one

---

display 17.2 **Common Ethical Problems**

Client's refusal of treatment/medications
Truth telling
Futile care
Participation in research protocols
Breaches in confidentiality
Incompetent or unethical practices by colleagues
Working over time when tired or forced to due to institutional issues

experiences as a result of moral suffering—is more common than anyone antici-pated. Pendry (2007) has defined moral distress as "the physical and emotional suffering that is experienced when constraints (internal or external) prevent one from following the course of action that one believes is right." Although not a new phenomenon, it is being increasingly studied. There is research to support that moral distress and outrage are the reasons why many nurses leave one job for another (Corley, Elswick, Gorman, & Clor, 2001) and why nurses may aban-don nursing for another profession. Moral outrage differs from moral distress in that outrage exists when a nurse observes immoral behaviors but does not participate in them.

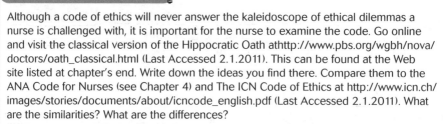

thinking critically

Although a code of ethics will never answer the kaleidoscope of ethical dilemmas a nurse is challenged with, it is important for the nurse to examine the code. Go online and visit the classical version of the Hippocratic Oath athttp://www.pbs.org/wgbh/nova/doctors/oath_classical.html (Last Accessed 2.1.2011). This can be found at the Web site listed at chapter's end. Write down the ideas you find there. Compare them to the ANA Code for Nurses (see Chapter 4) and The ICN Code of Ethics at http://www.icn.ch/images/stories/documents/about/icncode_english.pdf (Last Accessed 2.1.2011). What are the similarities? What are the differences?

Ethics and the Law

In Chapter 16, the laws and their relationship to nursing were explored. Ethical actions are above the law. Laws are what a given government defines as minimal acceptable behavior on the part of an individual or group. "Ethics delineate the highest moral standards of behavior" (Lachman, 2006, p. 4). Changes in the law are a result of changes in the values of society. Table 17.2 differentiates law from ethics. Laws cannot dictate what a person should do in every circumstance; they define what most individuals should do to protect the rights and property of others. They describe only the minimally acceptable standards.

table
17-2 .... LAW AND ETHICS

Ethics	Laws
Unclear, ambiguity exists	Clear rules of conduct
Individual	Impartial
Gray areas	Black and white
Individuals decide	Courts decide
Change with societal attitude changes	Do not keep pace with society
The right things to do	Doing things right
Ethics committee	Legal counsel
Ethical guidelines do not have a formal enforcement and law officers system	Regulated by authorized organizations

Ethics and Religion

Ethical actions go above and beyond religion. Religion is often the starting point for the development of moral thinking and virtues. As with laws, one "cannot assume that an accepted practice of certain religion is an ethical practice in every situation" (Wilkinson & Van Leuven, 2007, p. 1045). Religious beliefs have often led to wars and deaths of entire groups.

• NURSING ETHICS

According to Cherry and Jacob (2008) "nursing ethics is a system of principles concerning the actions of the nurse in his or her relationships with patients, patients' family members, other health care providers, policy makers, and society as a whole" (p. 118). Since nursing ethics start from personal values and morals, it is important that the nurse knows his/her personal philosophy about health care. A nurse, as with most other professionals, has two sets of ethics that are used to guide actions: personal and professional. Personal ethics are developed from values (see Chapter 13 for definitions) learned at an early age. Just like a code of ethics, they change and become more defined as the individual grows and is exposed to various circumstances throughout his or her life cycle. They provide the initial basis that professional ethics are built on. Professional ethics are explored and refined in nursing school and then put into action in the clinical environment when that student

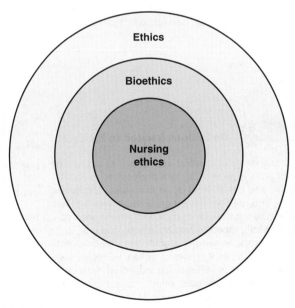

FIGURE 17.1 Model of ethics.

graduates and works as an LPN/LVN. As with the vignette, you as the LPN have already experienced basic professional ethics. You might find the vignette familiar regardless of your practice choice. You may already have firm opinions and feelings about placebos. But are they guided by ethical decision-making principles? Nurses are bound by law and their professional code of ethics to take a firm advocacy stance in an ethically justified manner.

Nursing ethics is a under the larger umbrella of bioethics (Fig. 17.1). Nursing ethics has evolved as nurses have become client advocates. The ethical decisions a nurse makes are far from the same in each case and are not black and white. No two situations about client care are clear and exactly alike because each patient is unique. The nurse needs to make ethical decisions based on professional standards and the ANA's (2001) *Code of Ethics for Nurses With Interpretive Statements.* During the nurse's education, she or he learns the technical skills needed to deliver competent care, but "if nursing care is to be competent, a balance between morality and science must be sought and understood" (Cherry & Jacob, 2008, p. 191). Although the *Code of Ethics for Nurses* provides a guideline to follow, nursing ethical dilemmas have such a diverse spectrum that it will not answer every situation.

In this chapter, we introduce theories and systems of ethics that have influenced the development of nursing ethics and factors that affect ethical decision making. Display 17.3 outlines definitions relevant to nursing ethics.

thinking critically

A nurse's ethical decision-making behavior comes from his or her past and is usually socially constructed by those important and influential people in our early development. Think reflectively about your past philosophy about life and health. Who was the most influential? Did it include a religious perspective? How does this influence your professional perspectives?

display 17.3   Definitions Related to Ethics

Code of ethics: Standards of conduct and values as defined by a profession; forms the basis for ethical decision making by a profession

Values: The ideals and beliefs held by an individual or group; usually influenced by family, society, and religion; have a great impact on behavior

Morals: An individual's standards of right and wrong; formed in childhood (see Chapter 2); also influenced by family, society, and religion

Bioethics: Ethical questions surrounding life and death; questions and concerns regarding quality of life as it relates to advanced technology

Ethical dilemma: A situation in which an individual must choose between two alternatives that are not desirable; often involves examining rights and obligations of particular individuals; choice frequently defended

• ETHICAL THEORIES

Ethical theory is a complex philosophical endeavor. This section is not meant to provide an in-depth examination of various ethical theories but rather to briefly present the primary ethical theories used for ethical decision making in nursing. In general, an ethical theory is used for the purpose of determining the rightness or wrongness of a particular situation. Due to the complex variety of individual situations, the nature of ethical decision making allows not just one theory to apply to each nursing dilemma. In nursing ethics, two systems or theories are predominant: teleology and deontology.

Teleology

Teleology has evolved from a humanistic and outcome-oriented approach to decision making. This system of teleology also is called utilitarianism theory (which refers to the end or outcome). Teleology has two principles: the greatest good for the greatest number and the end justifies the means. These principles are probably familiar to you, but in terms of ethical decision making, they need further examination. Teleology implies that the consequences of actions must be considered—that is, the benefits to many will outweigh the harm to a few. For instance, the allocation of funds may be determined by the number of individuals who benefit from a particular service. Recently, the United States has had several shortages of flu vaccine, causing this vaccine to be rationed to the young, physically debilitated, and health care workers. It was thought if these groups were vaccinated; the greatest good would come for the majority of society.

The advantage of using teleology is that the needs of the majority are considered. In this way, research is promoted when it involves finding the causes of a disease with which many are afflicted or finding treatments that will help many people and are of benefit to a particular company or research institute. The drawback of teleology is that the rights of individuals are not considered. The institution may have greater claim to conducting procedures or treatments without an individual being aware of alternatives; the premise is that the end justifies the means.

Deontology

The second theory that is often used for ethical decision making is called deontology. This system is based on moral principles and obligations and have evolved from Judeo–Christian origins and were further written about in the works of Immanuel Kant. The word "deon" comes from the Greek word "duty." When a nurse uses deontology, he or she is exercising duty to or a respect of others as the primary consideration. For example,

> A nurse might attempt to justify informing the spouse of a patient with a communicable disease against the patient's wishes in order to prevent cross-infection of the spouse. The nurse has a duty to protect the patient's confidentiality and also a duty to protect the public. She would need to inform the patient of her duty to report (mandated by the state). She should also encourage the patient to discuss it with his/her spouse. (Dahnke & Dreher, 2006)

One advantage of using the deontologic approach is that the rights of *each* person are considered. A second advantage is that the obligation to duty and moral thinking is foremost, so the decisions are the same for similar situations. However, it may become difficult to apply the deontological method when the consequence of the decision can be harmful to an individual. For example, the decision to maintain life for any patient regardless of the outcome (futile care) may be difficult when the patient is in constant pain, requiring many invasive and expensive procedures to survive in a vegetative state. Currently, one of the biggest ethical decisions in health care is health insurance for all. This is based upon the deontologic principle that health care should be available to all United States citizens but the dilemma is at what cost?

The Feminist Perspective

Although not a theory in itself, the feminists of the 1960s gave a different perspective to ethics—one might call this perspective "feminist ethics." They supported work done previously but believed that the predominately male perspective of the previous theorist (thought of a scientifically mediated and research based) did not fully explain the intense personal nature of the nurse–patient relationship. Feminists believed that virtues such as emotions, compassion, comfort, nurturing, intuition, and empathetic caring had a place in making ethical decisions. "Feminists argue that it is impossible to avoid being influenced by one's relationship. They see that influence as positive and believe that it should not be muted by an attempt to be objective—because objectivity is impossible anyway" (Wilkinson & Van Leuven, 2007, p. 1058). The problem with viewing ethical dilemmas from the feminist perspective is that it places women back into the subservient, stereotypical role of caregiver. This might also alienate men from entering the nursing profession because it emphasizes nursing as women's work (Williams, 1991).

thinking critically

Review the vignette at the beginning of the chapter. Using the ethics' theories described in the preceding pages, list the advantages and disadvantages of applying the system of teleology, deontology, and the feminist perspective to this situation when making a decision. Be specific regarding the impact on the client and the nurse.

Theoretically, selecting a system for ethical decision making should simplify the process. However, most of us do not necessarily use a particular theory to make an ethical decision and are influenced by many factors, not just a knowledge of ethical theory. Also, one ethical theory may not be appropriate to a given situation. The next part of this chapter examines factors that influence ethical decision making and then moves to a framework for ethical decision making that incorporates the use of ethical theory and recognition of various influences.

● FACTORS THAT INFLUENCE DECISION MAKING

As you further refine your process of studying ethical issues, you must recognize that many factors affect the way you think about something. These factors often overlap or are interdependent. They may also be dynamic because, in a particular situation, circumstances will influence the decision you make. The following section examines the factors that can influence ethical decision making.

Legislative and Judicial Factors

Societal thinking and the resulting legislative and judicial decisions have an obvious impact on the ethical decision-making process. For example, the issue of declaring death has been a dilemma in relation to technological advances. Formerly, the loss of cardiac and respiratory function was the deciding determinant for death. However, with greater abilities to maintain cardiac and respiratory function, medicine and society were compelled to redefine death. This resulted in the concept of brain death, which includes lack of receptivity and unresponsiveness, absence of movements or breathing, no reflexes, and a flat electroencephalogram reading. This definition is widely accepted by most states. The ethical issue for many nurses is related to their own beliefs about the dignity of life, the prolonging of a persistent vegetative state, the harvesting of donor organs from an individual who is brain dead, and supporting the family who may be asked to make decisions. The legality of brain death and declaration of donors has removed some of the uncertainties for nurses regarding ethical considerations.

Science and Technological Advances

In the preceding paragraph, the effect of technological advances on ethical decisions is described. The developments in science and technology have created ethical issues that were unheard of even 20 years ago. For example, the ability to artificially impregnate a woman who is past menopause has caused some governments to consider age limitations for women to bear children. Genetic engineering is a modern phenomenon that not only has the potential to harm humans by genetic alteration but also offers the hope of genetic engineering to conquer disease and organ loss. Fears related to this issue were only the stuff of science fiction a few years ago. These dilemmas created by science and technologies contribute to issues with which nurses are or will be involved. The duty to the client is often obscured by the need to promote science and progress.

Societal Influences

Chapter 2 discusses the development of moral reasoning, as theorized by both Kohlberg and Gilligan. The development of morals and values is influenced by the expectations of society. Changes in societal thinking affect a person's view of what is right and wrong. As an example, the women's movement, the gay rights movement, and the increasing call for an end to sexual harassment have had a great impact on behavior and society's views of what is acceptable. The rights of individuals have become more important; the demand for a say in a person's own care is seen as a right. Nurses and other health care providers are compelled to provide individualized and safe, competent care at all times. Situations that require an ethical decision may no longer seem as clear-cut as they once did.

Health Care Reform

The growing emphasis on cost control, managed care, shorter hospital stays, increase in client acuity, exploration of alternative health care provision, and other factors that are changing health care delivery has and will have a direct impact on ethical decision making. The discharge of clients to their homes when they are sicker and more vulnerable is of great concern. Issues related to the allocation of health care funds to those who need it most or who have the greatest potential to have a positive outcome are also ethically challenging. Nurses will continually face questions that make them examine their own values as they relate to providing quality care to clients and families.

Professional Values and Client Values

Values are the beliefs and concepts that individuals and groups hold as the most meaningful in their lives. These values have their origins in family, religious, and community ideals to which one is exposed early in life. Most of us can list what we believe is most important in our lives and what principles we use to make decisions.

Professional values are beliefs in relation to the work that a person does. Some of those values do not differ from personal values, and some may derive from a person's education for a particular profession. Several values guide the decisions that nurses make. These values are also called principles of nursing ethics (Display 17.4). These include beneficience, nonmaleficence, autonomy, justice, fidelity, and veracity.

BENEFICENCE

Beneficence is the duty to do good for the clients assigned to the nurse's care. This good includes technical competence, a humanistic and holistic approach. Examples of beneficence include handwashing, teaching, and maintaining isolation techniques. There may be a conflict when the nurse and the client differ about what is "good." When the nurse or another member of the health care team overrides the patient's desires, it is called paternalism.

---

display 17.4   **Principles of Nursing Ethics**

Beneficence: Actively do good
Nonmaleficence: Do no harm
Autonomy: The right to make decisions
Justice: Fairness to all people
Fidelity: Faithful to commitments
Veracity: Truth telling

NONMALEFICENCE

Nonmaleficence is the duty to do no intentional or unintentional harm to the client. It is at the opposite end of the spectrum from beneficence. It is difficult to discuss nonmaleficence without beneficence because the choice of treatment for a client may initially cause harm, although the outcome is potentially good. For example, a client with colon cancer undergoes a colostomy and endures the pain of surgery and the reality of a change in body image. In addition, she or he agrees to have chemotherapy and radiation therapy. Although harmed in many ways, the ultimate goal is for her or him to be cancer free. In some instances, this may be a difficult choice if the outcome is likely to be poor despite the treatment.

AUTONOMY

Autonomy is a client's right of self-determination or a freedom to make choices and decisions without opposition. Autonomy is based on the tenet that every competent person has the ability to determine their destiny. One egregious violation of autonomy was the Tuskegee Study of Untreated Syphilis in the black male. Poor African American men with syphilis were studied by medical researchers. They were not informed of the advent of treatment (penicillin) that would have prevented deformity and death but were left to continue in the study. Their rights to life were violated. Due to this and other research human rights violations, informed consent for research was pushed to the forefront. Nurses must respect each client's right to informed consent, even if the client's decision is in direct conflict with the nurse's.

JUSTICE

Justice is the obligation to be fair to all people, regardless of their age, gender, race, or other factors. You may recall that this is the first statement in the ANA's (2001) *Code of Ethics for Nurses* (see Chapter 4). Justice may be applied to the individual level in that each person has the right to fair and equitable treatment. One could argue that there is not fair access to health care in the United States with the gap between those that can afford care and those that cannot is widening. There is a different level of care for the underserved and even differences in care within individual insurance companies. Conflicts occur if there are limited health care resources or when fairness to one means discrimination to another.

FIDELITY

Fidelity is the duty to maintain commitments of one's professional obligations and responsibilities. It is the duty to keep promises and to act in the best interest of the patient. It requires meeting reasonable expectations. An example of fidelity occurs in the vignette. Janet Bieber is refusing to give the placebo for many reasons, one of them being that the patient is trusting the nurse to deliver pain medication. Other examples of fidelity would be to tell the patient you will be "right back" or "everything will be just fine" when you cannot make it back and everything may not turn out fine. Expectations of fidelity also include keeping the patient informed, teaching the client, and maintaining confidentiality. The bottom line is to not make promises you cannot keep.

NCLEX–RN *Might Ask* 17.1

The nurse is caring for a client with terminal cancer. The patient is seeking the truth about the prognosis of her disease, but her husband wants all health care workers involved to avoid talking about this illness. The nurse's duty to tell the truth in this situation is the principle of nursing ethics called

    A. Nonmaleficence.
    B. Beneficence.
    C. Veracity.
    D. Justice.

• *See Appendix A for correct answer and rationale.*

VERACITY

Veracity is the duty to tell the truth. Derived from beneficence, veracity means that truth should be told so the patient and family can understand it. An ethical dilemma may result from cultural issues when the family wants truths withheld from the patient, believing that they are acting in his or her best interest. How much information to provide to the patient can also present a problem. A prognosis can often become catastrophically overwhelming, as in the case of suicide as a result of a cancer diagnosis. Other times, it has a sound basis, such as when a family wants to know that a child is healthy but not the gender of their child after an ultrasound. The nurse is obligated to provide factual information to the client so that she or he may have autonomy. There are potential conflicts if the family or the physician withholds information from the client. The issues of beneficence and nonmaleficence can enter into this ethical conflict.

    The values described previously are some of the principles that guide the decisions that nurses make. A client's values may differ totally from the RN's values. There is not necessarily a right or a wrong decision, but there should be recognition that the client has a different value system. There can also be conflict if the client's decision will be harmful.

thinking critically

Review the ANA's *Code of Ethics for Nurses* in Chapter 4. Determine the value (described in the preceding paragraphs) that is addressed by each statement. Examine the additions to the *Code of Ethics for Nurses* (Display 17.5). What is the impact of these new additions? Are any values not addressed? Do you believe that any should be added? Discuss this with a group of your classmates and determine if these values are the same or different for LPN/LVNs.

The preceding material has described some of the influences involved in ethical decision making. The awareness that many factors are involved in an ethical decision should assist you in examining ethical issues more broadly and with less bias for a particular way of thinking. Letting go of former ways of thinking, not personalizing every issue, and working with emotional intelligence are particularly difficult. In your role transition from LPN/LVN, you are increasing your responsibility and obligation to be a client advocate. The increased responsibility requires that you demonstrate a greater understanding of ethical decision making. In the next section, you have the opportunity to do some group work with ethical decision making. Use the information you have learned to examine ethical dilemmas and develop strategies to make ethical decisions.

● ETHICAL DECISION MAKING

As implied, ethical theories are only important if they result in manifested behaviors. Putting them into practice requires the intellectual skills to think clearly and critically. Nurses have always used a problem-solving approach to provide care to clients. In the same way, a problem-solving approach can be used for ethical dilemmas and will incorporate the ethical theories described previously.

The method used to make ethical decisions generally involves the nursing process in the following steps:

1. Assessment: Identify the problem, and describe it. Determine what values are involved, who is involved, and who will be affected by the decision. Are there legal ramifications? Obtain as much information as possible to understand the situation. Recognize your own personal biases that might affect your assessment.
2. Diagnosis: A statement of the dilemma (after looking at all the data) will assist you in seeing the issue as concisely as possible.
3. Planning: List *all possible options* for solving the dilemma; do not get involved with determining the consequences at this point. This process is referred to as brainstorming. Identify any time constraints and your relationship to the situation. Examine the advantages and disadvantages of each option. Look at each option with the possibility of applying the teleological, deontological, and feminist perspective. Consider the effects on individuals for each option. Consultation with a more experienced nurse, nurse manager, nurse practitioner, or ethics committee may take place at this point. Evaluate similar cases.
4. Implementation: Make the decision and follow through on it.
5. Evaluation: Evaluate the decision in terms of effects and results. Evaluate your comfort with the decision. Have the outcomes been met or not?

NCLEX–RN *Might Ask* (17.2)

The RN is reviewing the expected outcomes in a case involving care of a terminally ill child. The nurse is using the step of the ethical decision-making process.

    A. Assessment.
    B. Diagnosis.
    C. Planning.
    D. Evaluation.

· *See Appendix A for correct answer and rationale.*

Using a methodology for solving ethical dilemmas may be awkward for you at first. The following situation provides some practice for you to apply the decision-making process.

EXAMPLE

Early on a Saturday evening, Patty L., a 25-year-old RN, was on her way to work a 12-hour shift at the local hospital. As she drove down a road about 2 miles from the hospital, a car came toward her rapidly, weaving from side to side. The road was narrow and not well lit. Eventually, the other car crossed onto her side of the road, hitting Patty's car on the driver's side and pushing her into a telephone pole. She was killed as a result of the two impacts. Patty had apparently tried to avoid the car, but the other driver was going too fast. The driver of the other vehicle (Billy K.) was not fatally injured but did sustain multiple orthopedic injuries and a closed head fracture. He was taken to the local hospital. Blood levels revealed that he was intoxicated at the time of the accident. Local police also stated that Billy was driving without a driver's license; it had been suspended for other charges of driving while under the influence of alcohol.

Both Patty and Billy had been brought to the local emergency room. Billy was taken to surgery and then admitted to the intensive care unit. Patty's body was identified by her roommate, also a nurse, who had been working on the maternity unit. She notified Patty's family and helped make initial arrangements for Patty's body to be moved to a funeral home in her hometown. Employees at the hospital were shocked and grief stricken; even those who had not known Patty were in anguish.

Two weeks later, Billy was moved to a step-down unit on the orthopedic unit. When Brian M., RN, arrived for his 11 PM to 7 AM shift, he was assigned to work in the stepdown unit. When he realized that he was assigned to Billy, he told the charge nurse that he refused to care for him: "I will not take care of the lousy drunk who killed a friend of mine; why did he live and she die? He should be taken out behind the hospital and shot." Brian was unaware that Billy's sister was near the telephone and heard the entire conversation.

You are the charge nurse. What is the best way to deal with this situation? You had assigned Brian to the care of Billy because of his expertise and because the other most experienced nurse had called in sick.

- Use the steps described for making an ethical decision.
- Write a statement for the ethical dilemma after you have identified the relevant facts for this situation. Do you need other information?
- Determine possible actions for this dilemma. Examine these choices in relation to teleology and deontology. How would a feminist perspective influence actions?
- What are the consequences of each action?
- What decision did you choose?
- What effect does this decision have on Billy, his sister, or the other nursing staff?
- In reviewing the ANA's (2001) *Code of Ethics for Nurses*, are there times when nurses may refuse an assignment?

display **17.5**   **Additions to the Code of Ethics for Nurses**

- The nurse must be focused on the client.
- The nurse has a duty to herself or himself.
- The nurse must commit to work on public policy.

There will be many ethical issues with which you as an RN may have to contend. Ellis and Hartley (2008) categorized issues that they think are relevant to RNs in their respective practices: those that are related to commitment to the client, commitment to personal excellence, and commitment to the nursing profession as a whole (Display 17.5). Dealing with ethical issues is never an easy task.

The ongoing challenge for all of us, grounded in history and tradition, is how everyday working relationships in complex health care systems can be shaped and influenced for effective and compassionate delivery of patient care and for respectful treatment of staff and employees. Respect for all persons as responsible, self-determining moral agents who are interconnected and interdependent citizens of the moral community of health care at a given point in time is fundamental.

Consider other ethical issues with which you may have to deal: observing inadequate care of a client, recognizing that you lack certain skills or knowledge for the job to which you are assigned, or observing a fellow nurse refusing to care for a client because that client is of a different race. Develop your own scenarios, and then use the framework for ethical decision making to make a decision and carry it out. Draw on your experiences as an LPN/LVN; dilemmas that you have faced in those roles will have a different impact as you move into the RN role.

● CONCLUSION

This chapter emphasizes that nurses have ethical responsibilities and need to acquire ethical knowledge. Ethical issues have a direct impact on the work nurses do. The decisions are not easy and promise to get more difficult as science and technology continue to advance. Having knowledge of an ethical framework for decision making assists the nurse to make decisions and carry out actions that are acceptable personally and professionally.

When making the transition from LPN/LVN to RN, students will begin to recognize that there are ethical consequences for the work that nurses do. If the nurse practices in an unethical manner, the issues are more relevant to what is right or wrong in particular situations. The most important concern for a nurse is the rights of clients, followed by the rights and responsibilities of the nurse's colleagues.

The nursing profession will continue to be challenged by changes in ethical issues. Society will be faced with dilemmas that have no answers. The role of government in determining legal answers for ethical questions will bring forth other issues for nurses. Awareness of your personal and professional values will assist you in clarifying ethical issues. Continuing self-growth and development will further enhance your ability to deal with and consider ethical dilemmas. Although you may hope you are never placed in a situation of conflict, it is likely to happen. Be informed. Be prepared. Be knowledgeable.

student exercises

Mrs. Smith is a 23-year-old woman who has had frequent episodes of nosebleeds, easy bruising, and one infection after another. After a bone marrow biopsy, Mrs. Smith, who is caring for her mother and ill father at home along with an 18-month-old infant, is visited by an oncologist and several residents. She is informed by the oncologist about her diagnosis of acute lymphocytic leukemia. She has a dazed look about her as the physician describes the next step of treatment, which will be aggressive chemotherapy. The physicians leave with the consent form signed, but when you question her, you realize she didn't hear a word of what transpired.

1. As the RN, would you consider this an informed consent?

2. From an ethical perspective, what are the items in her history that you would like to have more information about?

3. How would you proceed as the client advocate in this case?

References

American Nurses Association. (2001). *Code of ethics for nurses with interpretive statements*. Washington, DC: American Nurses Publishing.

Bosek, M., & Savage, T. (2007). *The ethical component of nursing*. Philadelphia, PA: Lippincott Williams & Wilkins.

Cherry, B., & Jacob, S. R. (2008). *Contemporary nursing: Issues, trends, and management* (4th ed.). St. Louis, MO: CV Mosby.

Corley, M., Elswick, R., Gorman., M., & Clor, T. (2001). Development and evaluation of a moral distress scale. *Journal of Advanced Nursing, 33*(2), 250–256.

Craven, R., & Hirnle, C. (2009). *Fundamentals of nursing: Human health and foundation* (6th ed.). Philadelphia, PA: Lippincott Williams & Wilkins.

Dahnke, M., & Dreher, H. (2006). Defining ethics and applying the theories. In: V. Lackman (Ed.), *Applied ethics in nursing* (pp. 3–13). New York, NY: Springer.

Ellis, J., & Hartley, C. (2008). *Nursing in today's world: Challenges, issues, and trends* (9th ed.). Philadelphia, PA: Lippincott Williams & Wilkins.

Lachman, V. (Ed.). (2006). *Applied ethics in nursing*. New York, NY: Springer.

Marquis, B., & Huston, C. (2009). *Leadership roles and management functions in nursing* (6th ed.). Philadelphia, PA: Lippincott Williams & Wilkins.

Pendry, P. (2007). Moral distress: Recognizing it to retain nurses. *Nursing Economics, 25*(4), 217–221.

Wilkinson, J., & Van Leuven, K. (2007). *Fundamentals of nursing: Theory, concepts and applications*. Philadelphia, PA: F. A. Davis.

Williams, C. (1991). *Gender differences at work: Women and men in nontraditional occupations*. Berkley, CA: University of California Press.

Suggested Reading

Arnstein, P. (2006). Placebos: No relief for Ms. Mahoney's pain. *AJN, 106*(2), 54–57.

Bjarnason, D., & Carter, M. (Eds). Legal and ethical issues: To know, to reason, to act. *Nursing Clinics of North America, 44*(4), 393–526.

Butts, J., & Rich, K. (2005). *Nursing ethics: Across the curriculum and into practice*. Sudbury, MA: Jones and Bartlett.

Day, L. (2006). Questions concerning the goodness of hastening death. *American Journal of Critical Care, 15*(3), 312–314.

Fry, S., Veatch, R., & Taylor, C. (2011). *Case studies in nursing ethics* (4th ed.). Sudbury, MA: Jones & Bartlett Learning.

Guido, G. (2006). *Legal and ethical issues in nursing* (4th ed.). Upper Saddle River, NJ: Pearson Prentice-Hall.

Malka, S. (2007). *Daring to care: American nursing and second-wave feminism.* Chicago, IL: University of Illinois Press.

Rushton, C. (2004). Ethics and palliative care in pediatrics. *AJN, 104*(4), 54–56.

Taylor, C., Lillis, C., & LeMone, P. (2009). *Fundamentals of nursing: The art and science of nursing care* (6th ed.). Philadelphia, PA: Lippincott Williams & Wilkins.

On the (WEB) *http://bioethics.net:* Site for the American Journal of Bioethics. (Last accessed 2.1.2011)

http://www.pbs.org/wgbh/nova/doctors/oath_classical.html: The Classical Version of the Hippocratic Oath. (Last accessed 2.1.2011)

http://cbhd.org/: Center for Bioethics and Human Dignity. (Last accessed 2.1.2011)

http://www.icn.ch/images/stories/documents/about/icncode_english. pdf: The ICN Code of Ethics for Nurses. (Last accessed 2.1. 2011) appendix

A

Answers to "NCLEX-RN Might Ask" Questions

• CHAPTER 1
NCLEX-RN Might Ask 1-1

Choice **B** is correct. **Rationale:** This is part of the conflict stage after the bliss of the honeymoon stage. Reintegration is characterized by hostility, withdrawal, and negative feelings. Resolution has four possible phases.

• CHAPTER 2
NCLEX-RN Might Ask 2-1

Choice **C** is correct. **Rationale:** The child's identification with her peer group is making adhering to a diet difficult. Trust versus mistrust is found in ages birth to 18 months. Industry versus inferiority is found in the 6- to 12-year age group and involves development of motor tasks and coping skills. Intimacy versus isolation is a job of the early adult who is developing intimate relationships.

NCLEX-RN Might Ask 2-2

The incorrect choice is **D. Rationale:** Be careful reading this because the stem (question) is asking for an incorrect answer. The professional role is merged with both personal and professional ideas. A, B, and C are acceptable according to Cohen's theory.

• CHAPTER 3
NCLEX-RN Might Ask 3-1

Choice **B** is correct. **Rationale:** A transformational change refers to a radical difference in how a group is handled as a result of the change. This is a planned change, so C and D are incorrect. There has been no mutual agreement by the stakeholders, so A is incorrect.

NCLEX-RN Might Ask 3-2

Choice **B** is correct. **Rationale:** A slight increase in vital signs and blood sugar are characteristic of stimulation of the sympathetic nervous system found in the alarm reaction stage. The changes are not normal and do not indicate those seen in resistance or exhaustion (which can lead to death).

NCLEX-RN Might Ask 3-3

Choice **B** is correct. **Rationale:** Refusing to look at the site and be involved in the dressings is the best answer. If the client had accepted the mastectomy, she would be involved in her care. Bargaining would be indicated by the client saying something like "If only I would have stopped smoking." Depression would be indicated by withdrawal behaviors.

• CHAPTER 4
NCLEX-RN Might Ask 4-1

Choice **C** is correct. **Rationale:** Discipline, devotion, and obedience in nursing do not have ancient or religious origins.

NCLEX-RN Might Ask 4-2

Choice **C** is correct. **Rationale:** The NLN is the only nursing association challenged with accrediting schools of nursing. The AMA is a governing body for physicians; the NSNA is a governing body for school nurses; and the ANA is involved with advanced certification and continuing education credits.

● CHAPTER 5
NCLEX-RN Might Ask 5-1

Choice **B** is correct. **Rationale:** Teaching a client how to irrigate his ostomy involves manipulating and practicing a new skill. Cognitive skills would be more about how and why the stoma functions. Affective learning would explore how the client feels about having the device and how it affects his lifestyle. Communication is not a learning domain.

NCLEX-RN Might Ask 5-2

Choice **D** is correct. **Rationale:** Because the LPN is a student studying to be an RN, she or he is held to the level of an RN.

● CHAPTER 7
NCLEX-RN Might Ask 7-1

The four main categories according to the NCLEX-RN test blue print are (a) safe, effective care environment, (b) health promotion and maintenance, (c) psychosocial integrity, and (d) physiological integrity.

● CHAPTER 8
NCLEX-RN Might Ask 8-1

Choice **A** is correct. **Rationale:** The nurse practice acts are regulations legislated by state law. They do not include permissive language. Policies and standards are proclaimed from national nursing organizations.

NCLEX-RN Might Ask 8-2

Choice **D** is correct. **Rationale:** When the RN is working with others, she is collaborating for client care. Independence and autonomy are working and making decisions alone. In the advocacy role, the RN would be working for the client.

NCLEX-RN Might Ask 8-3

Choice **D** is correct. **Rationale:** Only minimal safety and competency levels are demonstrated by the RN-level candidate when the NCLEX-RN test is successfully completed. Average, specialty, and excellent practice levels are not demonstrated by passing this examination.

● CHAPTER 9
NCLEX-RN Might Ask 9-1

Choice **A** is the *incorrect* statement. **Rationale:** Be careful; this is asking you to identify the *wrong* answer. Critical thinking involves recognizing and overcoming feelings as a basis for decisions. It also involves exploring options, problem solving, and not letting age, culture, or personal background influence decisions.

NCLEX-RN Might Ask 9-2

Choice **C** is correct. **Rationale:** C demonstrates that the student needs additional clarification. Critical thinking is based on facts and evidence and not how the student feels about a given situation.

● CHAPTER 10

NCLEX-RN Might Ask 10-1

Choice **A** is correct. **Rationale:** You are looking for the only *wrong* answer to this question. If the new nurse states that the nursing process is an extension of the medical plan, she or he needs additional help understanding that the nursing process is independent of the medical plan. The other choices are correct and are characteristics of the nursing process.

NCLEX-RN Might Ask 10-2

Choice **C** is correct. **Rationale:** Sleep pattern disturbance is the NANDA stem. Death of a spouse is the cause, and the last two parts are signs/symptoms of a sleep pattern disturbance. A has only two parts. B is correctly written but is not an actual diagnosis. D has only two parts and needs a third part that includes signs/symptoms.

NCLEX-RN Might Ask 10-3

Choice **D** is correct. **Rationale:** Airway problems always take top priority. C indicates as a "risk for" diagnosis; it can wait. A and B are lower in Maslow's hierarchy.

NCLEX-RN Might Ask 10-4

Choice **B** is correct. **Rationale:** This outcome stresses the immediate needs of the patient in that the problem is an airway one and needs a short target date. A does not relate to the nursing diagnosis but may be appropriate for a risk for Decreased Cardiac Output nursing diagnosis. C is related to the nursing diagnosis but is not a priority at this time. D is an intervention because it is an assessment.

● CHAPTER 11

NCLEX-RN Might Ask 11-1

Choice **B** is correct. **Rationale:** Active listening techniques let the client know the nurse is interested in what the client says and in the client as an individual. A and C are useful techniques for leading an interaction. D is incorrect: A nurse can be professional in appearance but can be cold and uncaring.

NCLEX-RN Might Ask 11-2

Choice **D** is correct. **Rationale:** Therapeutic interaction is done for the purpose of providing safe, effective nursing care. C is only part of the reason nurses use therapeutic techniques. B may not be necessary in a professional association. One of the goals for communication is to get the client to become more independent.

• CHAPTER 12

NCLEX-RN Might Ask 12-1

Choice **A** is correct. **Rationale:** Severe pain can block a client's concentration and decrease learning ability. B, C, and D are usually considered to be positive factors for effective learning.

NCLEX-RN Might Ask 12-2

Choice **B** is correct. **Rationale:** B is the correct answer and the easiest to do in the home setting. A is not practical, costs money, and may be demeaning to the client. C and D may also make the client feel inferior.

NCLEX-RN Might Ask 12-3

Choice **B** is correct. **Rationale:** The cause of the impaired communication is related to the client's learning need. A, C, and D are correct for the nursing diagnosis but do not clearly state a learning need.

• CHAPTER 13

NCLEX-RN Might Ask 13-1

Choice **B** is correct. **Rationale:** B is more global than A. A is only partly right. C ignores the problem and does not help the nurse. D shows that the nurse lacks cultural sensitivity.

NCLEX-RN Might Ask 13-2

Choice **D** is correct. **Rationale:** The nurse's ability to step outside her/his own culture to understand another is called cultural relativism. Enculturation is assimilating something outside one's culture. A and C are the opposite of cultural relativism

NCLEX-RN Might Ask 13-3

Choice **B** is correct. **Rationale:** The client speaks only Chinese. There are no data to support the etiologies of the other nursing diagnoses in this scenario.

• CHAPTER 14

NCLEX-RN Might Ask 14-1

Choice **B** is correct. **Rationale:** The first step in any decision-making process is assessment. A is incorrect because monitoring and assessing outside the normal is not the sole responsibility of the RN. C is incorrect because the nurse needs to trust members of the health care team. D is incorrect because the nurse cannot assume a task is completed. He or she is responsible for the level of care.

NCLEX-RN Might Ask 14-2

Choice **A** is correct. **Rationale:** B and C are strategies that make the nurse more efficient. D is a legal and ethical responsibility.

NCLEX-RN Might Ask 14-3

Choice **B** is correct. **Rationale:** This is a problem with interpretation of the RN's assignment. There are no data to support any of the other answers.

● CHAPTER 15

NCLEX-RN Might Ask 15-1

Choice **B** is correct. **Rationale:** This is the only answer that encompasses the characteristics of a professional. Although traditions are important, the RN must be willing to part with them if scientific research proves that traditional practices detract from client care. A, C, and D can be eliminated because they all include tradition.

NCLEX-RN Might Ask 15-2

Choice **C** is correct. **Rationale:** When a nurse tries to explain what the client's wishes are, s/he is acting in the role of advocate.

● CHAPTER 16

NCLEX-RN Might Ask 16-1

Choice **A** is correct. **Rationale:** This is a civil court case initially due to the accidental occurrence of this error. Although if the patient or family loses the case, in some instances, the case could be tried under criminal law. Intent is the determining factor.

NCLEX-RN Might Ask 16-2

Choice **A** is correct. **Rationale:** The state nurse practice acts define the scope of nursing practice. Professional organizations develop standards. Hospitals and physicians need to adhere to the practice acts and standards.

NCLEX-RN Might Ask 16-3

Choice **C** is correct. **Rationale:** To be informed comprehensively, the client needs to be informed about alternatives and about risks and benefits associated with the procedure the physician wants to perform. A client may withdraw consent at any time. The nurse has an ethical responsibility to the client to ensure that he or she understands the physician's explanations. Not all information gained from a client involves research. A research study would require special permission from the client.

● CHAPTER 17

NCLEX-RN Might Ask 17-1

Choice **C** is correct. **Rationale:** The nurse must tell the truth. The prognosis is something the client probably knows already but is attempting to confirm; she is ready to know if she asks. Nonmaleficence is the duty to do no harm, and beneficence is the duty to do good. Justice is fairness to all patients.

NCLEX-RN Might Ask 17-2

Choice **D** is correct. **Rationale:** In nursing diagnosis, the expected outcomes are evaluated, not the interventions (planning). A would be correct if the statement included gathering information about the situation. B would be correct if the nurse was clustering data to come up with a statement. C would be correct if the nurse was exploring alternatives and deciding on choices.

B

NANDA-Approved Nursing Diagnoses 2009–2011

This list represents the NANDA-approved nursing diagnoses for clinical use and testing.

Activity Intolerance
Activity Intolerance, Risk for
Activity Planning, Ineffective
Adult Failure to Thrive
Airway Clearance, Ineffective
Allergy Response, Latex
Allergy Response, Risk for Latex
Anxiety
Anxiety, Death
Aspiration, Risk for
Attachment, Risk for Impaired
Autonomic Dysreflexia
Autonomic Dysreflexia, Risk for
Bed Mobility, Impaired
Behavior, Risk-Prone Health (previously called "Impaired Adjustment")
Bleeding, Risk for
Body Image, Disturbed
Body Temperature, Risk for Imbalanced
Bowel Incontinence
Breast-Feeding, Effective
Breast-Feeding, Ineffective
Breast-Feeding, Interrupted
Breathing Pattern, Ineffective
Cardiac Tissue Perfusion, Risk for Decreased
Caregiver Role Strain
Caregiver Role Strain, Risk for
Cerebral Tissue Perfusion, Risk for Ineffective
Childbearing Process, Readiness for Enhanced
Comfort, Readiness for Enhanced
Communication, Impaired Verbal
Communication, Readiness for Enhanced
Conflict, Decisional
Conflict, Parental Role
Confusion, Acute
Confusion, Chronic
Confusion, Risk for Acute
Constipation
Constipation, Perceived
Constipation, Risk for
Contamination
Contamination, Risk for
Coping, Compromised Family
Coping, Defensive
Coping, Disabled Family

Coping, Ineffective
Coping, Ineffective Community
Coping, Readiness for Enhanced
Coping, Readiness for Enhanced Community
Coping, Readiness for Enhanced Family
Contamination, Risk for
Death Syndrome, Risk for Sudden Infant
Decision Making, Readiness for Enhanced
Delayed Development, Risk for
Denial, Ineffective
Dentition, Impaired
Development, Risk for Delayed
Diarrhea
Dignity, Risk for Compromised Human
Disproportionate Growth, Risk for
Distress, Moral
Disuse Syndrome, Risk for
Diversional Activity, Deficient
Electrolyte imbalance, Risk for
Energy Field, Disturbed
Environmental Interpretation Syndrome, Impaired
Failure to Thrive, Adult
Falls, Risk for
Family Therapeutic Regimen Management, Ineffective
Family Processes, Dysfunctional: Alcoholism
Family Processes, Interrupted
Family Processes, Readiness for Enhanced
Fatigue
Fear
Fluid Balance, Readiness for Enhanced
Fluid Volume, Deficient
Fluid Volume, Excess
Fluid Volume, Risk for Deficient
Fluid Volume, Risk for Imbalanced
Gas Exchange, Impaired
Gastrointestinal Perfusion, Risk for Ineffective
Gastrointestinal Motility, Dysfunctional
Gastrointestinal Motility, Dysfunctional, Risk for
Glucose, Risk for Unstable Blood
Grieving, Anticipatory
Grieving, Complicated
Grieving, Risk for Complicated
Growth and Development, Delayed
Growth, Risk for Disproportionate
Health Maintenance, Ineffective
Health-Seeking Behaviors (Specify)
Home Maintenance, Impaired

Hope, Readiness for Enhanced
Hopelessness
Human Dignity, Risk for Compromised
Hyperthermia
Hypothermia
Identity, Disturbed Personal
Immunization Status, Readiness for Enhanced
Incontinence, Functional Urinary
Incontinence, Overflow Urinary
Incontinence, Reflex Urinary
Incontinence, Risk for Urge Urinary
Incontinence, Stress Urinary
Incontinence, Total Urinary
Incontinence, Urge Urinary
Infant Behavior, Disorganized
Infant Behavior, Readiness for Enhanced Organized
Infant Behavior, Risk for Disorganized
Infant Feeding Pattern, Ineffective
Infection, Risk for
Injury, Risk for
Injury, Risk for Perioperative-Positioning
Insomnia
Intracranial Adaptive Capacity, Decreased
Knowledge, Deficient (Specify)
Knowledge, Readiness for Enhanced
Immunization Status, Readiness for Enhanced
Latex Allergy Response
Latex Allergy Response, Risk for
Lifestyle, Sedentary
Liver Function, Risk for Impaired
Loneliness, Risk for
Maternal/Fetal Dyad, Risk for Disturbed
Memory, Impaired
Mobility, Impaired Physical
Moral Distress
Nausea
Neglect, Unilateral
Neonatal Jaundice
Noncompliance
Nutrition, Imbalanced: Less Than Body Requirements
Nutrition, Imbalanced: More Than Body Requirements
Nutrition, Readiness for Enhanced
Nutrition, Risk for Imbalanced: More Than Body Requirements
Oral Mucous Membrane, Impaired
Pain, Acute
Pain, Chronic
Parental Role Conflict

Perioperative Positioning Injury, Risk for
Peripheral Neurovascular Dysfunction, Risk for
Peripheral Tissue Perfusion, Ineffective
Personal Identity, Disturbed
Poisoning, Risk for
Posttrauma Syndrome
Posttrauma Syndrome, Risk for
Power, Readiness for Enhanced
Powerlessness
Powerlessness, Risk for
Protection, Ineffective
Rape-Trauma Syndrome
Rape-Trauma Syndrome: Compound Reaction
Rape-trauma Syndrome: Silent Reaction
Relationship, Readiness for Enhanced
Religiosity, Impaired
Religiosity, Readiness for Enhanced
Religiosity, Risk for Impaired
Relocation Stress Syndrome
Relocation Stress Syndrome, Risk for
Resilience, Risk for Compromised
Resilience, Impaired Individual
Resilience, Readiness for Enhanced
Role Performance, Ineffective
Self-Care, Readiness for Enhanced
Self-Care Deficit, Bathing/Hygiene
Self-Care Deficit, Dressing/Grooming
Self-Care Deficit, Feeding
Self-Care Deficit, Toileting
Self-Concept, Readiness for Enhanced
Self-Esteem, Chronic Low
Self-Esteem, Situational Low
Self-Esteem, Risk for Situational Low
Self-Help Management, Ineffective
Self-Help Management, Readiness for Enhanced
Self-Mutilation
Self-Mutilation, Risk for
Self-Neglect
Sensory Perception, Disturbed (Specify: Visual, Auditory, Kinesthetic, Gustatory, Tactile, Olfactory)
Sexual Dysfunction
Sexuality Pattern, Ineffective
Shock, Risk for
Skin Integrity, Impaired
Skin Integrity, Risk for Impaired
Sleep Deprivation
Sleep Pattern, Disturbed

Sleep, Readiness for Enhanced
Social Interaction, Impaired
Social Isolation
Sorrow, Chronic
Spiritual Distress
Spiritual Distress, Risk for
Spiritual Well-Being, Readiness for Enhanced
Stress Overload
Sudden Infant Death Syndrome, Risk for
Suffocation, Risk for
Suicide, Risk for
Surgical Recovery, Delayed
Swallowing, Impaired
Therapeutic Regimen Management, Effective
Therapeutic Regimen Management, Ineffective
Therapeutic Regimen Management, Ineffective Community
Therapeutic Regimen Management, Ineffective Family
Therapeutic Regimen Management, Readiness for Enhanced
Thermoregulation, Ineffective
Thought Processes, Disturbed
Tissue Integrity, Impaired
Transfer Ability, Impaired
Trauma, Risk for
Unilateral Neglect
Urinary Elimination, Impaired
Urinary Elimination, Readiness for Enhanced
Urinary Incontinence, Functional
Urinary Incontinence, Overflow
Urinary Incontinence, Reflex
Urinary Incontinence, Stress
Urinary Incontinence, Urge
Urinary Retention
Unstable Blood Glucose, Risk for
Vascular Trauma, Risk for
Ventilation, Impaired Spontaneous
Ventilatory Weaning Response, Dysfunctional
Violence, Risk for Other-Directed
Violence, Risk for Self-Directed
Walking, Impaired
Wandering
Wheelchair Mobility, Impaired

From NANDA International (2009). *Nursing diagnoses: Definitions & classification 2009–2011*. West Sussex: Wiley-Blackwell.

INDEX

Note: Page numbers followed by *d* indicate displays; those followed by *f* indicate figures; those followed by *t* indicate tables.